Battle-scarred

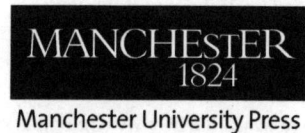

Manchester University Press

Politics, culture and society in early modern Britain

General Editors
DR ALEXANDRA GAJDA
PROFESSOR ANTHONY MILTON
PROFESSOR PETER LAKE
PROFESSOR JASON PEACEY

This important series publishes monographs that take a fresh and challenging look at the interactions between politics, culture and society in Britain between 1500 and the mid-eighteenth century. It counteracts the fragmentation of current historiography through encouraging a variety of approaches which attempt to redefine the political, social and cultural worlds, and to explore their interconnection in a flexible and creative fashion. All the volumes in the series question and transcend traditional interdisciplinary boundaries, such as those between political history and literary studies, social history and divinity, urban history and anthropology. They thus contribute to a broader understanding of crucial developments in early modern Britain.

Full details of the series are available at www.manchesteruniversitypress.co.uk.

Battle-scarred

Mortality, medical care and military welfare in the British Civil Wars

EDITED BY DAVID J. APPLEBY
AND ANDREW HOPPER

Manchester University Press

Published by Manchester University Press
Altrincham Street, Manchester M1 7JA

www.manchesteruniversitypress.co.uk

British Library Cataloguing-in-Publication Data
A catalogue record for this book is available from the British Library

ISBN 978 1 5261 2480 7 hardback

First published 2018

Typeset in 10/12 Scala by
Servis Filmsetting Ltd, Stockport, Cheshire
Printed in Great Britain by
CPI Group (UK) Ltd, Croydon CR0 4YY

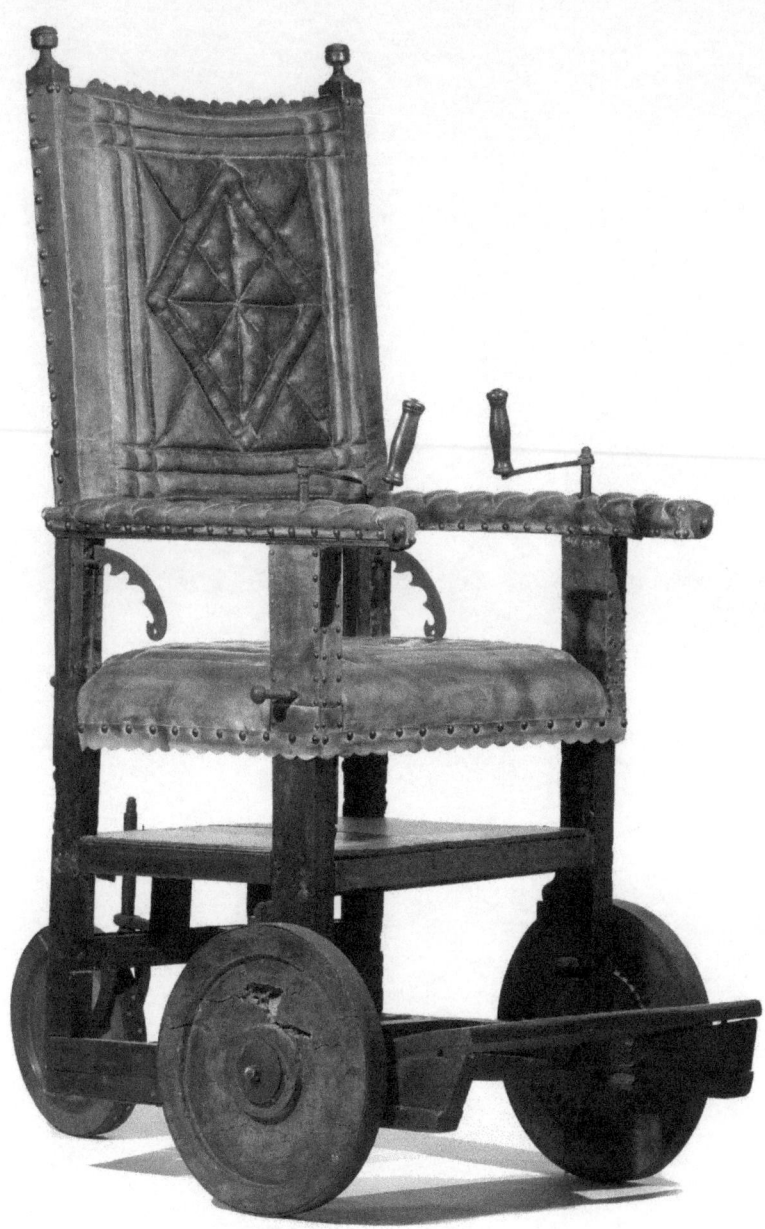

The wheelchair of Thomas, third baron Fairfax, the parliamentarian commander-in-chief (by kind permission of Tom Fairfax)

Contents

———◆———

Contents

List of figures and tables

FIGURES

TABLES

Notes on contributors

David J. Appleby has been Lecturer in Early Modern British History at the University of Nottingham since 2006. He is the author of *Black Bartholomew's Day: Preaching, Polemic and Restoration Nonconformity* (Manchester University Press, 2007), which was awarded the Richard L. Greaves Prize by the International John Bunyan Society in 2010. He has also written several articles on veteran politics and military welfare during the British Civil Wars and their aftermath. He is a Co-Investigator on the Arts and Humanities Research Council-funded project entitled 'Welfare, Conflict and Memory during and after the English Civil Wars'.

Ian Atherton is Senior Lecturer in History at Keele University. He is currently working on the memory of conflict, attitudes to the fallen, and burial and memorialisation as well as the history of early modern British cathedrals. He has written numerous articles on the civil wars in the Midlands and was the editor of *The 1630s: Interdisciplinary Essays on Culture and Politics in the Caroline Era* (Manchester University Press, 2006).

Eric Gruber von Arni is Honorary Visiting Fellow in the Centre for English Local History at the University of Leicester. Eric retired from his career in the British Army with the rank of Colonel in 1996, having served as the Army's Director of Nursing Studies at the Royal Army Medical College in London. He then undertook doctoral research into hospital care, surgery and military welfare during the civil wars and Interregnum at the University of Portsmouth. This research appeared in his first monograph, entitled *Justice to the Maimed Soldier* (Ashgate, 2001), which was followed by a sequel, *Hospital Care and the British Standing Army, 1660-1714* (Ashgate, 2006). Eric was Co-Guest Curator of the 'Battle-Scarred' exhibition at the National Civil War Centre.

Andrew Hopper is Associate Professor in English Local History at the University of Leicester. He is best known for his two monographs *Turncoats and Renegadoes: Changing Sides during the English Civil Wars* (Oxford University Press, 2012), and *'Black Tom': Sir Thomas Fairfax and the English Revolution* (Manchester University Press, 2007). He was Co-Guest Curator of the 'Battle-Scarred' exhibition at the National Civil War Centre. He is now an Academic Director of the National Civil War Centre and the Principal Investigator of the Arts and Humanities Research Council-funded project entitled 'Welfare, Conflict and Memory during and after the English Civil Wars'.

Stuart B. Jennings is Free Church Chaplain at the University of Warwick. He undertook a doctorate at Nottingham Trent University examining nonconformity in seventeenth-century Nottinghamshire. He is the author of numerous journal articles discussing Newark's civil-war experiences alongside his book *'These Uncertaine Tymes': Newark and the Civilian Experience of the Civil Wars, 1640–1660* (Nottinghamshire County Council, 2009).

Richard Jones is Associate Professor in Landscape History at the University of Leicester. His research examines the changing relationships between the people and the land in medieval England. He is the author of *The Medieval Natural World* (Routledge, 2013), and is the Principal Investigator of the Leverhulme Trust-funded project entitled 'Flood and Flow: Place Names and the Changing Hydrology of River Systems'.

Chris R. Langley is Senior Lecturer in Early Modern British History at Newman University. He is an expert on religion, the Covenanters and the Scottish experience of the civil wars. He is the author of *Worship, Civil War and Community, 1638–1660* (Routledge, 2015) and the editor of *The Minutes of the Synod of Lothian and Tweeddale, 1648–1659* (Boydell, 2016).

Ismini Pells is Postdoctoral Research Fellow and Project Manager of the Arts and Humanities Research Council-funded project entitled 'Welfare, Conflict and Memory during and after the English Civil Wars' at the University of Leicester. Before that she was an Associate Research Fellow in the Centre for Medical History at the University of Exeter on the Wellcome Trust-funded project, the 'Medical World of Early Modern England, Ireland and Wales, *c*. 1500–1715'. Her doctorate was awarded by the University of Cambridge in 2014 for research on the life and career of the parliamentarian general, Philip Skippon.

Erin Peters is Lecturer in Early Modern History at Gloucestershire University. She was awarded her PhD at the University of Worcester in 2015, and is the author of *Commemoration and Oblivion in Royalist Print Culture, 1658–1667*

(Palgrave Macmillan, 2017). She has also published several articles on trauma and the memory of the civil wars. Her long-term research encompasses an interdisciplinary study of the impact of civil war-related psychological trauma on medical and psychological theories between 1642 and 1681.

Stephen M. Rutherford is Senior Lecturer in Molecular Cell Biology in the School of Biosciences at Cardiff University. He is Deputy Director of Undergraduate Education and a National Teaching Fellow. Stephen teaches genetics, molecular cell biology, biotechnology and the history of the scientific method. Stephen also teaches an elective course to medical students on the history of military surgery.

Hannah Worthen is Postdoctoral Research Associate on the 'Gender, Place and Memory, 1400–1900' project at the University of Hull. Her PhD was awarded at the University of Leicester in 2017, funded by an Arts and Humanities Research Council Collaborative Doctoral Award with The National Archives. It examined the experiences of war widows in mid-seventeenth-century England, with special reference to Kent and Sussex. Hannah is a Trustee of the Battle of Worcester Society and the author of several articles on military welfare and war widows.

Preface and acknowledgements

———

Earlier versions of the chapters in this volume were presented as papers at the inaugural conference of the National Civil War Centre at Newark Museum on 7–8 August 2015. The conference was organised by Andrew Hopper, Stewart Beale and Hannah Worthen of the University of Leicester and was attended by over ninety delegates. As well as this volume, the conference also provided the springboard for a successful temporary exhibition at the National Civil War Centre focused on the same theme and entitled 'Battle-Scarred'. The exhibition ran in four rooms from March to October 2016, before being down-sized to two rooms for a further two years. Elements of it have since been made permanent. We are grateful to the National Civil War Centre for the title of this exhibition to lend its name to this volume. We are also grateful to the Wolfson Foundation for a grant to establish a Research Centre for Care, Welfare and Medicine during the British Civil Wars at the National Civil War Centre.

For their helpful comments and criticisms, the editors are grateful to the editors and readers of the Politics, Society and Culture in Early Modern Britain series at Manchester University Press. We would like to thank Viscount De L'Isle for his kind permission to cite the Foulis Manuscripts from his private collection. We are also grateful to the University of Leicester, Springhead Brewery and to the journal *Midland History* for grants that supported the inaugural conference of the National Civil War Centre. We would also like to thank Glyn Hughes, Team Leader for Collections, Kevin Winter, Exhibition and Collections Assistant and Carol King, Learning and Participation Officer at the National Civil War Centre, for their valuable assistance with organising the conference and exhibition from which this volume arose.

Abbreviations

BL   The British Library
Bodl.   Bodleian Library, Oxford
BRO   Berkshire Record Office
CALS   Cheshire Archives and Local Studies
CH   The copy of Gerard's *Herball* of 1636 owned by the Coopers of Thurgarton
CJ   *Journals of the House of Commons*
CSPD *Calendar of State Papers Domestic*
ERO   Essex Record Office
ESRO   East Sussex Record Office
HMC   Historical Manuscripts Commission
HMSO   Her Majesty's Stationery Office
JP   Justice of the Peace
KHLC   Kent History and Library Centre
LJ   *Journals of the House of Lords*
MP   Member of Parliament
NAO   Nottinghamshire Archives Office
NRO   Norfolk Record Office
NRS   National Records of Scotland
ODNB *The Oxford Dictionary of National Biography Online*
OHC   Oxfordshire History Centre
PCC   Prerogative Court of Canterbury
PROB   Probate Records
RPS   *The Records of the Parliaments of Scotland to 1707*
SHC   Somerset Heritage Centre
SP   The State Papers
SRO   Staffordshire Record Office

STC   Short Title Catalogue
TNA   The National Archives
Wing   Donald Wing, *Short-title catalogue of books printed in England,
       Scotland, Ireland, Wales, and British America and of English books
       printed in other countries: 1641–1700, Second edition, newly revised and
       enlarged* (New York, 1982).
WRO   Warwickshire Record Office

Introduction

David J. Appleby and Andrew Hopper

'Warr', Edward Calver declared in 1644, 'hath never seemed sweet to any but to the unexperienced, who, blinded with its florish and its glory, observe not the Tragicall events that doe attend it.'[1] Given that he was writing in the midst of the most extensive and sustained internecine fighting the British archipelago had ever seen, it was understandable that Calver should consider civil war to be the worst of all worlds. He had already observed at first-hand how political and religious tensions had caused friends, neighbours and relatives to take up arms against each other, with the result that 'all the obligations of friendship, and Nature lie cancel'd in one another's blood'.[2] The fighting became increasingly vicious in the years that followed. In 1646, after a series of reversals, Charles I surrendered to a Scottish Covenanter army gathered around Southwell in Nottinghamshire, and ordered all his followers to lay down their arms. He was eventually handed over to the English Parliament, but, although a prisoner, was able to divide his enemies and provoke a new civil war in 1648. In January 1649 a military junta within the parliamentarian alliance put Charles on trial for war crimes and high treason against the people of England. For a monarch to be thus condemned and publicly executed by his subjects was unprecedented; the regicide sent shockwaves throughout Europe. Far from ending the bloodshed it hardened existing enmities, and created fresh ones. Between 1649 and 1652 the death toll continued to mount, in Ireland, Scotland, England and finally in the Caribbean. A greater proportion of the British and Irish population perished in these conflicts than in both World Wars combined.[3]

The chapters which follow will show that royalist, parliamentarian and Covenanter leaders found it necessary to pay close attention to the lateral damage incurred during their military campaigns – not simply out of a sense of moral obligation, but in order to maintain public support for their respective war efforts. After the cessation of armed hostilities maimed sol-diers, war widows and orphans continued to feature in the respective agendas of the Commonwealth, the Protectorate and ultimately the restored Stuart monarchy, as each regime in turn tried to restore peace and harmony to a divided realm. For some time now, historians of the British Civil Wars have also been interested in these issues; indeed, several have come to view the developments that took place in military medicine and pension provision as significant episodes in the welfare history of Europe. *Battle-scarred* examines the human cost of the conflict, and the ways in which it left physical and mental scars on individuals and communities, and more broadly on the political culture of the British Isles.

This volume lies at the confluence of several rivers of historiography. It is a measure of the civil wars' pivotal significance to the national identities and political cultures of the United Kingdom and the Republic of Ireland that efforts to determine the causes and courses of the various conflicts, and the extent to which these were intertwined, have sparked such a variety of historiographical debates. These heated disputes began soon after the wars themselves, in the writings of rival participants.[4] There is still no consensus as to a collective name for these conflicts, or even whether a collective name is appropriate.[5] The term most familiar to the general public, 'the English Civil War', did not come into fashion until the late nineteenth century. It is still favoured today by some historians, and publishers nervous of confusing the book-buying public. Other scholars have fallen back on another established label, 'the English Revolution', for although that term carries the baggage of old Whig and Marxist metanarratives, the radicalism that countenanced the abolition of the monarchy was distinctively English. In recent decades terms such as the 'British Civil Wars' and the 'Wars in the Three Kingdoms' have been used by those who argue that Charles's failure to manage three disparate kingdoms was a prime cause of the conflict, and that events in each kingdom directly affected events in the others. The wars have now been placed in a wider Atlantic perspective, and the recent emergence of an ethnic history of the conflict has elicited a suggestion that it should be called 'the War of Five Peoples'.[6] We have chosen to use the term 'British Civil Wars' for this volume, despite the fact that most of the chapters are Anglocentric. The conference at which most of the contributors presented their initial findings included two excellent papers on Ireland, but both were already earmarked for publication elsewhere. Nevertheless, the interconnectedness of the differ-ent theatres of war is evident in several of the chapters that follow, not only in terms of military operations, but also with regard to the effects on politics, society and culture.

Until the mid-twentieth century most of the writing on the civil wars con-sisted of military and constitutional accounts, led by S. R. Gardiner's mag-isterial *History of the Great Civil War* (1886–93).[7] Alongside these national narratives antiquarian studies chronicled the conflict in the provinces.[8] In the

1960s these local histories metamorphosed into something more ambitious when Alan Everitt and others sought to explain the causes and conduct of the conflict in terms of gentry-led county communities and their relationship with the centre.[9] Clive Holmes and Ann Hughes, who famously provided a corrective to the county community model, were no less concerned with this relationship, although their studies stressed the primacy of national politics.[10] The chapters in this volume reflect these and other developments, which have served to enhance our understanding of the period.[11] Given that these were wars, however, it is important to consider how this volume stands in relation to wider historiographical trends in military history and the medical humanities.

Conflict has been an ever-present factor in human affairs, so it would seem to follow that war should be an important field of historical study. Why then do some surveys of the historian's craft fail even to mention war, much less military history?[12] And why should military historians – particularly those in the United States – so often complain of being belittled and shunned by academic colleagues?[13] It is not simply because war is hideous, for military historians would readily agree that it is; indeed, in the preface to his most famous work, *Fifteen Decisive Battles of the Western World*, the Victorian military historian Sir Edward Creasy intimated that those who revelled in war were either weak-minded or depraved.[14] The answer can be found in the cultural trauma of two World Wars, coupled with the democratisation of academe in the latter half of the twentieth century. Post-war governments in Britain, North America and several other countries sought to provide better educational opportunities for their respective populations after 1945. The establishment of new universities led to an expansion in the numbers of students, and these came from an increasingly diverse range of backgrounds. Many of these individuals eventually secured academic positions, which enabled them to promote the historical study of hitherto neglected social and ethnic groups.[15] Such aspirations, which fitted well with emerging post-modernist theory, led them to distrust traditional modes of history writing, which they saw as predicated on the activities and concerns of the political elite. Military scholars steeped in the Creasy paradigm of decisive battles, high politics and great leaders found themselves increasingly marginalised as more and more history departments were colonised by social and cultural historians. Of course, there was not simply an issue with the mode of military history, but also its subject matter. The situation became acute in the late 1960s when a strong anti-war movement emerged within Western academia, and students protested against American military involvement in Vietnam. Since the millennium, the superpowers' military interventions around the world and the attendant humanitarian disasters have revived such sentiments: academic military historians have been accused of lending respectability to industrial military complexes, and nurturing the public's morbid fascination with organised violence.[16] However, Ludmilla Jordanova has cautioned against neglecting this or any other historical specialism simply because the 'object of study or the manner in which it is pursued raises difficult issues or mobilises prejudices'.[17] Military history is a large tent, and academics have had to come to terms with the fact that it includes the purposely desensitised 'operational' history of the military academies on the one hand, and on the other a popular market which ranges from well-written analytical studies to near-pornographic narratives of violence.[18] Academic military history has undergone several transformations as a result of these pressures.

John Keegan's *The Face of Battle* (1976) has often been hailed as the catalyst for this process of refashioning. Although much of his book features fairly standard military narrative, Keegan certainly stimulated historians' interest in the impact of combat on individuals. He was not the first to venture into this area, for Bell Wiley had already written about the experiences of American Civil War soldiers in the 1940s.[19] That conflict also provided fertile ground for scholars to examine relationships between war and society: the so-called 'new military history', which emerged in the United States during the late 1970s. Shaffer's account of the struggles of African-American veterans and war widows to obtain equitable pensions from the Federal authorities is a recent example of this approach.[20] Nevertheless, the 'new military history' has attracted considerable criticism over the years. Stephen Morillo, while conceding that it helped rehabilitate war studies in university departments, hints that its original disciples presented themselves as social historians primarily to enhance their employability. His suspicion that they had sought to ingratiate themselves with academic colleagues by adopting a condemnatory tone in their publications echoes an earlier comment made by John A. Lynn, who described their terminology as 'apologetic'.[21] Practitioners of the 'new military history' have been accused of being uninterested in war, and some detractors have criticised them for focusing on veteran pensioners and prisoners-of-war, on the grounds that such individuals should be considered tangential to military studies. It was because these people could be viewed as victims, Lynn suggested, that the new military historians found it 'somehow more admirable to study them'.[22] Clearly, orthodox military historians had been stung by the dismissive and often sanctimonious attitudes they were then encountering within academe. At the same time they were genuinely concerned that military history was being diluted and adulterated. John Keegan had already expressed such anxieties in *The Face of Battle*, when he inferred from a review by Sir Michael Howard (that doyen of British military historians) that in the final analysis military history must be about combat.[23] It is instructive, therefore, to remember what Howard himself wrote in his introduction to *War in European History* (1976):

> But to abstract war from the environment in which it is fought and study its technique as one would those of a game is to ignore a dimension essential to the understanding, not simply of the wars themselves but of the societies which

fought them. The historian who studies war, not to develop norms for action but to enlarge his understanding of the past, cannot be simply a 'military historian', for there is literally no branch of human activity which is not to a greater or lesser extent relevant to his subject. He has to study war not only, as Hans Delbrück put it, in the framework of political history, but in the framework of economic, social and cultural history as well.[24]

In other words, combat cannot be properly understood without a context – and a multivalent context at that. Most medievalists and early modernists accepted this long ago, although they can be forgiven for wondering why colleagues working on modern wars sometimes seem to forget that life existed before the French Revolution. There is, for example, this astonishing statement in Keegan's *The Face of Battle*:

> It is really only in the English-speaking countries, whose land campaigns, with the exception of those of the American Civil War, have all been waged outside the national territory, that military history has been able to acquire the status of a humane study with a wide general readership among informed minds.[25]

It is remarkable that a statement which seeks to make a case for Anglophone particularity should overlook the myriad civil wars in Britain during medieval and early modern times, to say nothing of the numerous historical conflicts between the nations of the British archipelago. One of the aspects of early modern military historiography which does seem to have made an impression on historians of modern warfare is the debate concerning the early modern military revolution in technology, tactics and fortifications, and its role in state formation.[26] It should not be too much of a leap, therefore, to appreciate why contributors to this present volume consider that issues such as war-related mortality, medical care, desertion, pensions and welfare are highly relevant to the military revolution debate, because all had a significant impact on the state's capacity to wage war.

European historians have been less agitated by the 'new military history' than their American colleagues. One reason for this was that they found little in it that was actually new, another was that they viewed war-and-society studies as an expansion of traditional military history rather than its replacement.[27] M. S. Anderson has traced the beginnings of a European 'war-and-society' movement back to the 1960s, arguing that this was when scholars first began to question the efficacy of traditional military history:

> Although [military historians] had paid much attention to what armed forces did to one another in war, they normally showed little interest in how those armed forces related to the societies from which they were drawn and in what war itself – the experience of it while it was going on, the perhaps huge net effect of it once it was over – did to the societies which engaged in it.[28]

In fact, at least one historian had begun to consider these issues over half a century earlier. Sir Charles Harding Firth is best known as the author of

Cromwell's Army (1902), a comprehensive examination of the physical and mental world of parliamentarian soldiers. His research into the treatment of sick and wounded servicemen, and state provision for their demobilised comrades, was unprecedented. As one reviewer acknowledged at the time, these were subjects which historians had hitherto scorned to touch.[29] Firth's Victorian contemporaries tended to see even their own soldiery as a faceless mass, to be deployed (and written about) with no more sensitivity than moving pins on a map. He had perhaps first begun to think of common soldiers as individuals in the 1890s when editing the Clarke Papers. Reading the minutes of the Putney Debates between the rank-and-file and their commanders in 1647 (which had been recorded by William Clarke in his capacity as Secretary to the Council of the Army) Firth became intrigued by the 'agitators' who had been elected to represent their comrades in the debates. Such men required a very different scholarly approach from that used to study the political and social elite.[30] Firth's next publication, in 1901, was an article on the sick and wounded soldiers of the civil wars.[31] He returned to this theme in the following year, in *Cromwell's Army*. Later, looking back on his career, Firth expressed regret that he had not found the time to examine the impact of the civil wars upon civilian society. He had nonetheless produced a body of work that was ahead of its time, four decades before Trevelyan's *English Social History*, and sixty years before E. P. Thompson set out to rescue the working classes from the condescension of posterity.[32]

Despite Firth's innovative scholarship, publishers were slow to wean their readers off narratives which focused almost exclusively on generalship and strategy. Traditional military historians such as J. F. C. Fuller continued to dominate publishing catalogues until the end of the Second World War.[33] Nevertheless, Firth's legacy became increasingly evident when discussions of military medicine and welfare began to appear in academic works by the likes of Elizabethan scholar C. G. Cruickshank, and later still in popular histories of the civil wars written by Brigadier Peter Young and Wilfred Emberton.[34]

In recent years military historians have witnessed the emergence of a so-called 'third school', whose practitioners utilise a range of interdisciplinary approaches in order to examine armed conflict as a cultural phenomenon. Some might argue that culture has always been an important consideration for military historians: Hans Delbrück posited links between national cultures and ways of waging war well over a century ago, and numerous historians were still emphasising the importance of culture in shaping military practice in the 1970s and 1980s.[35] It fell to John Shy to lay the foundations of a theoretical framework for a cultural approach to the history of war in 1993.[36] Even the US military colleges have come to embrace the cultural turn, seeing in it an opportunity to enhance their 'operational' histories, and thereby gain a deeper understanding of the strategic cultures of friend and foe.[37]

Many critics of the war-and-society approach have proved receptive to this cultural turn. Even as he excoriated the 'new military history' in 1997,

Lynn declared culture and gender to be more profitable ways of analysing the military activity of the past.[38] Notwithstanding an instinctive suspicion of theory, his cultural approach consists of three strands: societal, military and strategic.[39] Ironically, the first strand in particular raises questions as to where 'society' ends and 'culture' begins; as discussions of plunder and rape in Lynn's own highly acclaimed *Women, Armies and Warfare in Early Modern Europe* (2007) illustrate.[40] The chapters in this present volume seek to explore those boundaries while investigating how cultural attitudes towards war (particularly civil war) were constructed, negotiated and maintained in seventeenth-century England and Scotland.

The collected essays in *Battle-scarred* investigate the capacity of the British peoples to cope with the traumatic events of the mid-seventeenth century, and with the physical, mental and cultural scars left in their wake. The dividing line between civilian and military communities was always blurred: apart from the fact that civilians and soldiers were invariably in close proximity to one another, most soldiers were not career professionals but, rather, civilians who had been induced to fight. Nevertheless, from the moment such individuals enlisted they were viewed in a different light. This volume is divided into three sections: Part I focuses on mortality and memorialisation; Part II offers several different perspectives on military medicine during the civil wars; Part III surveys the hidden human costs of war, including military-related disorder, psychological trauma and the complex issues associated with war relief.

In Part I Ian Atherton and Stuart Jennings consider how soldiers died, and what happened to their bodies. Whereas Atherton's chapter concentrates on battlefield fatalities, Jennings uses the royalist garrison of Newark as a prism through which to view the effects of epidemic disease. One question common to both chapters concerns the location of the physical remains. Huge numbers of dead must have been interred in individual graves or in mass burial pits after battles such as Marston Moor (where as many as 6,000 soldiers are thought to have died), and during numerous garrison epidemics.[41] That only a tiny fraction of these inhumations have so far been identified contrasts markedly with numerous discoveries associated with the Wars of the Roses. Osteoarchaeologists and forensic scientists know far more about medieval soldiers than those of the mid-seventeenth century (although the recent archaeological discovery of a mass grave containing soldiers killed at the battle of Lützen in 1632 may eventually help to redress this balance).[42] Both chapters contain intriguing suggestions as to why the bodies of civil-war soldiers remain largely unaccounted for. The practice in modern conflicts has been to construct and maintain battlefield cemeteries as sites of social memory and public commemoration. Atherton argues that this culture of memorialisation has encouraged archaeologists to rely heavily on later oral traditions when searching for civil-war battlefields and bodies. He proposes that they should pay more attention to seventeenth-century records and culture. By analysing contemporary records regarding the handling of

7

the slain, he contributes to ongoing debates regarding the nature and preservation of civil-war battlefields, and collective memories of the conflict. In
contrast to the care lavished on the bodies of the elite, and despite recent
historiography which argues that parish registers were strikingly inclusive
when recording mortality within civilian communities, Atherton concludes
that common soldiers were regarded as social outcasts even in death, and that
little effort was made to mark the site of their final resting place.

Atherton's findings dovetail neatly with Jennings' chapter on Newark.
Most soldiers spent their time occupying towns, patrolling and exploiting
the surrounding area, rather than fighting in large set-piece battles. Violent
death could come during a siege, or when conducting small-scale raids on
adjacent enemy territory, but even when they were besieged garrison troops
were far more likely to die of disease than anything else. Plague and other
epidemics regularly afflicted large towns in peacetime, particularly those
such as Newark, which lay astride important trade routes. In time of war
the presence of large numbers of troops made epidemics even more likely.
The risk was significantly higher when the soldiers came from outside the
area, as in October 1645 when Prince Rupert arrived at Newark with troopers from plague-ridden Bristol. Relations between civic authorities and garrison commanders were often complicated by arguments over resources and
housing, but outbreaks of dysentery, typhus or plague generally encouraged
cooperation. Jennings has analysed Newark's well-preserved civic archives
and what survives of the garrison's military records in order to reconstruct
the aetiology of disease in the town between 1642 and 1646. He finds that
Newark's civilian leaders were sensible of the military's need to maintain
discipline and combat effectiveness, while the royalist commanders acknowledged their moral obligation to protect civilian residents. Jennings explains
how responsibility for the measures to limit the spread of infection was
shared, how and where infected soldiers and civilians were treated, and who
met the cost of medical care and burial. He finds that while soldiers and civilians seem to have been treated equitably for the duration of their illness, they
were segregated after death. Consequently, whereas the burials of the town's
civilians were carefully recorded, the whereabouts of the military's burial
pits remain a matter of conjecture. Even in a staunchly royalist town such as
Newark, garrisoned largely by royalist troops recruited from the surrounding
area, soldiers remained a race apart.

Part II considers various aspects of military medicine during the civil
wars. The early modern period witnessed profound developments in medical
practice and theory. During the sixteenth century, medieval prohibitions on
dissection had been lifted, allowing practitioners such as Andreas Vesalius to
formulate a more accurate understanding of human anatomy. This offered
a corrective to the profession's widespread reliance on the theories of the
classical Greek physician Galen. These theories, which were largely based
on animal dissection, held that the body contained four 'humours' (blood,

yellow bile, black bile and phlegm), and that illness resulted from an imbalance between these fluids. Galen's notions were further challenged in the late sixteenth and early seventeenth centuries by the Swiss physician Paracelsus, and the Fleming Jan Baptist van Helmont, pioneers in the use of chemical medicines. Although iatrochemistry had not entirely superseded humoral theory by the end of the seventeenth century, it was indicative of a trend towards a more scientific approach based on experimentation and observation. The foremost representative of this trend in England before the civil wars was William Harvey – royal physician to both James I and Charles I – whose work on the function of the heart and blood circulation, *De Motu Cordis*, was published in Frankfurt in 1628. Harvey's findings met with a mixed reception, not least within the Royal College of Physicians, but his research and lectures had a profound effect on medical practice.

The historiography of medicine has undergone a transformation quite as dramatic as that experienced in military studies in recent decades. As Ian Mortimer has noted, medical practice in the sixteenth and seventeenth centuries can no longer 'be regarded as simply the low foothills before the steeper slopes of modern medical discoveries'.[43] Scholars such as Charles Webster and Roy Porter have successfully questioned the traditional view of early modern medical professionals as blundering amateurs, while Margaret Pelling has prompted us to re-evaluate the provision of medical care for those below the elite.[44] Mortimer himself has argued that there is evidence for a significant increase in medical usage from the mid-seventeenth century onwards, an argument with which Patrick Wallis has concurred.[45] Webster has provided a model for viewing the seventeenth century as a watershed in medical thinking, placing reforms in science and medicine within the wider movement for social reform fuelled by the apocalyptic and millenarian traditions of the so-called 'Puritan Revolution'.[46] While Webster's arguments have been questioned by Peter Elmer (who has shown that the drive for medical reform was shared by royalists and Anglicans) the historiography to date suggests that this was a key period in British medicine.[47]

The role the British Civil Wars played in the development of medicine – not least in increasing the demand for, and supply of medical care – remains largely underexplored. Harold Cook has argued that warfare was a primary factor in transforming medicine internationally, but suggests that as far as Britain is concerned the key period was at the end of the seventeenth century. By this interpretation, the restructuring of the British military establishment and attendant medical services after 1689 was undertaken in order to facilitate the large-scale Continental campaigns waged during the reigns of William and Anne. Cook's model implies that this restructuring acted as the catalyst for change, but he does acknowledge that some developments had their roots in earlier decades.[48] This makes it all the more imperative to encourage further study into how the medical profession reacted and adapted to the demands of the civil wars. Discussions on the subject have been hampered by the fact that it is only in recent years that the historical study of military medicine has begun to catch up with the rest of the medical humanities. C. H. Firth wrote in 1902 that he found the history of medical provision during the civil wars to be wholly inadequate; however, although he was keen to redress this deficiency he saw no reason to challenge the traditional view that early modern regimental surgeons were ignorant quacks.[49] Little progress had been made by 2001 when Eric Gruber von Arni sought to publish his work on parliamentarian military hospitals and nursing. During his researches Gruber von Arni was forced to contend with medical historians who held that warfare had had little effect on medieval and early modern medicine, and was therefore unworthy of study.[50] Since the millennium the situation has improved markedly, but there is still more to do as regards the early modern period. There are, nevertheless, reasons to be optimistic: firstly, although this present volume is devoted to the effects of land warfare, there is no doubting the huge strides which have been made in the study of early modern naval medicine by scholars such as Geoffrey L. Hudson.[51] It is also noteworthy that the Centre for Medical History at the University of Exeter saw fit to recruit a military specialist, Ismini Pells, into the team of their Wellcome Trust project, 'The Medical World of Early Modern England, Ireland and Wales 1500–1715', and that the Wolfson Foundation has funded the foundation of the Research Centre for Care, Welfare and Medicine at the National Civil War Centre in Newark.[52] Finally, it is a sign of progress that the issues discussed in Part II have now begun to seep into the mainstream histories of the civil wars.

   Stephen Rutherford's chapter focuses on the practicalities of military surgery, particularly the treatment of gunshot wounds. The rapid increase in the use of firearms in warfare led to profound changes in the balance of wound types by the end of the sixteenth century. Belying their popular image as incompetent butchers, many military surgeons appear to have been highly proficient, developing new techniques and surgical instruments in order to cope with an increasingly industrialised battlefield environment. Rutherford surveys the damage musket balls could inflict on the human body, and, using case studies and treatises authored by surgeons who served during the conflict, assesses how military surgery had developed by the mid-seventeenth century. English surgeons such as the parliamentarian James Cooke and the royalist Richard Wiseman were familiar with the latest European practices, and utilised an evidence-based approach reminiscent of modern practice. Rutherford considers the efficacy of their methods in the light of his detailed knowledge of modern biology, pathology and treatments. He finds that the techniques used by civil-war surgeons, and military surgical procedures, compare favourably with practices from the nineteenth century to the present day. Despite the fact that seventeenth-century medical practitioners knew nothing of microbiology, and little of the biological basis of physiology or wound-healing, Rutherford demonstrates that their procedures were often highly effective. Notwithstanding the lack of antibiotics, anaesthetics, hygienic environments and high-quality surgical steel, survival rates appear to have been impressively high. Rutherford concludes that in finding effective answers to the problems posed by the advent of gunpowder weapons, early modern practitioners should be seen as competent professionals who laid the foundations of modern surgery.

The man at the centre of Ismini Pells's chapter, Major-General Philip Skippon, received a near-fatal gunshot wound at the battle of Naseby in June 1645. At the height of the battle, a musket ball punched through his armour and penetrated his stomach, leaving him with an eight-inch wound. The extensive surviving documentation relating to the surgical operations and palliative care the general received allow for an unusually detailed medical case study. Using contemporary medical memoirs and treatises as a backdrop, Pells utilises original correspondence, financial accounts and hitherto unused material from Northampton General Hospital's archives to demonstrate that the episode reflected the best medical standards of the time. As she explains, there was more to this case than meets the eye: the fact that a particular faction within the parliamentarian alliance had substantial political capital invested in the general's recovery meant that the physicians and surgeons attending him were required to operate under considerably more pressure than usual.

Eric Gruber von Arni has been a leading light in the struggle to raise the profile of early modern military medicine, not least through his ground-breaking monograph *Justice to the Maimed Soldier*, which surveyed Parliament's military hospital provision and nursing during the civil wars.[53] He has gone on to produce further important studies on military medicine in the later seventeenth century.[54] In *Battle-scarred* Gruber von Arni focuses on royalist medical provision during the First Civil War, most especially military hospitals in the Oxford area. The fact that royalist hospitals are far less well documented than their parliamentarian counterparts perhaps explains why they have not previously been studied in any depth. Gruber von Arni begins by surveying the medical care provided for the royalist casualties injured at Edgehill in October 1642. He goes on to consider conditions in the Culham Hill Leaguer outside Oxford in 1643, before providing an assessment of the royalist military hospitals in and around Oxford. His findings leave no doubt as to the problems which faced Charles I and his advisors in the royalists' wartime capital. Supplies were often scarce, and overcrowding in the city created logistical, clinical and environmental problems. The chapter also examines royalist military hospital provision elsewhere in the country. Gruber von Arni concludes that, notwithstanding the imbalance in resources between the two sides, the royalists failed to give casualties the same priority as their parliamentarian enemies.

Richard Jones's chapter posits a number of links between the life-cycle of a famous Elizabethan reference work – John Gerard's *Herball, or, Generall*

Historie of Plantes (1597) – and the brutal realities of the civil wars. Gerard was a herbalist of repute in Elizabethan England, influential in the Barber-Surgeons' Company, and closely connected with Lord Burghley, but like so many early modern authors his work relied heavily on the efforts of predecessors. Nevertheless, his voluminous and expensive compendium was soon established as an essential reference work within the medical profession. Its popularity was boosted in 1633 by the publication of a revised and expanded edition, undertaken by the Yorkshire-born apothecary and physician Thomas Johnson. The work remained the most detailed and up-to-date commentary on the subject until Culpeper's *English Physician* appeared in the 1650s. For this reason, Jones is on safe ground in arguing that the 1633 edition informed the work of medical practitioners during the civil wars, and he demonstrates that many of the herbs and plants described therein were directly relevant to military medicine. Thomas Johnson's involvement with Gerard's *Herball* is therefore somewhat ironic: he went on to serve as a royalist field officer during the First Civil War, only to die of a fever in 1644 while recuperating from wounds suffered during a skirmish near Basing House.[55] Having established the historical context of the 1633 edition, Jones conducts a meticulous examination of a surviving copy, tracing its provenance through several generations of a Nottinghamshire family. The Coopers were noted royalists, and the head of the family, Sir Roger Cooper, was closely involved with the defence of Newark. The family home in Thurgarton hosted a small royalist garrison, and may conceivably have functioned as a military hospital for Newark. With this genealogical and historical information as a backdrop, Jones moves on to analyse the text, and more crucially the written annotations and manicules (pointing hands) in the margins. It is clear that this particular copy was consulted repeatedly for information on treatments of ailments commonly associated with siege warfare. Drawing the various strands of evidence together, Jones argues that the copy may very well have been utilised during the second siege of Newark in 1644.

Part III embraces both the cultural turn and war-and-society studies. The formation of collective memory is an important element in the process of shaping a society's political and military culture. In this, as in so many other things, modernists and early modernists have travelled the same road, mostly in blissful ignorance of each other's presence. There is now a healthy body of work on the complex relationships between war, societal culture, welfare and memorialisation in the modern world, underpinned by series such as Palgrave Macmillan's War, Culture and Society, and Manchester University Press's Cultural History of Modern War.[56] It is instructive, for example, to read Drew Gilpin Faust's account of how Confederate and Federal authorities developed protocols to manage the horrendous mortality of the American Civil War, both in terms of logistics and the maintenance of public morale.[57] Meanwhile, on the other side of the ridge, early modernists have been exploring similar issues in their own period. The recent historiography of the

British Civil Wars is rich in such studies, some predicated on the high politics at the centre, others on the social politics of the parish.[58] Just as Faust has uncovered a republic of suffering in the *post-bellum* United States, so the chapters here illustrate how the warring sides, and the civilian communities they administered, faced increasingly complex moral dilemmas and practical difficulties as the wars continued. If anything, these problems gained greater urgency after the fighting had ended. Not only had successive Commonwealth, Protectorate and Restoration regimes to deal with a divided society's collective sense of moral dislocation and mass bereavement, they had also to satisfy the expectations of thousands of maimed and impoverished officers and men, and an equally large army of widows and orphans. Furthermore, each regime in turn had to decide how to behave towards former enemies, thousands of whom had also been maimed, impoverished and bereaved – but who, as myriad petitioners emphasised, had been the agents of their own side's suffering.

David Appleby argues in his chapter that although the 'wandering soldier' was a stock figure in early modern literature, the deserters who haunted civilian communities have received little more than a passing mention in the historiography. It is also interesting that although there is now a rich historiography relating to early modern vagrancy, the civil wars are rarely discussed; indeed, the reader could be forgiven for assuming that war-related mortality between 1639 and 1652 reduced the floodtide of vagrants to a manageable trickle. Utilising local archives, state papers, plays, ballads and popular literature, Appleby argues that historians have seriously underestimated the political threat represented by the activities of thousands of deserters, escaped prisoners-of-war and counterfeit soldiers. The chapter shows how parish officials became adept at identifying different categories of unsupervised 'wandering soldiers'; an important skill, given that some could be extremely dangerous. Appleby challenges the received wisdom that demobilised veterans and deserters simply went home, arguing that thousands of conscripts had little incentive to do so. The chapter considers the economic dislocation which could be caused by such population displacement. Finally, Appleby scrutinises the efforts made by the authorities to manage the problem, and why, given the numbers involved, the old moral panics associated with vagabonds did not reoccur.

The chapter by Erin Peters investigates the public narration of psychological disability brought on by the lingering effects of combat trauma and memories of fear among soldiers and civilians during and after the civil wars. This is a particularly timely study given that psychologists specialising in modern post-traumatic stress disorder are beginning to explore the advantages of adding a historical dimension to their research.[59] Peters challenges conventional histories of psychiatry, which assume that medieval and early modern attitudes to mental illness were dominated by demonological concepts, and that the afflicted were treated in a cruel and inhumane manner as a consequence. A very different picture emerges from popular literature before, during and after the civil wars, with writers able to construct and disseminate remarkably sensitive psychological disability theories and narratives. These publications reflected a growing interest in the conceptualisation of psychological damage that was far removed from crude ideas of 'good' and 'evil'. Peters analyses the ways in which people attempted to understand their experiences of the civil wars, and the curative methods with which they attempted to treat the invisible wounds inflicted by those experiences. She argues that contemporary responses to the disabling nature of psychological trauma demonstrate that people were cognisant of the therapeutic value of attempting to construct publically available narratives. Peters concludes that the civil wars caused a popular understanding of the disabling and disfiguring nature of psychological damage to develop, which contrasted with the central authorities' insistence on viewing disability purely in terms of physical impairment.

Hannah Worthen's chapter reveals that seventeenth-century Kent was a very singular county. It did not experience any serious fighting within its borders during the First Civil War, but unlike most other counties within the so-called parliamentarian heartlands of south-east and eastern England it was always deeply divided along political and religious lines. This instability allowed royalists to exploit local grievances against parliamentarian rule and stage a full-scale insurrection in 1648. The memory of 1648, and increasing political fragmentation, made the task of restoring peace, order and harmony in Kent much more difficult, at the same time as the county's proximity to London made it imperative. Worthen explores the relationships between rulers and ruled through the administration of military welfare in the county between 1642 and 1680, focusing particularly on the petitions of maimed soldiers and war widows preserved in Quarter Sessions records. In doing so, she re-engages with Alan Everitt's famous (and famously contested) 'county community' model to assess whether local expediency or national policy exerted the greater influence on the administration of war relief.[60]

Criticisms that Everitt's model was too heavily predicated on the county elite have become more strident as civil-war historiography has swung towards the social history of the common people. However, Andrew Hopper's chapter shows that there will always be a need to study the mores of political and social hegemony. Hopper draws on petitions submitted by the widows and orphans of Parliament's military commanders, along with correspondence written by them or on their behalf, to show how they mobilised personal networks to agitate in their favour. Just as their dead menfolk would have done, widows were obliged to adopt strategies to safeguard their families, livelihoods and estates. Hopper investigates what conduct and deportment were expected of elite war widows and how strategic self-fashioning might elicit favourable responses from authority. The chapter questions how elite widows fared in comparison with those of the rank and file, before measuring their experiences against those of royalist officers' widows petitioning for relief after 1660. Hopper concludes by arguing that in several cases their involvement and sacrifice for the cause transformed some widows into significant political figures.

In the final chapter, Chris Langley provides a wider British perspective by investigating the charitable campaign undertaken on behalf of Scottish prisoners-of-war held in England during the 1650s. The New Model Army took large numbers of Scots Covenanters prisoner at the battle of Dunbar in September 1650, most of whom were subsequently transported to Tynemouth Castle and Durham in England. Despite the disruption caused by the ongoing English invasion, Scottish Kirk leaders organised countrywide collections to enable the prisoners to purchase food and other essentials. Letters from Edinburgh arrived in parishes around Scotland, updating communities on the whereabouts and living conditions of their imprisoned servicemen, and requesting donations. There was an enthusiastic response, although only a proportion of the money reached the prisoners. Langley argues that ministers realised that this networking might serve as a way to heal differences within the Kirk and the wider Scottish political nation. As a result, their letters pointedly omitted references to the prisoners' previous political affiliations or the divisive issue of Charles II. Eventually the campaign merged into other movements aimed at unifying (Protestant) Scotland, and constructing a coherent opposition to English occupation. Langley concludes that the Kirk's charitable venture was not only successful in raising money, but made an important contribution to a wider political debate about what it meant to be a good Covenanter.

Battle-scarred, then, presents an integrated and multi-faceted survey of the 'Tragicall events' that attended the British Civil Wars, and how they affected English and Scottish people across the social spectrum. The historiography behind the topics covered by this volume is, in most cases, still very much in its infancy; as we are still in the process of framing the questions, this volume is necessarily a reconnaissance. It explores several promising avenues of research, which, it is hoped, will broaden the scope of civil-war studies. In *War in England, 1642–1649* (2008) – an outstanding example of recent scholarship on the mental landscape of the conflict – Barbara Donagan has ventured the rather pessimistic observation that 'the English civil war [*sic*] is of only moderate interest to military historians'.[61] It is true that the conflict did not inspire any great innovations in military technology, strategy or tactics; neither did the limited scale of the campaigns enable commanders such as Prince Rupert or Thomas Fairfax to establish reputations to match those of Gustavus Adolphus and Count Tilly in the Thirty Years' War.[62] Scholars who see military history solely in terms of combat can indeed safely ignore the civil wars. However, as discussed earlier, the finest military historians have invariably sought to take a more sophisticated approach.[63] Those who subscribe to a more inclusive military history can learn much from the innovations in administration and oversight which emerged during the conflict, particularly as these developments had an influence on British military and political culture – a culture which took on a global significance by the end of the seventeenth century.[64] Additionally, the conflict stimulated marked improvements in military medicine, and the quality of institutional care bestowed on maimed soldiers and war widows in seventeenth-century England compared favourably with that provided elsewhere in Europe. While few of the contributors to *Battle-scarred* would describe themselves as military historians, all intend that their work should complement and enhance the military and political history of the civil wars, not dilute or replace it. Above all, the editors' aim is to help bring about that 'complete-picture' history, which many military historians have themselves called for.[65] At the same time, we remain mindful of Barbara Donagan's comment that 'every war is miserable in its own way', and we note John A. Lynn's warning against creating a 'universal soldier' (or a universal surgeon, deserter, prisoner or war widow). Above all, we concur with Jeremy Black's observation that 'culture is dynamic, not static, as both a reality and as an analytical process'.[66] If the British Civil Wars teach us anything it is that culture – like history – is a malleable product.

NOTES

1 BL, Thomason E1150(3), E. Calver, *England's Sad Posture* (London, 1644), preface.
2 *Ibid.*
3 I. Gentles, *The English Revolution and the Wars in the Three Kingdoms, 1638–1652* (Harlow: Pearson Longman, 2007), p. 436.
4 J. Rushworth, *Historical Collections*, 8 vols (London, 1659); B. Whitelocke, *Memorials of the English Affairs* (London, 1682); E. Ludlow, *The Memoirs of Edmund Ludlow*, 3 vols (Vevay, Switzerland, 1698–99); E. Hyde, earl of Clarendon, *The History of the Rebellion and Civil Wars in England Begun in the Year 1641*, 3 vols (London, 1702–4). A critical survey of the early histories of the conflict can be found in C. H. Firth, 'The development of the study of seventeenth-century history', *Transactions of the Royal Historical Society*, 7 (1913), 25–30.
5 J. Morrill (ed.), *The Nature of the English Revolution* (London: Longman, 1993), p. vii.
6 L. Bowen, 'Rediscovering difference: nations, peoples and politics in the British Civil Wars', *History Compass*, 4:5 (2006), 847. The pioneer in this field was M. Stoyle, *Soldiers and Strangers: An Ethnic History of the English Civil War* (New Haven, CT: Yale University Press, 2005).
7 S. R. Gardiner, *The History of the Great Civil War*, 4 vols (London: Longmans, 1886–93).
8 A. Kingston, *East Anglia and the Great Civil War* (London: Stock, 1897); J. Willis Bund, *The Civil War in Worcestershire, 1642–1646* (Birmingham: Midland Educational Co. Ltd, 1905); E. Broxap, *The Great Civil War in Lancashire, 1642–1651*

(Manchester: Manchester University Press, 1910); A. C. Wood, *Nottinghamshire in the Civil War* (Oxford: Clarendon Press, 1937).

9   A. Everitt, *The Community of Kent and the Great Rebellion, 1640–60* (Leicester: University of Leicester Press, 1966); A. Fletcher, *A County Community in Peace and War: Sussex, 1600–1660* (London: Longman, 1975); J. Morrill, *Cheshire, 1630–1660: County Government and Society during the English Revolution* (Oxford: Oxford University Press, 1974).

10 C. Holmes, 'The county community in Stuart historiography', *Journal of British Studies*, 19:2 (1980), 54–73; A. Hughes, 'The king, the Parliament, and the localities during the English Civil War', *Journal of British Studies*, 24:2 (1985), 236–65.

11 C. Hill, *The World Turned Upside Down: Radical Ideas during the English Revolution* (London: Temple Smith, 1972); C. Hill, *The English Bible and the Seventeenth-Century Revolution* (London: Allen Lane, 1993); R. Cust, 'News and politics in early seventeenth-century England', *Past & Present*, 112 (1986), 60–90; J. Raymond, *The Invention of the Newspaper: English Newsbooks 1641–1649* (Oxford: Clarendon Press, 1996).

12 A recent example is P. Claus and J. Marriott (eds), *History: An Introduction to Theory, Method and Practices* (London: Routledge, 2012).

13 D. Showalter, 'A modest plea for drums and trumpets', *Military Affairs*, 39:2 (1975), 71; J. Lynn, 'The embattled future of academic military history', *The Journal of Military History*, 61:4 (1997), 778, 780–3; R. Citino, 'Military histories old and new: a reintroduction', *American Historical Review*, 112:4 (2007), 1070.

14 E. Creasy, *Fifteen Decisive Battles of the Western World* (3rd edn, London: Richard Bentley, 1852), p. vii.

15 S. Morillo, with M. Pakovic, *What Is Military History?* (Cambridge: Polity Press, 2006), p. 39.

16 Morillo, *What Is Military History?*, pp. 38–9, 41; J. Chambers II, 'The new military history: myth and reality', *The Journal of Military History*, 55:3 (1991), 395.

17 L. Jordanova, *History in Practice* (2nd edn, London: Hodder Arnold, 2006), p. 176.

18 See N. Dixon, *On the Psychology of Military Incompetence*, quoted in R. Holmes, *Acts of War: The Behaviour of Men in Battle* (London: Cassell, 1985), pp. 4–5.

19 B. Wiley, *The Life of Johnny Reb* (Baton Rouge, LA: Louisiana University State Press, 1943); B. Wiley, *The Life of Billy Yank* (Indianapolis, IN: Bobbs-Merrill Co., 1952).

20 D. Shaffer, *After the Glory: The Struggles of Black Civil War Veterans* (Lawrence, KA: University Press of Kansas, 2004).

21 Morillo, *What Is Military History?*, pp. 39–40; Lynn, 'The embattled future of academic military history', 784.

22 Lynn, 'The embattled future of academic military history', 784; Citino, 'Military histories old and new', 1070; R. Browning, 'New views on the Silesian Wars', *Journal of Military History*, 69:2 (2005), 522–3.

23 J. Keegan, *The Face of Battle* (London: Jonathan Cape, 1976), p. 29.

24 M. Howard, *War in European History* (Oxford: Oxford University Press, 1976), pp. ix–x.

25 Keegan, *The Face of Battle*, p. 55.

26 C. Rogers (ed.), *The Military Revolution Debate: Readings on the Transformation of*

Early Modern Europe (Boulder, CO: Westview Press, 1995); Citino, 'Military histories old and new', 1077–8.

27 D. Dunn (ed.), *War and Society in Medieval and Early Modern Britain* (Liverpool: Liverpool University Press, 2000), p. 1.

28 M. Anderson (ed.), *War and Society in Europe of the Old Regime 1618–1789* (Stroud: Sutton Publishing, 1998), p. 5.

29 C. H. Firth, *Cromwell's Army: A History of the English Soldier during the Civil Wars, the Commonwealth and the Protectorate* (London: Methuen, 1902), chapter 11; F. Harrison, 'Review of *Cromwell's Army*, by C. H. Firth', *English Historical Review*, 18:69 (1903), 170.

30 W. Clarke, *The Clarke Papers*, ed. C. H. Firth, 4 vols (Camden Society, new series, 1891–1901), I, p. 285.

31 C. H. Firth, 'The sick and wounded of the Great Civil War', *Cornhill Magazine*, 3rd series, 10 (1901), 289–99.

32 I. Roots, 'Firth, Sir Charles Harding (1857–1936)', *ODNB*; G. Trevelyan, *English Social History* (London: Longman, 1942); E. Thompson, *The Making of the English Working Class* (London: Victor Gollancz, 1963), p. 12.

33 J. Fuller, *The Generalship of Ulysses S. Grant* (London: John Murray, 1929); J. Fuller, *Grant & Lee: A Study in Personality and Generalship* (London: Eyre & Spottiswoode, 1933); J. Fuller, *The Decisive Battles of the Western World and their Influence upon History*, 3 vols (London: Eyre & Spottiswoode, 1954–56).

34 C. Cruickshank, *Elizabeth's Army* (Oxford: Oxford University Press, 1946), especially chapter 11 'The medical service'; P. Young and W. Emberton, *The Cavalier Army: Its Organization and Everyday Life* (London: Allen and Unwin, 1974).

35 Howard, *War in European History*, p. x; Morillo, *What Is Military History?*, p. 43; A. Marwick (ed.), *The Study of War and Society: Thucydides to the Eighteenth Century* (Bletchley: Open University Press, 1973), pp. 15–17.

36 J. Shy, 'The cultural approach to the history of war', *The Journal of Military History*, 57:5 (1993), 13–26.

37 W. Pruett, 'A history of the organizational development of the Continental Artillery during the American Revolution' (US Army Command and General Staff College, unpublished MA thesis, 2008), pp. 131–41; J. Black, *War and the Cultural Turn* (Cambridge: Polity Press, 2012), pp. 27, 152.

38 Lynn, 'The embattled future of academic military history', 784–9.

39 J. Lynn, *Battle: A History of Combat and Culture* (rev. edn, New York: Basic Books, 2003), pp. xv, xix, xx.

40 J. Lynn, *Women, Armies and Warfare in Early Modern Europe* (Cambridge: Cambridge University Press, 2007), pp. 150–9.

41 P. R. Newman and P. R. Roberts, *Marston Moor, 1644: The Battle of the Five Armies* (Pickering: Blackthorn Press, 2003), p. 124.

42 N. Nicklisch, F. Ramsthaler, H. Meller and S. Friederich, 'The face of war: trauma analysis of a mass grave from the Battle of Lützen (1632)', *Plos One*, 12/5 (2017); e0178252. https://doi.org/10.1371/journal.pone.0178252 (accessed 31 August 2017).

43 I. Mortimer, *The Dying and the Doctors: The Medical Revolution in Seventeenth-Century England* (Woodbridge: Boydell, 2009), p. 1.

44 C. Webster, *The Great Instauration: Science, Medicine and Reform 1626–1660*

(London: Duckworth, 1975); R. Porter, *Disease, Medicine and Society in England 1500–1860* (Basingstoke: Macmillan, 1987); M. Pelling, *The Common Lot: Sickness, Medical Occupations and the Urban Poor in Early Modern England* (Harlow: Longman, 1998).

45 Mortimer, *The Dying and the Doctors*, pp. 204–11; P. Wallis and T. Pirohakul, 'Medical revolutions? The growth of medicine in England, 1660–1800', *Journal of Social History*, 49:3 (2016), 510–31.

46 Webster, *The Great Instauration*.

47 P. Elmer, 'Medicine, religion and the puritan revolution', in R. French and A. Wear (eds), *The Medical Revolution of the Seventeenth Century* (Cambridge: Cambridge University Press, 1989), pp. 10–45.

48 H. J. Cook, 'Practical medicine and the British armed forces after the "Glorious Revolution"', *Medical History*, 34 (1990), 26.

49 Firth, *Cromwell's Army*, pp. 251, 254–5.

50 E. Gruber von Arni, *Justice to the Maimed Soldier: Nursing, Medical Care and Welfare for Sick and Wounded Soldiers during the English Civil Wars and Interregnum, 1642–1660* (2nd edn, Nottingham: Partizan Press, 2015), p. 2.

51 G. L. Hudson (ed.), *British Military and Naval Medicine, 1600–1830* (New York: Rodopi, 2007); G. L. Hudson, 'The relief of English disabled ex-sailors c. 1590–1680', in C. A. Fury (ed.), *The Social History of English Seamen, 1485–1680* (Woodbridge: Boydell, 2012), pp. 229–52.

52 http://humanities.exeter.ac.uk/history/research/centres/medicalhistory/pro jects/earlymodernmedicine (accessed 18 April 2017).

53 E. Gruber von Arni, *Justice to the Maimed Soldier: Nursing, Medical Care and Welfare for Sick and Wounded Soldiers during the English Civil Wars and Interregnum, 1642–1660* (1st edn, Aldershot: Ashgate, 2001).

54 E. Gruber von Arni, *Hospital Care and the British Standing Army, 1660–1714* (1st edn, Aldershot: Ashgate, 2006); E. Gruber von Arni, 'The medical resources of William III's English Army during the Nine Years' War', *Journal of the Society for Army Historical Research*, 85:342 (2007), 126–45.

55 C. King, 'Johnson, Thomas (1595x1600–1644)', *ODNB*.

56 For example, C. Reardon, *Pickett's Charge in History and Memory* (London: University of North Carolina Press, 1997); P. Fussell, *The Great War and Modern Memory* (Oxford: Oxford University Press, 1977); J. Watson, *Fighting Different Wars: Experience, Memory and the First World War in Britain* (Cambridge: Cambridge University Press, 2004); E. Rosenberg, *A Day Which Will Live: Pearl Harbor in American Memory* (Durham, NC: Duke University Press, 2003); J. Anderson, *War, Disability and Rehabilitation in Britain: Soul of a Nation* (Manchester: Manchester University Press, 2011).

57 D. Gilpin Faust, *This Republic of Suffering: Death and the American Civil War* (New York: Vintage Books, 2009), p. xviii.

58 B. Worden, *Roundhead Reputations: The English Civil Wars and the Passions of Posterity* (London: Allen Lane, 2001); J. Mills (ed.), *Cromwell's Legacy* (Manchester: Manchester University Press, 2012); G. L. Hudson, 'Negotiating for blood money: war widows and the courts in seventeenth-century England', in J. Kermode and G. Walker (eds), *Women, Crime and the Courts in Early Modern England* (London, University College, 1994), pp. 146–69; D. J. Appleby, 'Unnecessary persons?

Maimed soldiers and war widows in Essex 1642–1662', *Essex Archaeology and History*, 32 (2001), 209–21; M. Stoyle, 'Memories of the maimed: the testimony of Charles I's former soldiers, 1660–1730', *History*, 88:290 (2003), 204–26.

59 Professor Jamie Hacker Hughes at Anglia Ruskin: www.anglia.ac.uk/news/research-detects-ptsd-3000-years-ago (accessed 20 April 2017).

60 Everitt, *The Community of Kent and the Great Rebellion*.

61 B. Donagan, *War in England, 1642–1649* (Oxford: Oxford University Press, 2008), p. 2.

62 *Ibid.*, p. 3.

63 Howard, *War in European History*, pp. ix–x.

64 Donagan, *War in England*, p. 3.

65 Citino, 'Military histories old and new', 1081; Black, *War and the Cultural Turn*, pp. 148–9; Browning, 'New views on the Silesian Wars', 522–3; Howard, *War in European History*, pp. ix–x.

66 Donagan, *War in England*, p. 1; Lynn, *Battle*, p. xiii; Black, *War and the Cultural Turn*, pp. 3, 43.

Part I

—————

Mortality

Chapter 1

———◆———

Battlefields, burials and the
English Civil Wars

Ian Atherton

The idea that 'military care' extends beyond death to the treatment of the war dead is not new, though the forms it has taken have varied over time. Roger Boyle's 1677 military treatise advised a victorious general to look after the wounded and prisoners, and see 'his Dead honourably buried'. Similar ideas can be found in a number of sixteenth-century military manuals, and can be traced back at least as far as the Graeco-Roman world.[1] While the absence of discussion of burial in most manuals is striking, some did advise that burial of the dead was both a moral duty and good policy, since soldiers would be more likely to risk their own lives if they believed that they too would receive an honourable burial.[2] Such claims drew upon concerns for a decent burial, which scholars have noted as a significant pressure in early modern society, reflected in popular concerns about burial and funerals, as well as in the denial of burial in consecrated ground as a punishment for a variety of criminals and social outcasts from excommunicates to suicides.[3] 'Decent' or 'proper' burial meant interment in a designated burial place (usually a church or churchyard) in a shroud or coffin, usually in a single grave, with the body laid on its back and orientated east-west, accompanied by customary religious and social rites. Many Protestant writers tried hard to square the circle of biblical precedent for decent burial, alongside the teachings of reformed theology which were often allergic to ideas of sacred space, and general Christian ideas that the fate of the body after death did not affect the passage of the soul in the afterlife. Typically, Protestants resorted to claims that decent burial showed a proper regard for others and, as John Dunster, one of Archbishop Abbot's chaplains, put it, 'manifesteth our Faith and Hope of the Resurrection'. Failure to accord a corpse proper burial was variously criticised as 'inhumane and barbarous crueltie', 'impiety', or as treating Christians like carrion or swine, unless it was a deliberate act to show 'great indignation against sin'.[4] Wills reveal that hopes for proper burial extended to the lower levels of society, with testators setting out their desired burial location, or at least requesting 'decent' or 'Christian burial'.[5]

Elite burials during the civil wars reflected these ideas, continuing pre-war customs. Most spectacularly, the earl of Essex's funeral in 1646 was on a quasi-royal scale,[6] but elaborate heraldic funerals were not uncommon in war-time Oxford. Richard Symonds recorded five, such as that of Lord John Stewart, fatally wounded at Cheriton in 1644. His body, carried 'in an open chariot with his Coates of Armes' and accompanied by heralds and the queen's troop of horse, processed into Oxford where it was met by the senior herald and the king's troop of horse; the body was borne into Christ Church by colonels, with other officers carrying his armour; burial was on the south side of the quire next to the grave of his brother Lord D'Aubigny.[7] Officers killed on the battlefield might hope to have their bodies recovered for burial in the family vault, as Captain John Horsey of Clifton Maybank, killed while besieging neighbouring Sherborne Castle, was given a funeral 'after a martiall manner' and buried in Sherborne abbey among his ancestors in August 1645.[8] Death at a much greater distance from the family vault need pose no obstacle to the elite. When the earl of Lichfield was killed at Rowton Heath in September 1645 his body was marched by the victorious parliamentarians with a guard of horse and foot to a pre-arranged point where it was met by a comparable royalist military guard who processed into Chester garrison; the body was then embalmed awaiting collection. The earl's master of horse, a prisoner at Nantwich, obtained a pass to bury his lord and, after the surrender of Chester in February 1646, carried the corpse to Oxford where it was buried on 1 March in Christ Church cathedral next to his two brothers, lords Stewart and D'Aubigny.[9] Embalming the bodies of noble casualties to allow burial later was not uncommon: the body of Lord Brooke, killed while besieging Lichfield cathedral on 2 March 1643, was embalmed by the family's surgeon, James Cooke, probably at Coventry, and buried in the family vault at Warwick a few weeks later.[10] The social convention of fulfilling the deceased's wishes about burial placed a heavy burden on others that only the most extreme circumstances obviated. Bishop Robert Wright of Coventry and Lichfield died in Eccleshall Castle (one of his episcopal residences) in the summer of 1643, requesting burial in either Lichfield cathedral or Wadham college. When the royalist garrison fled in August on news of a parliamentarian advance, they took very little of the castle's provisions with them, but they did attempt to take Wright's corpse, only to abandon it on the drawbridge in panic as the enemy neared.[11]

If such proceedings were exceptional, officers might still expect that their bodies would be identified and given decent burial in the nearest church or churchyard. The morning after Marston Moor, the royalist prisoner Sir Charles Lucas was made to walk the battlefield to identify the bodies of royalist officers from among the dead lying on the field, all of which had already been stripped by the victors: one he recognised by a bracelet woven from his lover's hair, while other gentlemen were said to be readily distinguishable by their 'smooth, white Skins'.[12] A dead officer could expect a military funeral: Francis Markham's military treatise had described the formalities of such a send-off, with the ensign-bearer trailing his colours behind the corpse and then tossing them up and displaying them after the burial.[13] How far such rituals were followed is not known, but where financial accounts of officer funerals survive, they suggest elaborate affairs, such as the £11 3s 2d expended by Sir William Brereton's forces on the funeral of Major Robert Jackson, killed at Farndon Bridge in February 1645.[14] Just as elite prisoners were exchanged, so were their dead bodies.[15] A further sign that elite corpses were usually treated with the same respect during the war as in peacetime are the consequences of those dramatic occasions where such respect was not shown. When the body of Sir Edmund Verney was not found after the battle of Edgehill, stories began circulating that his ghost stalked the battlefield.[16] The lack of proper burial for Verney was accidental, but for the earl of Northampton, killed at Hopton Heath, it was initially deliberate, and provoked an outcry. Sir John Gell tried to ransom his corpse in exchange for the Parliament's captured artillery. The outraged royalists refused, and though the earl's body was not returned, Gell was forced to make some concessions to sentiment, taking the body to Derby, having it embalmed and then buried eleven weeks later in the vault of the earls of Devonshire in All Saints' church.[17] Pre-war practices for the elite continued in commemoration, with monuments and tombs recalling their service and sacrifice, though these were often not erected until after the Restoration. A memorial to Colonel Richard Bolles, killed at Alton in December 1643, with an inscription lauding his civil-war service, was erected by a relative in Winchester cathedral only in 1689. Even the middling sort might remember and commemorate their relatives who died in the wars. Nathaniel Friend, yeoman and schoolmaster, sought out the grave of his brother John, a parliamentarian quartermaster who had died of smallpox in 1645, paid for a gravestone in 1676 and visited it two years later.[18]

What of the corpses of the ordinary dead? In theory the same peacetime principles of decent burial applied. An army that made an orderly retreat from a defeat typically carried away its dead and wounded together in carts;[19] sometimes a truce was arranged between the two sides for the recovery of the dead, particularly during a siege where the opposing armies remained facing one another, as at Lyme Regis in 1644.[20] Relatives might search the bodies for their loved ones, as Sarah Frampton hunted through the night for her four brothers among the dead clubmen after the battle of Hambledon Hill in August 1645.[21] War, however, modified the customary treatment of the dead. Bodies left on a battlefield, the wounded and the dead, were routinely stripped, often within hours, sometimes even in the midst of a battle. Sir Adrian Scrope, left for dead on the battlefield of Edgehill, later explained his survival on the grounds that he had been promptly stripped, for the frost that night staunched the bleeding of his naked body.[22] Stripping the dead and dying was mainly an act of plunder used, as at Naseby, to reward the victorious troops, but occasionally items of military or propaganda value turned up, such as the crucifix and rosaries reportedly found on dead royalists at Caversham Bridge in May 1643.[23] When parliamentarians quit the siege of Banbury in September 1644, they desired to leave with the bodies of their dead; the defenders agreed, on condition that the plunder of all corpses lying within pistol shot of the castle walls should belong to them. They stripped the bodies and delivered them to the town's market place for collection; among the booty for the royalists were 120 arms and a collection of scaling ladders.[24] Prompt stripping of the dead, of course, rendered any attempts to distinguish friend from foe much harder.

The most detailed account we have of clearing an early modern battle-field comes not from the civil wars but from the battle of Sedgemoor, 1685. According to the parish register of Westonzoyland, only sixteen royal troops were reported killed: five of them were buried in the church, the remaining eleven in the churchyard; none were named. Monmouth's followers appear to have been buried where they fell. Captain Edward Dummer of the royal artillery recalled that some of the rebels were buried by the victorious soldiers on the battlefield, while those who died as they fled were buried by the countryfolk. Adam Wheeler, drummer in the Wiltshire militia, claimed that the local inhabitants gave an account to the minister and churchwardens of Westonzoyland of 1,384 dead and buried, along with many more as yet unfound in the cornfields. Nevertheless, they noted only 'about 300' of Monmouth's forces killed 'upon the spott' in their parish register. Wheeler also claimed to have seen 174 dead rebels lying in one heap about to be buried by locals in a pit.[25] Andrew Paschall, rector of neighbouring Chedzoy, provided a detailed account of the battle, including a map which noted, 'Slain in the moor and buried in one pit 195'.[26] A week after the battle a royal army officer, Colonel Percy Kirke, ordered local parishes to impress plough-teams and men, at their own expense, to rebury many interred on the moor in a shallow mass grave by erecting 'a mount' over them.[27] It seems likely that the forced employment of locals by the victorious army hastily to bury the dead where they fell was commonplace in the civil wars as it was at Sedgemoor forty years later; certainly, it is known that local inhabitants buried the dead at Edgehill and Marston Moor, and were apparently ordered to do so after the first battle of Newbury.[28]

The application of customary principles about decent burial became a weapon of the propaganda war, with both sides comparing their decent treatment with their opponents' inhumanity. After the first battle of Newbury the royalists alleged that Essex neglected the dead, forcing locals to undertake burial, and contrasted the king's 'pious care' in his order to the mayor of Newbury to oversee burial.[29] Both sides claimed that the other hastily threw their own corpses into pits, ditches, rivers and wells rather than give them proper burial.[30] For royalists, such claims were lent weight by the absence of a ceremony of burial in the 1645 Directory of Public Worship and allegations that sectaries believed that 'a Ditch or a Dunghill [was] thought as fit for Burial, as any Sepulcher'.[31] Both sides also alleged that the other desecrated tombs. Royalists claimed that roundhead soldiers broke into the Lucas vault in Colchester, scattering bones and wearing the corpses' hair as hatbands or bracelets, while Richard Symonds's diary of the royal army's progress is filled with accounts of tombs smashed by roundhead soldiers. Parliamentarians meanwhile alleged that cavaliers exhumed and broke into Brilliana Harley's coffin looking for jewels.[32] Irish Protestants made frequent allegations that Roman Catholics denied Protestant dead Christian burial, proclaiming them heretics, and accusing them of burying their Protestant victims in ditches, sandpits, sawpits or the sea, or leaving their corpses unburied to be eaten by crows and dogs.[33] Deliberate mutilation of the enemy's dead was not unknown before the civil wars, a practice echoing punishment of the corpses of certain criminals. It had been practised in the brutal wars in Tudor Ireland, for example, as well as, according to English sources, on the English dead at the battle of Bryn Glas, 1402, when Welsh women allegedly cut off the genitalia and noses of the English dead and placed them in their mouths and anuses. The incident was known to early modern audiences through mentions in Holinshed's *Chronicles* and Shakespeare's *Henry IV Part One* (I.i.41–6).[34] It was also not unknown in Ireland in the 1640s.[35] The French Wars of Religion, meanwhile, witnessed many incidents of the deliberate mutilation of corpses.[36] All these cases involved heightened ethnic hatred or the almost total collapse of social and political order. Nevertheless, no incidents of the deliberate mutilation of corpses on the battlefield are known from the civil wars in England,[37] where ethnic animosities did not, perhaps, run as strongly and where order was largely maintained in local communities. Nevertheless, the fear that dead bodies might be desecrated in the heat of battle led one royalist preacher to caution soldiers against 'wreak[ing] ones furie upon a dead carkas' as 'a most barbarous, cowardly thing, and odious to God'.[38]

Counting the dead was also a weapon of war, since the arithmetic of death (probably much exaggerated) constituted one way of claiming or magnifying victory. Both sides complained that the other hid their dead by burying them in secret places in order to disguise the true extent of their losses,[39] a tactic advised by some contemporary military manuals.[40] Counting was skewed by the conventions of social hierarchy, for one dead name of quality outweighed countless numbers of unnamed rank-and-file casualties. The parliamentarian chronicler John Vicars contrasted a list of 97 dead royalists (noblemen, officers and gentlemen) with 29 eminent parliamentarian dead as an 'Ocular Map' of the extent of the king's defeat in the wars. Commoner casualties were not included.[41] Moreover, the arithmetic of death was not even the principal way in which victory was measured, for lists of named prisoners taken at a battle occupied far more space on the printed page, and hence no doubt counted for more, than lists of the dead.[42] The modern equivalent of these lists are the famous casualty figures computed by Charles Carlton, that the civil wars in Britain saw unequalled numbers of dead in proportion to the total population – around 85,000 killed in combat in England, besides those who died from disease.[43]

Carlton's figures are often used to argue for the significance of the civil wars, but I wish to highlight them in another way. Where one might expect to see the war dead filling up page after page of parish registers, there is barely a mention. Estimates of the numbers killed at the battle of Hopton Heath in March 1643 varied widely from around 100 to 600, with modern scholarship suggesting 300–500 killed and wounded.[44] All of the registers from the surrounding parishes survive, but they record the burials of only three soldiers killed in the encounter. The battlefield lay in the parish of St Mary's, Stafford, and though the registers survive from 1643, they show only a typical number of burials in March 1643, none of which can be tied to the battle.[45] A similar case is Edgehill, where only fifteen burials can be found in local parish registers.[46] Comparable exercises for other civil war battles are difficult because registers are often missing or have obvious gaps; individual soldiers can only be identified if they were so described or noted as having died in a particular fight; while mass casualties may be revealed only in a sudden increase in the numbers of burials, such as in Cirencester, where the only indication in the register of Rupert's storming of the town on 2 February 1643 is the burial of sixteen persons (only two of them labelled as 'souldier'), on 5 February.[47] Some of these problems are illustrated by the first battle of Newbury, fought on 20 September 1643. The parish registers for Enborne, whose constables were ordered by Essex to bury the dead, do not survive before 1665. While those for Newbury are extant, there are no entries between 12 August and 1 October, leaving no signs of either the sixty cart-loads of dead and wounded reportedly carried into the town or the king's order to the mayor to organise burial. The Newbury churchwardens' accounts, meanwhile, show payments of £6 10s 5d for the purchase of shrouds and for burials of soldiers in the church, churchyard and on the battlefield at Wash Common.[48] These many problems, however, cannot account for most of the absence of burials, where many a register of a parish in the midst of the fighting shows no trace of the war whatsoever. So, where are all the bodies?

The straightforward answer is that they are probably buried on the battlefields themselves, as some at least of the Newbury dead were. Contemporary reports describe bodies being buried, often in mass graves rather than singly, on battlefields and, during sieges, in defensive works, or indeed in any available space. At Birmingham in 1643 it was supposed that many attacking royalists were buried in the defensive ditches they stormed; after the first battle of Newbury it was reported that thirty royalists were buried in one pit on the battlefield; after an attack on Marlborough, the king's forces buried their dead 'in severall places in the fields about the Town'.[49] Very few such burials have been found, even though finding the bodies remains the holy grail of conflict archaeology. One set of mass graves that has been excavated and linked to the civil wars is at York: ten post-medieval mass graves, each containing between four and eighteen bodies, most of them adult men, none showing unhealed battle trauma.[50] The investigating archaeologists suggested that they were parliamentarian troops who succumbed to disease while besieging York in 1644. For our purposes, three factors stand out. The first is the burial location. Seven of the pits were within the walls of All Saints' church, the remaining three just outside the church walls; and yet the church was disused and partially ruined, having been abandoned a century earlier. The archaeologists speculated that the site was chosen so that the bodies still lay in consecrated ground, but it is as likely that the spot was simply a vacant plot; two parliamentarian soldiers marching to the relief of Manchester in 1642 were buried in a bowling alley adjacent to an alehouse, suggesting that convenience rather than consecration governed the choice of burial place.[51] Second, the bodies lay in parallel rows, almost all orientated the same way, but they were not placed in the customary Christian fashion on their back: most lay face down or on their sides. Perhaps the corpses were shrouded and then rolled into pits. And third, the connection to the civil war is purely a supposition. Indeed, dating such burials is notoriously difficult without either associated finds or expensive radiocarbon dating.

The romance of the civil war means that any burial in the vicinity of a civil-war site is likely to be identified as a casualty of war. Any lump or bump on a battlefield has generally become, in popular memory, a mass grave. Mounds upon Wash Common at Newbury were, by the late nineteenth century, remembered as marking the site of mass graves from the first battle of Newbury; they are now determined rather to be a barrow cemetery of the Neolithic or Bronze Age.[52] Local memories about mass graves are often highly misleading. Guided by them, neither Edward FitzGerald at Naseby in the 1830s nor modern archaeological science at Sedgemoor have had much success in locating mass graves.[53] Modern archaeology has succumbed to the cult of the war dead and is likely to be misled into supposing any 'deviant burials' to be soldiers. In fits of romantic speculation, skeletons recovered from castles at Aberystwyth, Beeston, Nottingham, and Sandal have all been proclaimed to be civil-war dead despite the absence of strong supporting evidence; indeed, later radiocarbon dating of the Nottingham skeleton (carried out in 2016) suggested that it was buried *c.* 1500.[54]

Apart from the possible case of York, only two civil-war mass grave sites have been scientifically excavated. In 2001 two mass graves at Carrickmines Castle south of Dublin were found, containing at least twenty-one bodies, including women and children. They were determined to be some of those put to the sword by the Protestant troops who stormed the castle in March 1642. None of the bodies were orientated east-west in the traditional manner but some at least were laid in rows; at least one was buried face down.[55] In 2013 between seventeen and twenty-eight bodies were found in two pits at Durham Castle. Dating techniques and scientific analysis of their origin show they were Scottish soldiers captured at Dunbar in 1650. These were among the 1,700 Covenanters imprisoned at Durham who died from wounds, disease and ill treatment. The bodies were tipped into pits, jumbled together and tightly packed; the pits may have been left open while the bodies accumulated. All suggests disposal of bodies with little or no ceremony and no regard to notions of 'decent' burial.[56] These cases indicate that mass burials of common soldiers and ordinary civilians who died through or during the fighting were carried out with less care and reverence than peacetime norms dictated.

Why have the masses of civil-war dead proved so elusive? One answer is that there have been few modern archaeological excavations of any battlefield. Moreover, despite the folk memory of large mass graves (which finds echoes in toponyms such as 'Graveground Coppice' at Edgehill), it is more likely that the dead were buried where they fell in many shallow graves rather than parishes going to the expense of carrying all the dead to a central point for burial. Much of the killing probably took place over a wide area when an army broke and fleeing infantry were cut down by cavalry, leaving a trail of destruction for several miles (four at Naseby).[57] Comparisons should not be made with medieval battle-graves that have been excavated, such as at Visby (1361) and Towton (1461), for before the Reformation ideas about praying for the dead meant that there was considerable pressure to gather the bodies into a small area that might then be proclaimed consecrated ground (as at Agincourt, 1415) or to exhume the dead later and re-inter them in a churchyard (as at Towton).[58]

Some explanation for the missing war dead can be found if we return to parish registers. Recent work by Adam Smyth has shown the many ways in which parish registers were a genre of life writing, a central part of a Protestant means to 'record and remember the dead' following the abolition of purgatory, a written form of communal memory.[59] Smyth sees registers as dramatically inclusive; he emphasises the attention paid to marginal people who were often given a more detailed description or greater textual space than respectable parishioners; and he underlines the ways that registers responded to the high mortality of plague by linking entries into a narrative 'to create a heightened sense of society'. He does not consider registers and the civil wars, and it is striking how those wars challenge all three of Smyth's conclusions.

The exclusion of common soldiers from burial registers, otherwise so inclusive, is, as we have already seen, particularly marked. It was not the function of a register only to record those buried in the parish church and churchyard, thereby excluding battlefield burials, for it was not uncommon for registers to record burials both in other churches,[60] and elsewhere in the parish in unconsecrated ground.[61] Soldiers buried on the battlefield could have been included in parish registers just as some excommunicates or plague victims, buried in fields, were.[62] And occasionally such burials were noted: the register of Staindrop recorded the burial of William Joplin, 'slaine at the seidge of Raby Castle', on 27 August 1648 and then added 'Mem. Many souldiers slaine before Raby Castle, which were buried in the parke and not registered'.[63] But many more soldier burials were not recorded, their exclusion a considered omission, not inherent in the nature of the burial register.

Barbara Donagan's alternative explanation for the absence of soldiers – that normal procedures of burial and recording were overwhelmed by major battles – can also be dismissed.[64] The war certainly caused many problems of registration, but those cannot explain all the missing war dead. While a major battle no doubt made naming the dead impossible, it did not preclude counting them, and it is clear that parish clerks and others regularly totted up the numbers killed locally. Indeed the best estimates of the numbers killed at both Edgehill and Marston Moor were believed to come from the locals who had buried the dead. After Marston Moor (the bloodiest battle of the civil wars in England), John Vicars noted that 'the Countrymen (who were commanded to bury the dead Corps) told us, they, for certaine, buried 4150 bodies'.[65] Most civil-war engagements were far smaller and the numbers killed were by no means too great to be recorded in a parish register. Moreover, despite the dislocations of war, clerks and clergy often took great care during the war to ensure their records were as complete as possible, noting gaps and filling them retrospectively.[66] The minister of Horningsham in Wiltshire buried two soldiers from Weston in Somerset killed in 1644 while fighting in his parish; the following year he sent the details of their deaths to their home parish and his letter was entered into Weston's register.[67] The peacetime concern for the proper auditing of mortality continued during the war. The city of Oxford even published weekly bills of mortality during the wars.[68] Finally, it is important to note that the tribulations of war did not always prevent the keeping of financial accounts, which sometimes referred to the costs of burying soldiers. Despite siege and epidemic, the Newark churchwardens kept full accounts throughout the war, recording payments for winding sheets and inkles (tapes to tie the winding sheet) for a handful of soldiers in 1643 and 1644, and for 'passing Bells and making of souldiers graves' in 1645. The omission of soldiers in the parish register (where only twenty-eight officers and four common soldiers were recorded) was not therefore the result of administrative confusion.[69] Rather, it was a deliberate choice. It is instructive to compare the local response to plague epidemics, where only in the most severe epidemics were parishes overwhelmed and unable to record burials or forced to abandon traditional burial practices – practices which parishes surrendered much more willingly and consciously in the face of civil-war deaths.[70]

Occasionally, registers do give soldiers the greater textual space that Smyth has noted for other types of marginal people, recording not just the mere fact of burial but other details of their rank, regiment, circumstances of their death, or whether they supported the King or the Parliament. The Bunbury register, for example, records the burial of fifteen soldiers between 1643 and 1649, merely noting three as 'soldier' but giving additional details for the remaining twelve such as their regiment or troop, and whether they came from the garrison in Beeston Castle within the parish. Even anonymous soldiers might be described at length, such as 'A soldier slain by his fellow shooting at an other soldier that had been plundering at Richard Vernon's in Bunbury', buried on 30 March 1645.[71] Nonetheless, registers tend to give greater textual space to civilian victims of violent death during the wars than to soldiers. The Bunbury register also recorded the burial of Ralph Coddington in September 1643, 'shot through for saveing his own horse from the theft of a soldier who came from the [Castle]' and 'Richard Robinson of Alpraham wounded and dying there of by Chester soldiers' in March 1644. The Wolverhampton register notes the burial on 14 June 1644 of 'John Harrison, of Willenhall, killed by ye Parliament Souldiers in Monmore field', while Brewood has 'John Wourt, slaine at Bromehall by a Souldier' and Ellastone noted 'Hugh Poyser of Stanton, who was killed by Captain Watson's Souldiers in the night'.[72] These biographical details, preserving some memory of the civil wars as a violent conflict while ignoring the many more soldiers who died in the wars, reflect other ways in which many parish registers were used to record and preserve a memory of the wars. Key national events are sometimes noted. The register of Gayton noted 1640 as the year the Scots invaded England and took Durham and Newcastle-upon-Tyne, and also as the year of 'a great parliament' where Strafford, Laud, Finch and Windebank were prosecuted, while 1641 was the year 'the papists Rebells did rise in Ireland & did give Energie to killing & burning many townes'.[73] Such records were in part designed as reminders to repentance: after describing the battle of Edgehill, the Alrewas register added, 'O Lord give us grace to amend our lives'; a similar comment was added after the note of a fire in the village which destroyed two houses and a barn – national and local events could be seen in parallel as divine warnings.[74] The wars were typically remembered in parish registers as a time of disruption, turmoil and problems: 'This year / Brewtons ffeare / 1641' in the Bruton register. Stanton Lacy headed each of 1643, 1644 and 1645 with a Latin tag or verse, each one noting the times as ones of robberies, sedition or a deep abyss of misery, while in 1650 the register merely pleaded in Latin, 'Give peace O Lord we have exhausted ourselves'. Rotherby gave briefer headings to a number of years: 1643 was 'Bellum!', 1644 was 'Bellum! Interruption, Persecution!', while each year from 1649 to 1654 was 'Sequestration!'[75] While a few registers recorded the deliverance of the community from their enemies (such as Barnstaple and Beverley),[76] most comments viewed the war as a traumatic and terrible interruption into the fabric of the community, be it the nation or the parish; moreover, it was almost always an interruption from outside. That mindset helps to explain the exclusion of soldiers, often troublesome outsiders, from parish registers which preserved the memory of the community's dead. Those registers which were most likely to note large numbers of burials of soldiers are those of garrisons. The two parishes in Dudley recorded the burial of forty-two soldiers; most or all probably came from the garrison of Dudley Castle, for many had local names. Ludlow recorded the burials of fifty named soldiers, again presumably the majority of these came from the castle and were probably local.[77] Similarly, the register of Nantwich recorded the burial of 190 soldiers, but the chronology of the burials suggests that none of these were those royalists who besieged the town in the winter of 1643–44, nor those royalists defeated at the battle of Nantwich on 25 January 1644.[78] It would appear as if local soldiers were recorded in the parish registers, while soldiers from beyond the community were likely to be excluded. Entry in a parish register was a record of inclusion within the community, even for the marginalised and anonymous such as vagrants. But rarely for soldiers.

Despite all the early modern pressures for decent burial and a record of name and burial in the strikingly inclusive parish register, common soldiers were typically buried where they fell, kept away from the churchyard and excluded from the parish register. They might subsequently be remembered long after the wars had ended, and thereby reabsorbed into the communal fabric, as Richard Gough recalled the names and lives of eighteen men from Myddle who went off to fight.[79] Or their names might be remembered by their officers or within their regiment or troop, a body which functioned as a community of memory, as Mark Stoyle has argued, as Captain Henry Westby recorded in his account book the names of three of his troop killed at Marston Moor, as well as payments for the funeral of another of his troopers who died earlier in 1644.[80] But they were very often deliberately excluded from the institutionalised social memory of the parish, the burial register. The wounded of the civil war preserved the memory of the conflict on their bodies,[81] but the names of the rank-and-file dead had little part to play in parishes' memory of the wars. The chapters in this volume demonstrate early modern society's attempts to integrate the wounded back into communities (and the limits of those attempts); but during the wars themselves the common soldier was in death the ultimate social outcast.

NOTES

1 Wing / 0499, R. Boyle, *A Treatise of the Art of War* (London, 1677), p. 205; STC (2nd edn) / 11625, W. Garrard, *The Arte of Warre* (London, 1591), p. 338; T. Styward, *The Pathwaie to Martiall Discipline* (London, [1581]), p. 142; G. Dennis (ed.), *The Taktika of Leo VI* (Washington, DC: Dumbarton Oaks, 2010), p. 543; STC (2nd edn) / 18815, Onasander, *Of the Generall Captaine, and of His Office* (London, 1563), p. 108. I am grateful to David Appleby, Andrew Hopper, Ann

Hughes and participants at the Mortality, Care and Military Welfare during the British Civil Wars conference at Newark, 7–8 August 2015, for help and guidance in the preparation of this chapter.

2 STC (2nd edn)/23413.5 Styward, *Pathwaie*, p. 142; also STC (2nd edn)/20116, J. di Porcia, *The Preceptes of Warre* (London, 1544), sig. [H5r].

3 C. Gittings, *Death, Burial and the Individual in Early Modern England* (London: Routledge, 1988), p. 60; D. Cressy, *Agnes Bowker's Cat: Travesties and Transgressions in Tudor and Stuart England* (Oxford: Oxford University Press, 2000), pp. 116–37; S. Tarlow, *Ritual, Belief and the Dead in Early Modern Britain and Ireland* (Cambridge: Cambridge University Press, 2013), pp. 38–43, 52–4.

4 STC (2nd edn)/7355 J. Dunster, *Prodromus* (London, 1613), pp. 27–8; BL, Thomason E158(19), H. Spelman, *De Sepultura* (London, 1641), pp. 1–2; J. Cosin, *Works*, ed. J. Sansom and J. Barrow, 5 vols (Oxford: John Henry Parker, 1843–56), I, pp. 25–6; Cressy, *Agnes Bowker's Cat*, p. 119.

5 V. Harding, 'Burial choice and burial location in later medieval London', in S. Bassett (ed.), *Death in Towns: Urban Responses to Dying and the Dead 100–1600* (Leicester: Leicester University Press, 1995), p. 122.

6 J. Adamson, 'Chivalry and political culture in Caroline England', in K. Sharpe and P. Lake (eds), *Culture and Politics in Early Stuart England* (Stanford, CA: Stanford University Press, 1993), pp. 191–3.

7 BL, Harleian MS 965, fos. 1v–2v.

8 Wing / S5070, J. Sprigg, *Anglia Rediviva* (London, 1647), p. 82; J. H. Bettey, 'Horsey family', *ODNB*.

9 J. B. (ed.), 'John Byron's account of the siege of Chester 1645–1646', *Cheshire Sheaf*, 4th series, 6 (1971), 10–11; HMC, *The Manuscripts of His Grace the Duke of Portland* (London: HMSO, 1891), I, p. 282; WRO, Z65/2.

10 Wing / C6012, J. Cooke, *Mellificium Chirurgie* (London, 1648), p. 382; P. Styles (ed.), 'The genealogie, life and death of the right honourable Robert Lorde Brooke', in R. Bearman (ed.), *Miscellany I* (Publications of the Dugdale Society, 31, 1977), p. 191. I am grateful to Maureen Harris for discussions about embalming.

11 J. Hall (ed.), *Memorials of the Civil War in Cheshire* (Lancashire and Cheshire Record Society, 19, 1889), pp. 73–5; A. G. Matthews, *Walker Revised* (Oxford: Clarendon Press, 1948), p. 4.

12 BL, Thomason E312(3), J. Vicars, *Gods Arke Overtopping the Worlds Waves* (London, 1646[5]), p. 276; BL, Thomason E2(1), *A Continuation of True Intelligence*, no. 5, 10 June–10 July (London, 1644), pp. 7–8.

13 STC (2nd edn)/17332, F. Markham, *Five Decades of Epistles of Warre* (London, 1622), p. 76.

14 R. N. Dore (ed.), *The Letter Books of Sir William Brereton*, 2 vols (Lancashire and Cheshire Record Society, 123, 128, 1984–90), I, pp. 256–7, 332.

15 Dore (ed.), *Letter Books*, II, p. 272; BL, Thomason E312(3), Vicars, *Gods Arke*, p. 99; BL, Thomason E69(15), H. Foster, *A True and Exact Relation of the Marchings of the Two Regiments of the Trained Bands of the City of London* (London, 1643), sig. B2.

16 BL, Thomason E85(41), *A Great Wonder in Heaven* (London, 1642[3]); BL, Thomason E86(23), *The New Yeares Wonder* (London, 1643).

17 S. A. H. Burne, 'The battle of Hopton Heath, 1643', *Collections for a History of*

Staffordshire (Staffordshire Record Society, 1936), p. 183; J. C. Cox, *The Parish Registers of England* (London: Methuen, 1910), p. 192.

18 C. Illingworth, *A Topographical Account of the Parish of Scampton* (London, 1810), pp. 63–4; S. Porter (ed.), 'The biography of a parliamentarian soldier', *Transactions of the Bristol and Gloucestershire Archaeological Society*, 108 (1990), 131–4.

19 BL, Thomason E69(15), Foster, *True and Exact Relation*, [sig. B4r]; BL, Thomason E40(1), [E. A.,] *A Fuller Relation of the Great Victory Obtained (Through Gods Providence) at Alresford* (London, 1644).

20 BL, Thomason E50(25), *A Letter from the Right Honourable Robert Earl of Warwicke ... with an Exact Diurnall of All the Most Speciall and Remarkable Passages which Have Hapned during the Siege of Lyme* (London, 1644), pp. 8–9.

21 T. S. Evans (ed.), *The Life of Robert Frampton Bishop of Gloucester* (London: Longmans, 1876), p. 20.

22 J. Gwynne, *Military Memoirs*, [ed. W. Scott] (Edinburgh, 1822), pp. 42–3; J. Aubrey, *Brief Lives*, ed. O. L. Dick (Jaffrey: David Godine, 1999), pp. 128–9.

23 BL, Thomason E348(1), J. Vicars, *Magnalia Dei Anglicana* (London, 1646), p. 163; BL, Thomason E101(2), *Certaine Informations*, no. 16, 1–8 May (London, 1643), p. 127.

24 BL, Thomason E13(14), *Mercurius Aulicus*, 39th week, 28 September (Oxford, 1644), pp. 1180–[1181].

25 SHC, D/P/w.zoy/2/1/3, rear; W. MacDonald Wingfield, *The Monmouth Rebellion: A Social History* (Totowa, NJ: Barnes & Noble, 1980), p. 70; H. E. Marden (ed.), 'Iter bellicosum: Adam Wheeler his account of 1685', *Camden Miscellany XII* (Camden Society, 3rd series, 18, 1910), p. 164.

26 C. D. Curtis, 'Battle of Sedgemoor', *Notes & Queries for Somerset and Dorset*, 28 (1968), 15–21.

27 SHC, A/CTP//7/3.

28 Wing/C359, W. Camden, *Britannia*, ed. E. Gibson (London, 1695), col. 509; BL, Thomason E312(3), Vicars, *Gods Arke*, p. 275; BL, Thomason E69(18), *Mercurius Aulicus*, 38th week, 23 September (Oxford, 1643), pp. 530–1.

29 BL, Thomason E69(18), *Mercurius Aulicus*, pp. 530–1. See also BL, Thomason E300(15), J. Taylor, *The Generall Complaint of the Most Oppressed, Distressed Commons of England* ([Oxford, 1645]), p. 7.

30 BL, Thomason E348(1), Vicars, *Magnalia Dei Anglicana*, p. 470; BL Thomason E69(15), Foster, *True and Exact Relation*, sig. [B4r]; Burne, 'Battle of Hopton Heath', p. 184.

31 BL, Thomason E293(10), *A Dirge for the Directory* (Oxford [London], 1645), p. 2; Wing/D2492A, W. Dugdale, *A Short View of the Late Troubles in England* (Oxford, 1681), p. 561.

32 HMC, *The Manuscripts of the Duke of Beaufort, and Others* (London: HMSO, 1891), p. 28; BL, Thomason E1202(2), *The Loyall Sacrifice* ([London], 1648), pp. 87–9; C. E. Long (ed.), *Diary of the Marches of the Royal Army* (Cambridge: Cambridge University Press, 1997), pp. 21, 92, 102, 222; HMC, *Calendar of the Manuscripts of the Marquis of Bath. Vol. I* (London: HMSO, 1904), p. 33.

33 Trinity College Dublin, MS 812, fos. 202v, 240v; MS 816, fo. 184v; MS 820, fo. 12v; MS 821, fos. 1, 3; MS 826, fo. 160r; MS 830, fo. 41v; MS 833, fo. 1r; MS 834, fo. 169r; BL, Thomason E141(30), H. Jones, *A Remonstrance* (London, 1642),

pp. 9, 22, 36, 59, 65–6; B. Mac Cuarta, 'Religious violence against settlers in South Ulster, 1641–2', in D. Edwards, P. Lenihan and C. Tait (eds), *Age of Atrocity: Violence and Political Conflict in Early Modern Ireland* (Dublin: Four Courts Press, 2007), pp. 167–9. I am grateful to Jane Ohlmeyer for drawing my attention to Irish cases.

34 STC (2nd edn)/5235.2, T. Churchyard, *A General Rehearsall of Warres* (London, 1579), sig. Qiiiv; TNA, SP63/48, fo. 57i; J. Clarke and D. Preest (eds), *The Chronica Maiora of Thomas Walsingham, 1376–1422* (Woodbridge: Boydell, 2005), p. 322; STC (2nd edn)/13569, R. Holinshed, *The Third Volume of Chronicles* (London, 1587), p. 528.

35 BL, Thomason E238(17), *A Trve Relation of Such Passages and Proceedings of the Army of Dublin ... Since the Death of Sir Charles Coote* (London, 1642), p. 2; Wing/ C6824, J. Cranford, *The Teares of Ireland* (London, 1642), pp. 54–5, 63–4.

36 S. Carroll, *Blood and Violence in Early Modern France* (Oxford: Oxford University Press, 2006), pp. 170–81; Natalie Zemon Davis, 'The rites of violence: religious riot in sixteenth-century France', *Past and Present*, 59 (1973), 82–3.

37 Perhaps the nearest was the slashing of the faces of royalist women camp followers after Naseby, but that was practised on the living, to mark them as whores: Mark Stoyle, 'The road to Farndon Field: explaining the massacre of the royalist women at Naseby', *English Historical Review*, 123:503 (2008), 895–923.

38 BL, Thomason E53(19), E. Symmons, *A Militarie Sermon* (Oxford [London], 1644), p. 26.

39 Wing/P597, *A Particular Relation of the Action before Cyrencester* ([Oxford], 1642[–3]), p. 14; BL, Thomason E245(8), T. B., *Marleborowes Miseries* ([London], 1643), p. 7.

40 R. Ward, *Animadversions of Warre*, 2 books (London, 1639), II, p. 66; Wing/ F2244A, S. Julius Frontinus, *The Stratagems of War* (London, 1686), pp. 96–7.

41 BL, Thomason E348(1), Vicars, *Magnalia Dei Anglicana*, pp. 468–70, 474–5.

42 See BL, Thomason E262(9), *Perfect Passages of Each Dayes Proceedings in Parliament*, no. 34, 11–18 June (London, 1645), pp. 270–2, where the list of those captured at Naseby occupies over five columns, while those killed less than one.

43 C. Carlton, 'The impact of the fighting', in J. Morrill (ed.), *The Impact of the English Civil War* (London: Collins & Brown, 1991), pp. 18, 20. Carlton has subsequently revised his figures slightly to 86,000 combat deaths: C. Carlton, *This Seat of Mars: War and the British Isles, 1485–1746* (New Haven, CT: Yale University Press, 2011), pp. 146–7.

44 S. Shaw, *The History and Antiquities of Staffordshire*, 2 vols (London, 1798–1801), I, general history, p. 54; BL, Thomason E94(15), *Speciall Passages and Certain Informations*, no. 33, 21–28 March (London, 1643), p. 270; BL, Thomason E247(26), *Mercurius Aulicus*, 19–25 March (Oxford, 1643), p. 148; BL, Thomason E94(11), *Certain Informations*, no. 10, 20–27 March (London, 1643), p. 80; BL, Thomason E247(10), *A Perfect Diurnall*, no. 40, 20–27 March (London, 1643); BL, Thomason E94(14), *Kingdomes Weekly Intelligencer*, no. 13, 21–28 March (London, 1643), p. 100; BL, Thomason E94(18), *A Continuation of Certaine Speciall and Remarkable Passages*, no. 38, 23–30 March (London, 1643); BL, Thomason E99(18), *The Battaile on Hopton-Heath* ([Oxford], 1643), pp. 3–4; 'English Heritage Battlefield Report: Hopton Heath 1643' (1995), www.english-heritage.

org.uk/caring/listing/battlefields/battle-of-hopton-heath (accessed 27 February 2015).

45 *S. Mary's and S. Chad's Stafford* (Staffordshire Parish Register Society, 1936), p. 264; *Sandon* (Staffordshire Parish Register Society, 2014), p. 53; SRO, D975/1/1.

46 C. J. Ribton-Turner, *Shakespeare's Land Being a Description of Central and Southern Warwickshire* (Leamington: Glover, 1893), p. 336, n. 1.

47 Gloucestershire Archives, PFC 86 IN 1/2.

48 BRO, D/P51/1/1; Newbury parish register transcript; W. Money, *The First and Second Battles of Newbury and the Siege of Donnington Castle during the Civil War, 1643–6* (2nd edn, London: Simpkin, Marshall, 1884), pp. 60, 62, 64. A few scattered entries in other registers also show how the wounded died along the route of the two retreating armies: BRO, D/P108/1/1; D/P3/1/1.

49 BL, Thomason E100(8), *Prince Ruperts Burning Love to England* (London, 1643), p. 7; BL, Thomason E69(15), Foster, *True and Exact Relation*, [sig. B4r]; BL, Thomason E245(8), T. B., *Marleborowes Miseries*, p. 7.

50 L. McIntyre and G. Bruce, 'Excavating All Saint's [sic]: A medieval church rediscovered', *Current Archaeology*, 245 (2010), 30–7.

51 W. Beaumont (ed.), *A Discourse of the Warr in Lancashire* (Chetham Society, 1st series, 62, 1864), p. 8.

52 Money, *Battles of Newbury*, p. 64; L. V. Grinsell, 'An analysis and list of Berkshire barrows. Part I. Analysis', *Berkshire Archaeological Journal*, 39 (1935), 183; West Berkshire Historic Environment Record, MWB1550 www.heritagegateway.org.uk/Gateway/Results_Single.aspx?uid=MWB1550&resourceID=1030 (accessed 3 August 2015). In the mid-eighteenth century they were thought to be civil-war defensive works, not graves: *Bibliotheca Topographica Britannica*, 8 vols (London: John Nichols, 1780–90), IV, p. 84.

53 A. Terhune and A. Terhune (eds), *The Letters of Edward FitzGerald*, 4 vols (Princeton, NJ: Princeton University Press, 1980), I, pp. 351, 357, 365, 517; T. Pollard and N. Oliver, *Two Men in a Trench II: Unlocking the Secrets of British Battlefields* (London: Michael Joseph, 2003), pp. 168–72.

54 Articles about Aberystwyth Castle on the Ceredigion County Council online press cuttings page, www.ceredigion.gov.uk/index.cfm?artcileid+10096 (accessed 8 July 2016); P. Ellis (ed.), *Beeston Castle, Cheshire: Excavations by Laurence Keen & Peter Hough, 1968–85* (Swindon: English Heritage, 1993), pp. 120–2; C. Drage, *Nottingham Castle: A Place Full Royal* (Nottingham: Transactions of the Thoroton Society, 93, 1989), pp. 75, 78, 135; 'Lost half of human skeleton to be excavated from Nottingham Castle grounds', http://nottstv.com/human-skeleton-excavated-nottingham-castle-gounds/ (accessed 1 June 2016); information from Scott Lomax, Nottingham City archaeologist, to whom I am grateful for discussions of the skeleton; L. Butler, *Sandal Castle, Wakefield* (Wakefield: Wakefield Historical Publications, 1991), pp. 87–8.

55 M. Clinton, L. Fibiger, and D. Shiels, 'Archaeology of massacre: the Carrickmines mass grave and the siege of March 1642', in Edwards, Lenihan and Tait (eds), *Age of Atrocity*, pp. 192–203.

56 Scottish Soldiers research blog, http://community.dur.ac.uk/scottishsoldiers/ (accessed 19 July 2016).

57 BL, Thomason E288(28), *A More Exact and Perfect Relation of the Great Victory*

... in *Naisby Field* (London, 1645), p. 4; BL, Thomason E312(3), Vicars, *Gods Arke*, p. 134; BL, Thomason E245(8), T. B., *Marleborowes Miseries*, p. 7. Metal-detector surveying of Marston Moor has revealed the extent of the battlefield and how the fighting shifted across the field. P. R. Newman and P. R. Roberts, *Marston Moor: The Battle of the Five Armies* (Pickering: Blackthorn Press, 2003).

58 V. Fiorato, A. Boylston and C. Knüsel (eds), *Blood Red Roses: The Archaeology of a Mass Grave from the Battle of Towton AD 1461* (Oxford: Oxbow, 2007); M. Cassidy-Welch, 'Grief and memory after the battle of Agincourt', in A. Villalon and D. Kagay (eds), *The Hundred Years War (Part II). Different Vistas* (Leiden: Brill, 2008), pp. 133–50; T. Sutherland and S. Richardson, 'Arrows point to mass graves: finding the dead from the battle of Towton, 1461 AD', in D. Scott, L. E. Babits and C. M. Haecker (eds), *Fields of Conflict: Battlefield Archaeology from the Roman Empire to the Korean War* (Washington, DC: Potomac, 2009), pp. 167–8.

59 A. Smyth, *Autobiography in Early Modern England* (Cambridge: Cambridge University Press, 2010), especially pp. 192–8.

60 Compare the record of the burial of Captain Edward Dod in St Oswald's, Chester, in the register there with a copy in the register of Malpas, his home parish: CALS, P29/1/1, 27 February 1642/3, and Malpas register transcript, PAR/MAL.

61 Hertfordshire Archives, D/P 111/1/3, noting burials in the Quaker burial ground from 1682; S. G. R. Barratt, *A Short History of Totteridge* (London: Elliot Stock, 1934), p. 117, noting burial 'in the field of R. N.'

62 For a case of an excommunicate's burial in a field, nonetheless with the burial recorded without comment in the register, see Lincolnshire Archives, PAR/1/4, 28 August 1667 and *Gazetteer and Daily Advertiser*, 7 June 1783.

63 Cox, *Parish Registers*, p. 196.

64 B. Donagan, 'The casualties of war: treatment of the dead and wounded in the English Civil War', in I. Gentles, J. Morrill and B. Worden (eds), *Soldiers, Writers and Statesmen of the English Revolution* (Cambridge: Cambridge University Press, 1998), p. 129.

65 Bodl., MS Wood D 4, fol. 148r; Wing/C359, Camden, *Britannia*, col. 509; BL, Thomason E312(3), Vicars, *Gods Arke*, p. 276.

66 Hertfordshire Archives, Flamtsead parish register transcript, s.a. 1647; J. Nussey (ed.), *The Parish Register of Birstall. Volume 2: 1636–1687* (Yorkshire Archaeological Society, Parish Register Section, 152, 1987), p. 17; East Riding Archives, PE69/1, s.a. 1645–46, 1649, 1651; Cox, *Parish Registers*, p. 197.

67 SHC, D/P/w.as/2/1/1.

68 F. Madan, *Oxford Books ... Vol. 2. Oxford Literature 1450–1640, and 1641–1650* (Oxford: Clarendon Press, 1912), pp. 491, 499.

69 NAO, PR/24,810; S. B. Jennings, *'These Uncertaine Tymes': Newark and the Civilian Experience of the Civil Wars, 1640–1660* (Nottingham: Nottinghamshire County Council, 2009), pp. 82–3. I am grateful to the Reverend Dr Stuart Jennings for discussions about Newark.

70 V. Harding, 'Burial of the plague dead in early modern London', in J. A. I. Champion (ed.), *Epidemic Disease in London* (London: Centre for Metropolitan History Working Papers, 1, 1993), pp. 53–64.

71 CALS, P40/1/1.

72 *Wolverhampton* (Staffordshire Parish Register Society, 1932), p. 195; *Brewood*

(Staffordshire Parish Register Society, 1906), p. 119; *Ellastone* (Staffordshire Parish Register Society, 1907), p. 128.

73 SRO, D705/ADD/1.

74 *Alrewas Parish Registers 1547–1670* (Staffordshire Parish Register Society, 2003), pp. 95–6, 98.

75 D. Hayward (ed.), *The Registers of Bruton, Co. Somerset. Volume I. 1554–1680* (London: The Parish Register Society, 60, 1907), p. 156; *Shropshire Parish Registers. Diocese of Hereford. Vol. IV* (Shropshire Parish Register Society, 1903), pp. 58–60, 61, 63; T. F. Thiselton-Dyer, *Old English Social Life as Told by the Parish Registers* (London: Elliot Stock, 1898), p. 8.

76 C. Boddington and K. Holt (eds), *The Parish Register of Beverley St Mary. Volume 2. 1637–1689* (Yorkshire Archaeological Society, Parish Register Series, 173, 2008), p. 275; T. Wainwright (ed.), *Barnstaple Parish Register of Baptisms, Marriages and Burials 1538 A. D. to 1812 A. D.* (Exeter: James G. Commin, 1903), burials, p. 63.

77 *St Edmund Dudley 1540–1646* (Staffordshire Parish Register Society, 2001), pp. 95–101; *Dudley St Thomas* (Staffordshire Parish Register Society, 1997), pp. 89–95; *Ludlow* (Shropshire Parish Register Society, 1912), pp. 421–8.

78 CALS, P120/4525/2.

79 R. Gough, *The History of Myddle*, ed. D. Hey (Harmondsworth: Penguin, 1981), pp. 71–5, 171–2, 268, 271–2.

80 M. Stoyle, '"Memories of the maimed": the testimony of Charles I's former soldiers, 1660–1730', *History*, 88:290 (2003), 204–26; Sheffield Archives, OD/1420, [fols 12r, 26r].

81 I. Atherton, 'Remembering (and forgetting) Fairfax's battlefields', in A. Hopper and P. Major (eds), *England's Fortress: New Perspectives on Thomas, 3rd Lord Fairfax* (Farnham: Ashgate, 2014), pp. 111–12.

Chapter 2

Controlling disease in a civil-war garrison town: military discipline or civic duty? The surviving evidence for Newark-upon-Trent, 1642–46

Stuart B. Jennings

The treatment and containment of epidemic disease proved to be a contentious and difficult area of governance for civic authorities across much of England during the sixteenth and seventeenth centuries. The 1604 Plague Act, which superseded the Statutes previously issued by the Privy Council, had given local authorities and JPs more coercive powers to isolate infected individuals and a clearly defined set of procedures for dealing with outbreaks of plague.[1] The outbreak of civil war in 1642 created new challenges, with many towns being occupied and garrisoned by both sides. Alongside plague, typhus was increasingly virulent over the civil-war period as the movement of armies across the land and the close confinement of large numbers of people behind defensive walls during winter months facilitated the further spread of infection.

The relationship between military and civil jurisdiction in such circumstances, especially with regard to the treatment and isolation of infected soldiers and civilians when such disease appeared, has proven difficult for historians to discern or define. Issues of responsibility and questions relating to medical care, finance and infection control were areas of potential conflict between both sets of authorities. Many of the castles and fortified manors around which towns and settlements developed were not of sufficient size or design (having functioned as private residences prior to the war) to accommodate all the garrison troops. As these were often the major stone buildings in a town, their large halls and storerooms housed gunpowder and provisions rather than troops, while ordinary soldiers were usually billeted in the homes of townsfolk. The intermingling of military personnel and civilians made control and containment of epidemic disease particularly problematic. 'Pesthouses' built by civic authorities to quarantine the sick were often too small to accommodate both soldiers and civilians, giving rise to problems as to where the respective groups should be housed, and who was to care for them.

Understanding the complexity of arrangements between military and civilian authorities is further complicated by the scarcity of surviving contemporary evidence. This is especially true of military records, which were often accidentally lost during the fighting and bombardments, or deliberately destroyed prior to surrender. This, coupled with the unique local arrangements made in each garrison, has made an assessment of overall policy fraught with difficulty for the historian. Royalist garrison documents are particularly scarce in this respect, as by the end of 1645 the King's cause was clearly in decline and many commanders chose to be rid of such incriminating evidence. Where such documents do survive they are usually incomplete and consist primarily of accounts and assessments rather than books of orders and instructions.[2]

This chapter, which builds upon the author's earlier research into borough records, will focus on the Nottinghamshire town of Newark-upon-Trent. Newark remained an undefeated royalist garrison from 1642 through to May 1646, when it was ordered to surrender by the King.[3] This chapter will explore the relationship between military and civilian jurisdiction in regard to epidemic disease, drawing upon evidence within the surviving civic records. Newark is fortunate to have extensive borough and parish records surviving from the period, which include minutes, bills of payment, churchwardens' accounts, private papers and letters. Alongside these there remains a small, but not insignificant number of military documents and a regimental account book for 1644–45, although the garrison accounts and records appear to have been destroyed prior to the surrender. It is rare for such a quantity of documents to survive, and that they survived at all is probably due to the fact that plague was raging in Newark at the time of surrender, thereby discouraging the victorious allies from either entering, remaining long in the vicinity or removing anything from the town.[4] That so many diverse records have survived is particularly fortunate given that Newark was a focus of sustained violence throughout the First Civil War. This was because the possession of the town was of immense strategic importance to both sides.

Newark lay at the conjunction of three key transport routes linking southern England with the important northern towns of Hull, York and Newcastle. The first of these routes was the Great North Road, which ran from London to York and on to Edinburgh. Just outside the town, the road was intersected by the old Roman Fosse Way, which ran from Exeter in the south-west to the city of Lincoln. The third route was the River Trent, an arm of which passed directly in front of Newark Castle's walls. This was the main artery for goods travelling to and from Nottingham to the port of Hull via the Humber estuary. At Newark, the first crossing of the Trent by a bridge south of the Humber was also to be found, again adding to the town's strategic significance.[5]

Large numbers of travellers passed along these major routes, and the fact that a large proportion frequented Newark's markets, and regularly required accommodation in the town, meant that from the fifteenth century increasing numbers of coaching inns were built there. Many of these timber-framed buildings can still be seen around the market place today. During the war years from 1642 to 1646 several of these served as barracks for officers and men.[6] From its earliest beginnings, therefore, a close relationship was forged between the crown (based in the castle), commerce and travel. These links made Newark Castle an important place to garrison from the start of the conflict. It was to be the local royalist gentry who were to seize the initiative and secure the town for the King in the autumn of 1642.

Newark Castle had reverted to royal control at the Reformation, and was leased by the crown to a succession of tenants before Charles I gave it to his queen Henrietta Maria, as a wedding gift. Over the previous century a succession of aristocratic tenants, of whom William Cecil, Lord Burghley was the most significant, had spent large sums of money turning the castle into a comfortable country house, inserting extra fireplaces, large windows and constructing additional smaller rooms for accommodation. Burghley spent over £400 on the fabric in 1607 alone. This alteration of use was to have consequences for the defensive function of the castle. As early as 1536, complaints had been sent to Henry VIII that the castle had 'scant lodgings for a 100 men and no water'.[7] When the town came to be garrisoned at the end of 1642, the castle was not able to accommodate the majority of the soldiers. The symbiotic relationship between castle and town, which developed over several centuries, was therefore to become a significant factor in its success as a royalist garrison over the course of the First Civil War. Matters were to be further exacerbated during these years by the fact that the county gentry who made up the royalist Commission of Array were not only based in Newark, but also physically accommodated there for much of the war and often occupied the prime accommodation.

In 1603, James I stayed at the castle and was entertained by the town on his progress from Edinburgh to London to be crowned King of England. He further visited the castle in 1612, 1614, 1616 and 1617, while his son Charles I made several visits, both at the start of his reign and during the course of the war. The frequency of these visits suggests that the castle fabric remained in good repair and enjoyed a degree of comfort suitable for a royal visitor.[8]

By 1640, Newark was predominantly a town of homogeneous, low-roofed timber-framed houses, some still retaining large gardens. Like other medieval towns it was laid out with a well-planned regularity. The medieval walls remained largely complete, but in places were in a ruinous condition and required much attention and finance to repair. The town gates provided access but their narrow entrances and the confined streets beyond caused considerable congestion, especially on market days when large numbers made their way to the market place at the heart of the town. Within the walled town there were a few stone buildings, the most prominent being the castle, the parish church and the Magnus School. Thomas Magnus, a wealthy churchman, had founded Newark Grammar School in 1527 and his stone-built schoolroom in Appleton Gate today houses the National Civil War Centre. This school hall witnessed many a frantic meeting between the military governor, mayor and aldermen over the course of the war, especially during the three sieges of Newark.[9]

Charles I chose Nottingham to be the rallying point for his followers to assemble, raising his Royal Standard at Nottingham Castle on 22 August 1642. Of the royalist forces mustered across Nottinghamshire, a substantial number originated from the Newark area. These units included a foot regiment raised by the MP for Grimsby, Gervase Holles (who was resident in Newark at the time) and a cavalry regiment raised by John Bellasis from his estates at Holme near Newark and in Yorkshire. A further infantry company was raised by Captain William Staunton of Staunton who was promoted to Colonel after Edgehill. Staunton parish lay approximately seven miles south of Newark.[10] All of these forces left the county with Charles and were present at the battle of Edgehill, leaving Nottinghamshire largely devoid of royalist troops. Not until the arrival of Sir John Henderson (sent to control the region by William Cavendish, earl of Newcastle with around 4,000 horse in December 1642) was Newark finally secured for the King and a royalist garrison established. The first siege of Newark occurred soon after when East Midland parliamentarians attacked the town between 27 and 28 February 1643.[11] A muster held in Newark on 29 May 1643 identified the garrison strength as consisting of thirty-eight troops of horse and dragoons, amounting to around 2,000 men, the origin of the Newark Horse. This appears to have remained the garrison's core strength throughout most of the war until its surrender in May 1646, when 1,500 to 1,700 soldiers were allowed to march out.[12] This final number (even after plague had cut a swathe through the garrison) had been inflated further at the end of 1645 by an influx of men, mainly officers, arriving from vanquished royalist garrisons. At the point of surrender, soldiers in these other garrisons were usually given leave either to return to their homes under licence or march to the next remaining royalist garrison, which in many cases was Newark. The fact that towards the end of the war, locally raised regiments commanded by local officers, such as Staunton and Bellasis, also ended up back at Newark eased some of the tensions that quartering may have caused in the town. It should also be noted that around 1643 a town regiment was raised from among the citizens, for whom payments are recorded in the borough accounts.[13]

Alongside the presence of a regular garrison of around 2,000 men, the town of approximately 2,200 civilians also had to accommodate the arrival of large numbers of troops who habitually accompanied important royalist visitors. On 16 June 1643, Queen Henrietta Maria arrived at Newark with supplies and an army of around 4,500 soldiers. She stayed in the town for just over a week before going on to Oxford to reinforce her husband's army.[14] On

21 March 1644 Prince Rupert arrived outside Newark with a force of around 6,400 horse and foot to break the second siege. After his victory against the parliamentarian besiegers, he remained in Newark for several days, seeking both to consolidate his gains and allow his army to recover.[15] Finally on 4 October 1645, Charles I arrived at Newark with a force of just under 1,500 soldiers to reorganise and restructure the garrison. All of these additional troops had to be quartered in and around the town, and in the case of Rupert's wounded soldiers, cared for in the aftermath of combat.[16]

As the garrison's accounts fail to survive (probably deliberately destroyed before Newark's surrender in May 1646), it is to the surviving civic and ecclesiastical records that the historian must turn in order to reconstruct how the town and garrison authorities coordinated medical provision for the wounded, and supervised infection containment when epidemic disease appeared. The churchwardens' accounts for 1643 (year ending 24 March 1644) and 1644 (starting 25 March 1644) give us an insight into what was happening after the lifting of the second siege by Rupert. An undated bill for the period 1644 to January 1646, but probably dating from the aftermath of the fighting in 1644 and filed among the town rental accounts, records that the Corporation paid £1 'to a surgion'. This individual may well have been working alongside the garrison surgeons attending wounded soldiers quartered in civilian homes.[17] Where such soldiers succumbed to their wounds, especially if cared for in the homes of the poorest civilians, the churchwardens' accounts clearly record that the town met the costs incurred for burial, though these had to be sanctioned by the mayor.

Superficially the entries in Table 2.1 seem self-explanatory, but they raise some interesting questions. First and foremost, the burial of these soldiers was not recorded in the parish burial registers. Those registers only record the burial of twenty-eight officers and four ordinary soldiers during the entirety of the First Civil War. This suggests that garrison soldiers were buried in a

Table 2.1 Burial payments for soldiers in the Newark churchwardens' accounts

To John Gill by Mr Maiors command for a winding sheet & Inkle for a soldier wch died at his house	2s 6d
To Mr Maior for a winding sheete and inkle for one of Prince Rupert's soldiers	2s
To Mr Johnson for the like by Mr Maiors appointment	2s
To Mis[tress] Atkinson ffor two sheets 2s 8d and for an inkle and to a poore woman for winding two soldiers 8d in total	3s 4d
To Walker and Yoxall for passing Bells and macking of souldiers graves by Mr Maiors command	3s 4d
To Ralph Walker for grave making at Mr Maiors command	2s
[15 August 1644] For a winding sheet for a souldier by Mr Maiors command	2s

Source: NAO, Newark churchwardens' accounts, 1640–60, PR/24,810

military plot away from the parish graveyard, the records or details of which were the responsibility of the military. Given the carefully maintained registers, which certainly recorded stranger civilian burials in the town, and even during the epidemics attempted (though not without some oversight and omission) to record most interments, it seems a little unfair to attribute carelessness or indifference to the keeper of the registers. Why record payments for burials but not the burials themselves? When we come later to look at Newark's typhus and plague epidemics, a separate military burial plot appears to be the most likely explanation for this phenomenon.

In the aftermath of the second siege of 1644, the surviving records indicate that two protocols were established. The first was that as well as quartering the troops the civilian authorities assumed some responsibility for the treatment of sick and wounded soldiers. Secondly, and most unexpectedly, subject to the authorisation of the mayor and Corporation, the town sought to meet the additional financial burdens that were incurred, rather than leave individual households to foot the bill. Following the breaking of the second siege, the Corporation was in a generous mood. The large sum of £5 10s 6d was made over to 'Prince Rupert's trumpeters and his servants at the raising of the siege', so the additional unspecified costs of care and burial charges amounting to 17s 2d were not large in the grand scheme of celebrations and payments.[18] The payment of monies to a Mistress Atkinson, and through her on to 'a poor women for winding of corpses', again suggest that the policy of meeting this need attracted the support of the highest levels of civic society across Newark. This woman, probably of some social significance given the title attributed to her, may have been related to Thomas Atkinson who was Newark's mayor from 1641 to 1642. These fragments of surviving entries suggest that a tentative agreement was in place between the military and civilian authorities on medical logistics following periods of fighting, even before typhus and plague really gained a foothold at the end of 1643 and into 1644.

The medical and care arrangements which evolved following periods of siege and fighting were to be seriously challenged by the arrival of epidemic diseases in the town during the later years of the war. Accommodated across the town inns and quartered in people's homes, soldiers were as vulnerable to infection as the civilian population. A lack of resources and physical space for isolation and treatment meant that the governor and mayor were required to coordinate their response. In the absence of the garrison accounts, specifics are hard to identify but preserved in the surviving borough and ecclesiastical accounts and minutes, there are tantalising glimpses of what may have happened.

The first major epidemic to be recorded in the registers at Newark appears to have been typhus, which appeared over the winter of 1643–44.[19] Garrison soldiers were far from immune to this infection but they fail to appear in the parish registers. Typhus was an infection transmitted by human body lice and was commonly associated with overcrowding and dirt, and was to be found in most early modern field armies. One of the reasons typhus was particularly virulent over the winter months was that the cold weather discouraged people from bathing and changing their clothes (not that the poorest inhabitants had spare sets to change into), causing the lice to proliferate. Once infected, the patient developed a fever, leading to a stupor with extraordinary headaches and red pustules resembling fleabites to appear over the body of the sufferer. The demographic and seasonal character of the disease makes it easier to identify within a parish from the burial registers. The winters of 1644 and 1645 were extremely harsh in the Midlands, with the River Trent freezing over and floating ice causing considerable damage to the town's wooden bridges.[20] Particularly worrying for the military authorities was the fact that while mortality rates for children from typhus were relatively low, it was potentially lethal for adults, especially malnourished and exhausted soldiers. The first outbreak, identified within the burial registers (see Figure 2.1), began towards the end of 1643 and became particularly virulent over the course of the second siege from 29 February through to 21 March 1644. While the registers clearly show that typhus was raging through the civilian population, killing citizens across the social spectrum, they fail to record the burial of any ordinary troopers, listing only the interment of two captains and one colonel over the periods of the epidemic. Garrison troops inside Newark were affected, but it is not immediately apparent why their deaths were not recorded in the generally well-kept parish registers. With the successful lifting of the second siege, Prince Rupert and his 6,000-plus soldiers remained in and around Newark to recover and regroup, intensifying the overcrowding and squalor that further fuelled the typhus then raging in the town. In the three weeks after Rupert's arrival a further nineteen burials (almost certainly typhus, and all civilians), were recorded in the register, more than the monthly totals for the previous three months. The escalation of the typhus epidemic may well have been a contributory factor in Rupert's sudden departure from Nottinghamshire with his army, passing up the chance to attack the parliamentarian garrison of Nottingham.[21]

The parish registers also clearly suggest that there were further typhus outbreaks over the winter of 1645–46, prior to the arrival of the plague at the end of 1645.[22] The three outbreaks between them probably accounted for the mortality of between 12 to 15 per cent of the town's pre-war civilian population. A failure to record the burials of ordinary soldiers makes it impossible to quantify with certainty the impact upon the garrison, but it is reasonable to assume a similar pattern of mortality for the soldiers. If this were the case, then the garrison itself would have lost approximately 240 to 300 of its soldiers over the three-year period 1643–45 to typhus alone.

Treatment of typhus usually consisted of isolating the patient and treating the fever (which lasted between nine to twelve days) with a mixture of herbs, infused drinks and bloodletting, while keeping the sufferer cool in the hope that the fever would break before it proved lethal.[23] Newark's small

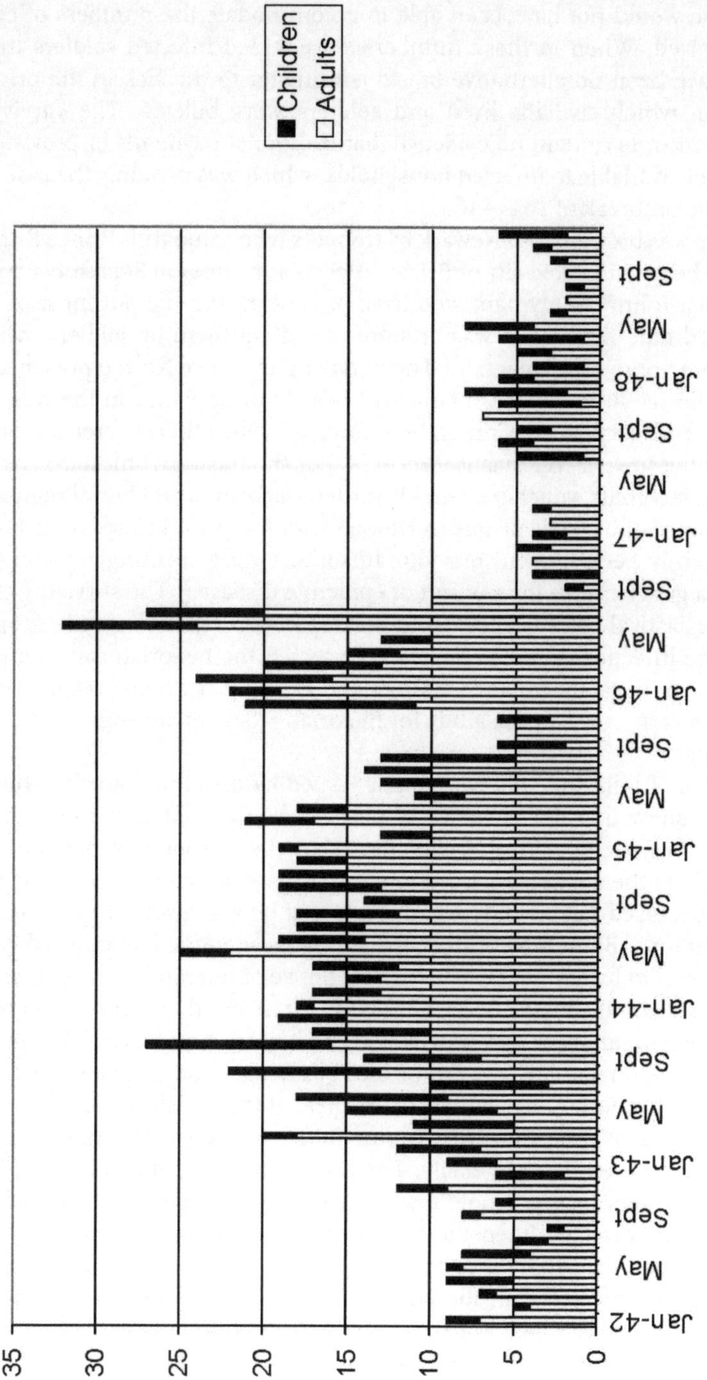

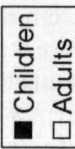

Figure 2.1 Burials in Newark, 1642–48

pesthouse would not have been able to accommodate the numbers of civilians involved. When to these numbers were added infected soldiers there would have been no alternative but to administer to the sick in the private houses in which civilians lived and soldiers were billeted. The surviving borough records contain no evidence that additional payments or provisions were made available to infected households, which was certainly the case for the plague outbreak of 1645–46.

Plague was brought into Newark by troopers who came with Prince Rupert from the heavily-infected city of Bristol after its surrender in September 1645. The diarist John Twentyman, who lived at Newark throughout most of the war, noted that 'the plague was brought in among them by soldiers, which came from some other places'.[24] The surviving evidence for the presence of plague and its subsequent containment is only to be found in the recently available and catalogued Corporation records, with other references to be found in the town's ecclesiastical records. For the most part these consist of plague orders, bills, vouchers, churchwardens' accounts and burial registers. The presence of bubonic plague in Newark over the period 1645–46 has only been recently been proven; previous historians were seemingly content to see it as a generic term for any sort of epidemic disease.[25] The surviving civic and ecclesiastical records allow us to develop both a chronology and geography of the infection and also a context in which the historian can interpret a number of separate military matters and logistics. In many respects this makes Newark a useful case study for historians to compare with other cities and towns.

A series of bills and vouchers, many issued by the churchwarden Robert Gonison, show that the presence of plague was first noted in the autumn of 1645. On 6 October 1645 (Julian calendar) the Corporation paid out the sum of £1 'to the doctors for searching the corps at William Hayes'. The fact that the deceased was not named suggests that he was a soldier quartered at Hayes's house. By mid-November the numbers identified as infected were high enough to justify the pest or 'visited' house of quarantine to be opened, and monies amounting to £4 4s 2d to be spent in less than a month on oats, coals, candles, salt, beer and watchers at the house. A note scribbled on the back of this bill recorded that the various sums spent on plague relief came from the 'collection money on fast dayes' held at the parish church.[26]

With the arrival of warmer weather in March 1646, the epidemic re-emerged with even more intensity. The Corporation responded by reissuing its plague orders for the whole town, including the instruction that where infection was detected 'then their house may be forthwith shut up, and a guard set upon the same, to prevent the further spread of such infection'.[27] The numbers infected with the pestilence again proved to be too great for Newark's small pesthouse to cope. Over the next few months those unfortunate enough to be infected with the plague were locked up in their own homes in an effort to contain its spread. Watchmen were appointed to make sure that those shut up in quarantined houses did not wander abroad spreading the contagion. The watchmen were paid 8d per day for watching through the daytime and 10d for watching through the night. Any soldier billeted in a home that had the infection would almost certainly have been isolated with the rest of the household, to make sure that he did not infect other garrison troops. A period of statutory isolation lasting for six weeks after the last plague death in a house had been prescribed by the 1604 Plague Act prior to the war but in the chaos of the final siege the governor may not have been able to spare the affected troops for that length of time.[28] An undated voucher recorded: 'A Bill for bread for the vizitted for barnebee gate and norgate and the towne to me Samuel Cole – £4 16s 6d.'[29]

Another bill, filed in the same batch of papers, records the additional sum of £2 2s being spent on beer being delivered to these 'visited households' around the same time. Both Barnby Gate and North Gate were poor but densely-populated areas at this time, being adjacent to the outer defences constructed prior to the start of the third siege. Houses beyond the defensive perimeter had been demolished and many of the inhabitants were moved into these parts of the town. During the final siege, numerous garrison soldiers were quartered in these areas, in the homes of Newark's poorest citizens, placing them at the epicentre of the unfolding catastrophe. The garrison officers were generally billeted in the coaching inns and taverns and were thus slightly removed from the main areas of infection. From the accounts of Colonel William Staunton we know that many of the non-commissioned officers were billeted at the Angel Inn while Staunton and his senior officers were accommodated separately at the Old White Hart Inn.[30] Even in war, social divisions were strictly observed. As the third siege tightened, soldiers could no longer be quartered in outlying parishes, as some of Staunton's troopers had been prior to the arrival of the Scots. They too had to be accommodated within the defensive works, adding to the sheer volume of humanity crammed into a decreasing area of habitation and increasingly exposed to plague.

For the military historian, these surviving records raise at least three key questions. Firstly, who bore the expense of provisioning the quarantined soldiers? Secondly, who watched over them? Thirdly, given the absence of burial entries in the registers, what happened to those soldiers who succumbed to the pestilence? Many issues relating to the provisioning of quarantined households remain unresolved. Surviving evidence for Newark strongly indicates that the civic authorities met some of the expenses related to the provisioning of basic goods such as oats, bread and beer, but whether this was for the whole household or whether soldiers shut up in the household were supplied via garrison provisions is far from clear. It is also unclear as to what other provisions might have been supplied to households under quarantine, especially given that the town was besieged and there was certainly rationing of much of that which may have been available. If the household had to buy other goods, given the shortage of coin in Newark this would have been problematic for many of the town's poorer households.

For the military governor, the key concern was to halt the spread of pestilence among the garrison. The conditions of 'free quarter' varied slightly from place to place across the country, and even between succeeding governors in the same garrison. They were shaped by prevailing local circumstances, but it usually involved the provision of some food and drink. Given this overlap of responsibility, it may well have been that the Corporation and Newark's governors reached some form of agreement relating to assessment and provision for infected, quarantined troops across the town. The fact that after the war ended in 1646 there was little recorded in the town minutes relating to outstanding debts or payments further supports this.[31]

The surviving evidence at Newark itself does not provide a definitive answer to this issue, but what does survive suggests that the potential for friction between military and civilian authorities over quarantine and burial did not result in large amounts of angst and paperwork in Newark. Certainly the survival of these rare civilian records – quite unique for a royalist garrison – helps to highlight the sorts of issues that a close proximity of garrison and town could, and often did, generate.[32]

This absence of substantial burial entries for the ordinary soldiers in the garrison, though officers from local families are occasionally recorded, is not unique to Newark. As Ian Atherton details in the previous chapter, this is a nationwide phenomenon. In the context of Newark, where the survival of some borough and ecclesiastical records add further context, this may imply that at Newark this particular area of military jurisdiction remained firmly under the control of the garrison commander. In many ways this makes military sense, for the death of soldiers had implications for regimental strength, pay and rotas of duty across the siege defences. In both the deployment of forces and the logistics of provisions, it was essential for officers to have a firm awareness of their company's strength. Even in the face of an epidemic, coupled with a major siege, this would be a responsibility they would not willingly surrender to the civilian authorities. Likewise quartermasters would require such information. An officer's focus upon mortality rates across their company though was as much an operational concern as a humanitarian one.

If the parish graveyard was filling up with civilian interments – and churchwardens' accounts indicate this was the case for the last two years of the war, with regular payments over 1645 and 1646 for 'dressing the church yard' – a military operation to collect and bury dead soldiers in a military pit would have facilitated easier monitoring and less points of friction with civilian authorities regarding payments and grave spaces. The new plot in Appleton Gate, identified in the plague orders of 1646, is a good candidate for this missing pit. It is very possible that a more remote pit nearer the southern defences of Millgate was dug. Memories of this pit probably led to the area being reused later during Newark's plague outbreak of 1665.[33]

Research by Joan Dils on Berkshire mortality rates and epidemics for the period 1642–46 suggests this was also the case for that county. She too has noted the virtual absence of military burials across seventy-four Berkshire parishes and offers the conclusion that pits were constructed for military casualties either on the field of conflict or possibly beyond the local parish churchyard.[34] Other garrisons such as Banbury clearly record the burial of soldiers in the churchyard during the outbreaks of plague over the civil-war period. Fifty-eight soldiers were recorded in the burial registers as part of the overall total of 225 interments in the parish churchyard during the 1644 plague epidemic. The pre-war annual mortality rate for the parish was between thirty to ninety-eight burials, reflecting the sort of mortality crisis that was also engulfing Newark over the period 1645–46.[35] Where the churchyards were clearly the place of burial and the registers survive, entries for soldiers can often be found recorded in them, and even where the name of the deceased is unknown, 'a soldier buried' is entered. This was certainly the case for the parish registers for St Peter's in the neighbouring parliamentarian town of Nottingham. During the siege of York, numerous burials of soldiers were recorded in the burial registers of the city parishes but there were also known burial pits for soldiers beyond the city walls. Several mass graves were found just outside York's walls in 2008, which contained the skeletons of 113 civil-war soldiers who had probably fought and died for Parliament during the siege of York in 1644.[36] These examples, both local and from across England, all add weight to the suggestion that a military pit was established at Newark over the period 1644–46, maintained by the garrison, but sometimes utilising the services and skills of a minister, gravediggers and other able-bodied civilians of the town, thus freeing up garrison soldiers for the defences.

Diseases such as typhus and plague were a scourge for both urban and rural communities over much of the early modern period. Treatments during such outbreaks typically consisted of a combination of isolation and fumigation. One contemporary view about the transmission of infectious disease was that it was spread by miasma, 'stinking vapours by which the air is putrefied'.[37] The smell of graveyards, unburied corpses and stagnant pools (of which there were many in and around Newark during the final siege) were claimed by contemporary medical practitioners to be the main source for plague infections. Only by the burning of incense and perfumes across the whole of the infected area could the potential effects of miasma be counteracted. Town, garrison and defensive works in the vicinity of infected quarters would all need to be fumigated. It is not surprising, therefore, to find within the Corporation papers a surviving bill for such fumigating and purging agents (see Table 2.2), though the quantities involved would suggest it was more for use in public buildings than across the whole town.

The antidote may well have been kept as a medical secret but it is likely that the hawthorn, marigold flowers, mithridate and syrup of maidenhair

Table 2.2 Payments for fumigation by Newark's corporation

An Ante dote	6s 8d
Harthorne and Marygold flowers	2s 0d
The Ante dote	6s 8d
The same Agayne	6s 8d
Frankinscence	1s 0d
fumeing powder	4s 6d
A Cataplasme	3s 6d
Mithridate & Syrup of maydenhare	1s 0d
A Perfumeing powder	4s 6d

Source: NAO, Newark Borough Misc., DC/NW D6.75/C46/4

were mixed up into a treacle and given to the infected person as a form of theriac medicine.[38]

This type of response to epidemic disease was intensive and demanding in times of peace. Therefore its implementation across the whole town during conflict, scarcity and siege would have been especially problematic. Differing chains of authority, civic and military, had to cooperate with each other, but in order to impose a strict quarantine, and, indeed, to ensure continuity, it was important for someone to lead and coordinate the response. Newark's surviving civic records clearly demonstrate that, even in the midst of war, the borough and ecclesiastical authorities sought to implement the long-held traditions and practice of control in place since the start of the century. The lack of surviving evidence from the military garrison makes it difficult to make definitive claims for their response in the face of typhus and plague. As this chapter has shown, however, issues of billeting and quartering, quarantining and provisioning recorded in the surviving civic papers suggest that separating soldiers from civilians in a cramped, besieged and densely populated garrison town was virtually impossible: soldiers and their needs often creep into the civic records. There is sufficient evidence to indicate that at Newark the garrison commander (the last of whom was John Bellasis, from a local gentry family) was content to leave the logistics of quarantine, quartering, provisioning and monitoring of the plague in the hands of the borough officials who had considerable experience of handling such matters. The governor had the option of tinkering with the deployment of his troops, most obviously by extending the periods of service on the sconces and defensive perimeter for uninfected soldiers in order to limit movement and the possible further spread of the infection. All this hard work in containing the epidemic was to be undone by Newark's surrender. The withdrawal of the Scottish besiegers allowed the citizens to flee the town and carry the infection with them into the neighbouring rural parishes.[39]

The town of Newark was neither unusual nor unique in its experience of being garrisoned, besieged (albeit three times) and visited by plague and disease over the course of the British Civil Wars; towns and cities as diverse as Bristol, Gloucester, Exeter, Banbury, Lichfield and Colchester, and in Ireland

Drogheda and Wexford, all experienced similar events.[40] As with Newark, surviving military records and accounts are scarce for these places and make no mention about containment and treatment across town and garrison. This has generally led historians to do little other than use civic records for basic demographic data to confirm the presence of plague or typhus within a community. This case study of Newark, using its civic and ecclesiastical records, demonstrates that often glimpses of the interactions between military and civilian authorities can be inferred from previously underutilised archives (where they survive). It is hoped that this chapter will provide both a template and an encouragement for future historians to revisit the history of such garrisoned towns and further explore the vexed issue of jurisdiction in the face of indiscriminate epidemics.

NOTES

1 P. Slack, *The Impact of Plague in Tudor and Stuart England* (Oxford: Oxford University Press, 1985), pp. 199–226.

2 M. Bennett, S. B. Jennings and M. Whyld, 'Two military account books for the Civil War in Nottinghamshire', *Transactions of the Thoroton Society*, 100 (1996), 107–21; I. Atherton, 'Royalist finances in the English Civil War: the case of Lichfield Garrison, 1643–1645', *Midland History*, 33:1 (2008), 43–67.

3 S. B. Jennings, *'These Uncertaine Tymes': Newark and the Civilian Experience of the Civil Wars, 1640–1660* (Nottingham: Nottinghamshire County Council, 2009).

4 Bennett, Jennings and Whyld, 'Two military account books', 116–21.

5 Jennings, *'These Uncertaine Tymes'*, pp. 6–17.

6 J. Mordan, *Timber-Frame Buildings of Nottinghamshire* (Nottingham: Nottinghamshire County Council, 2004).

7 P. Marshall and J. Samuels, *Guardian of the Trent: The Story of Newark Castle* (Nottingham: Nottinghamshire County Council, 1997), pp. 37–9.

8 Jennings, *'These Uncertaine Tymes'*, pp. 6–7.

9 *Ibid.*, pp. 8–10.

10 Bennett, Jennings and Wilde, 'Two military account books'.

11 BL, Thomason E84(6), *Special Passages*, 27 December–3 January (London, 1643). See also A. C. Wood, *Nottinghamshire in the Civil War* (East Ardsley: EP Publishing Ltd, 1971), pp. 30–2, 38–43.

12 Royal Commission on Historical Monuments, *Newark on Trent: The Civil War Siege Works* (1964), p. 24.

13 Jennings, *'These Uncertaine Tymes'*, pp. 46–7.

14 C. Brown, *Annals of Newark-upon-Trent Comprising the History, Curiosities and Antiquities of the Borough* (London: H. Sotheran, 1879), p. 118.

15 BL, Thomason E39(8), *A Brief Relation of the Siege of Newark*, 26 March (London, 1644).

16 Jennings, *'These Uncertaine Tymes'*, pp. 32–3.

17 NAO, Newark Borough Miscellaneous Papers, DC/NW D6.75/H24, bundle 5.

18 NAO, Newark Borough Miscellaneous Papers, chamberlains' accounts, 1644, DC/NW D6.75/C28.

19 For a fuller discussion of this, see S. B. Jennings, '"A miserable, stinking infected town": pestilence, plague and death in a civil war garrison, Newark 1640–1649', *Midland History*, 28 (2003), 51–70.

20 Jennings, *'These Uncertaine Tymes'*, pp. 66–8.

21 L. Hutchinson, *Memoirs of the Life of Colonel Hutchinson*, ed. N. H. Keeble (London: Phoenix, 2000), pp. 157–9.

22 NAO, Newark parish registers, 1642–46, PR/27,256–27,257.

23 A. Cunningham and O. P. Grell, *The Four Horsemen of the Apocalypse: Religion, War, Famine and Death in Reformation Europe* (Cambridge: Cambridge University Press, 2001), pp. 270–2.

24 University of Nottingham Manuscripts and Special Collections, The Mellish Papers, Twentyman Manuscript.

25 Jennings, 'A miserable, stinking infected town', 51–70.

26 NAO, Newark Borough Miscellaneous Papers, DC/NW D6.75/C46/7. A different or later hand has dated this bill December 1646 but Goniston was churchwarden only up to March 1646. He died of the plague in June 1646.

27 NAO, Newark Borough Council Minutes, 1640–60, DC/NW/3/1/1, Plague Orders 1646.

28 NAO, Newark Borough Council Minutes, Plague Orders, 1646.

29 NAO, Newark Borough Miscellaneous Papers, DC/NW D6.75/C46/9.

30 Bennett, Jennings and Whyld, 'Two military account books', pp. 107–21.

31 NAO, Newark Borough Council Minutes, 1640–60, DC/NW/3/1/1.

32 The surviving accounts of the royalist garrison at Lichfield fail to address any of these practical issues at all. See Atherton, 'Royalist finances in the English Civil War', 43–67.

33 Brown, *Annals of Newark*, p. 190.

34 J. Dils, 'Epidemics, mortality and the civil war in Berkshire, 1642–46', in R. C. Richardson (ed.), *The English Civil War: Local Aspects* (Stroud: Sutton, 1997), pp. 145–55.

35 C. Creighton, *A History of Epidemics in Britain*, 2 vols, reprinted edition (Cambridge: Cambridge University Press, 2014), I, pp. 556–7.

36 P. Wenham, *The Great and Close Siege of York, 1644* (Kineton: Roundwood Press, 1970), pp. 132–9. For recent archaeological digs of such pits see www.bbc.co.uk/news/uk-england-york-north-yorkshire-14027148 (accessed 22 November 2016).

37 Slack, *The Impact of Plague*, pp. 26–32.

38 *Ibid.*, pp. 30–3.

39 See especially S. B. Jennings, 'The anatomy of a civil-war plague in a rural parish: East Stoke, Nottinghamshire, 1646', *Midland History*, 40:2 (2015), 201–19.

40 See especially M. Stoyle, *From Deliverance to Destruction: Rebellion and Civil War in an English City* (Exeter: University of Exeter Press, 1996); Wenham, *The Great and Close Siege of York, 1644*; J. Lynch, *For King and Parliament: Bristol and the Civil War* (Stroud: Sutton, 1999); R. Sherwood, *The Civil War in the Midlands, 1642–1651* (Stroud: Sutton, 1992); A. R. Warmington, *Civil War, Interregnum and Restoration in Gloucestershire, 1640–1672* (London: Royal Historical Society, 1997); J. Wroughton, *An Unhappy Civil War: The Experience of Ordinary People in Gloucestershire, Somerset and Wiltshire, 1642–1646* (Bath: Lansdown Press, 1999); Atherton, 'Royalist finances in the English Civil War'.

Part II

——

Medical care

Chapter 3

———

A new kind of surgery for a new kind of war: gunshot wounds and their treatment in the British Civil Wars

Stephen M. Rutherford

This chapter aims to evaluate the validity of the medical practice of the early modern military surgeon. Significant progress has been made, in recent years, in researching the social impact of medicine in the post-Renaissance period. Considerable attention has been paid to the role and social status of medical practitioners,[1] the impact of medical care for the dying,[2] the role of women in medical care (both as practitioners and nurses),[3] the accessibility of medicine to the less wealthy,[4] and the changing interface between medicine and folk superstitions and religion.[5] However, as Nancy Siraisi notes, it is difficult to evaluate clearly the efficacy of medical practitioners.[6] This is due to a lack of reliable evidence of the symptoms, diagnosis, treatment and outcomes of individual cases. This chapter aims to evaluate the impact of early modern surgical practice via two approaches: firstly, by evaluating the validity of the methodologies used from a biological and biomedical perspective; secondly, by placing early modern surgeons in a broader context, and highlighting the extent to which the pioneering medical procedures developed during this period continued in their use over subsequent centuries.

Despite Roy Porter's assertion that the surgical art 'did not undergo revolution until the nineteenth century', sixteenth- and seventeenth-century medical practice shows clear paradigm shifts in understanding and methodologies compared to previous centuries, and clear indications of laying foundations for future practice.[7] Texts published by surgeons of this period reveal a high level of understanding of physiology, anatomy, hygiene and medical practice. Several seventeenth-century medical texts remained in active use for many decades after they were written, and many techniques described by these authors did not change substantially for centuries thereafter. Indeed, the approach exemplified by some of the authors of medical texts from the period shows clear parallels to present-day 'evidence-based medicine', for example, the approach of basing medical practice on observed positive outcomes and research.[8] Through developing an evidence base, and presenting cases that were both effective and less-so, the approach of these surgeons is directly analogous to modern-day medical practice. In broader studies of the history of surgery, early modern surgeons often are either largely ignored,[9] or dismissed as unskilled and primitive butchers, whose horrifying and unsanitary procedures, undertaken while the patient was still conscious, were just as likely to kill as cure.[10] However, evidence suggests high levels of training and competence among early modern medical practitioners.[11] This chapter will show that many of the approaches used by seventeenth-century surgeons do have a solid basis in medical science, and that they remained in use – and largely unchanged – for considerable periods afterwards, up to the present day.

Some of the most significant advances in surgical practice in the early modern period appear to have been made by military surgeons. The cliché that war drives innovation was certainly true of the British Civil Wars, regarding medical practice.[12] These advancements were likely driven by necessity, from the high numbers of casualties, and facilitated by the repetitive nature of the battlefield wound-types themselves. Wounds that would be unfamiliar to the civilian surgeon would be commonplace for their military counterparts. In particular, military surgeons were afforded the opportunity to compare their treatments between patients, and test new approaches. They could therefore develop their practice constantly, and the published writings of military surgeons from this period demonstrate the abundant use of an evidence-base for their medical methods.

This chapter will highlight some of the surgical procedures used during the civil wars, evaluate their biomedical validity, and situate early modern military surgeons in context with the ongoing development of military surgical practice. The sudden increase in the use of firearms in infantry warfare in this period would have shaped military surgeons' practice and required effective remedies.[13] Therefore this chapter will focus primarily on the methods used to treat injuries caused by firearms.

THE SURGEON

Alongside the physician and apothecary, the surgeon (sometimes termed barber-surgeon) was one of the recognised medical professions in the seventeenth century.[14] Physicians (doctors) were well educated, and attended to 'physic', the science of maintaining the body's homeostatic balance. Apothecaries purveyed chemicals and medicines, usually as prescribed by the physician. Apothecaries also provided their own medical advice, supplying a cheaper alternative for medical care than the physician. Surgeons focused on the treatment of injuries, and any operation which involved cutting the patient open or spilling blood (amputation, surgery or blood-letting); also setting limbs, dentistry, and curing injury-related conditions such as gangrene, septicaemia or sepsis. The surgeon's role was traditionally associated with the barber, and in many societies across Europe, the combined role of barber-surgeon was the norm. However in England and Scotland, despite often being joined administratively by a single guild, it was common for the roles of barber and surgeon to be separate.[15] By the 1640s, barbers and surgeons had enjoyed Royal Guild status for a century in a regulated profession.[16] Military surgeons were attached to regiments or garrisons, and were a mixture of civilian and professional military surgeons. Richard Wiseman was particularly disdainful of the errors that civilian surgeons would make, based on their inexperience of wounds.[17]

Surgeons usually learned their trade through apprenticeship, and accounts of surgeons refer to subordinates and surgeons' mates who assisted the qualified surgeon, and may subsequently have moved on to their own independent practice.[18] Although eminent sixteenth-century surgeons Thomas Gale, William Clowes, and John Woodall each lamented the poor state of education among young surgeons, the training of surgeons does appear to have been extensive, supported by the circulation of texts and study of anatomy. The study of anatomy through cadaveric dissection was a commonly-accepted practice for medical practitioners.[19] The exceptional accuracy of engravings in mid-seventeenth-century surgical texts showing musculoskeletal, circulatory and nervous system anatomy could only have been gained through cadaveric dissection.

Seventeenth-century surgeons were potentially well-trained professionals. Although there were clearly some in the profession with poor or dangerous practices, there was a self-regulating professional infrastructure to promote good practice within the profession. Although there were several surgeons of note during the British Civil Wars, the two most relevant to this analysis each authored printed texts of significant longevity: James Cooke, and Richard Wiseman.

James Cooke (d. 1693–94) was surgeon to the Greville family, Warwick, from 1638, and served Robert, second baron Brooke until Brooke's death at the first siege of Lichfield in 1643.[20] Cooke served as a surgeon throughout the wars, becoming a Baptist minister in later years. He published *Mellificium Chirurgiae, or the marrow of many good authors* in 1648, and his *Mellificium Chirurgiae, or the Marrow of Chirurgery* (1655) was reprinted six times before 1717. Cooke references several patient cases, and his *Select Observations on English Bodies* (1657), a translation of the work of the late Dr John Hall of Stratford-upon-Avon, was based on over a thousand recorded cases.[21]

Richard Wiseman (c. 1620–76) became the wartime surgeon to Charles, Prince of Wales, and was later present at the battle of Worcester.[22] Wiseman was appointed Sergeant Surgeon to the King in 1660, remaining so until his death in 1676, and he appears to have been financially successful.[23] Wiseman also worked collaboratively with many other contemporary surgeons.[24] Wiseman published two major works, *A Treatise of Wounds* (1672) and *Severall Chirurgicall Treatises* (1676, renamed *Eight Chirurgical Treatises*, 1696). Like Cooke's works, these were also of significant impact (the latter receiving five reprints, up to 1734). Ballingall's *Outlines of Military Surgery* (1844), for example, used Wiseman as its main authority on gunshot wounds.[25] Wiseman's texts also make extensive use of examples of patients treated. What makes Wiseman of particular note is his reference to cases that did not have positive outcomes, and his suggestions as to why they failed. This evidence-based approach identifies Wiseman as a reflective practitioner, rather than a passive employer of traditional practices.

Another English author of particular note to this chapter is John Browne (1642–1702). Browne was not active during the civil wars, but his works reference several examples of cases from the period. Continental European surgeons also had a significant impact, especially the French military surgeon, Ambroise Paré, who revolutionised surgery during the latter sixteenth century.[26] Paré died in 1590; however, his pioneering works were published in English during the early to mid-1600s and so had a direct impact on English practitioners during the civil wars. Wiseman frequently describes Paré's procedures, suggesting a strong influence. Wilhelm Fabry (1560–1634; also known as *Guilelmus Fabricius Hildanus*), and Johannes Scultetus (1595–1645), were German surgeons who each made significant advances in surgical practice that are still used today.[27] Both had works translated into English and are referenced in writings by former civil-war surgeons. Each of these authors adopted evidence-based practice, and referred extensively to examples of patient cases.[28]

CORE MEDICAL UNDERSTANDING

Contemporary medical practitioners were still strongly wedded to many traditional theories, such as those of Galen or Aristotle. In particular, physic rested heavily on the four humours (blood, yellow bile, black bile and phlegm), whose natural balance was the key to good health. Practices such as bleeding and cupping were still taken as effective methodologies, and belief in these approaches continued well into the nineteenth century. However, the writings of many seventeenth-century authors display a critical stance on numerous traditional practices, and dissatisfaction with established authorities. This scepticism is unsurprising, given the context of the intellectual developments in natural science during the period, to which these practitioners – certainly Wiseman at the court of Charles II – were exposed. The level of understanding of physiology and anatomy in the printed surgical texts is extensive and generally accurate. Understanding of physiology is often couched within terms that the authors would have understood. For example, the importance of blood flow was referred to as maintaining 'heat', as the concept of oxygenated blood was not known.

Gangrene, and its more severe form *sphacelus*, were recognised and their causes understood, despite a lack of knowledge of the physiological causes. Both involved the restriction of 'heat' (blood flow) to the affected part of the body, either by the over-tight torsion of a bandage, tourniquet or ligature, frostbite, sepsis from foreign matter in a gunshot wound, or damage from a wound or concussion.[29] Over-tightening of bandages was identified as a particular danger when affixing a splint to a broken limb. Gangrene was easily recognised by the body part going pale (as if it had been scalded) and then black. The remedy for the condition was to try to encourage blood flow by scarification of the tissue, and to cut away the dead matter. By the rate of blood flow and the nature of the blood being released, the surgeon would be able to ascertain the progression of the gangrene.[30] Left untreated, gangrene, and the ensuing *sphacelus*, were fatal, and the death would be a painful one. Wiseman wrote of one patient he had attended too late: 'he died howling'.[31]

Seventeenth-century surgeons understood the impact of infection, although the role of pus was misunderstood. 'Laudable pus' was seen as a means of cleansing the wound, referred to as 'digestion', rather than as a discharge of waste matter.[32] Despite this, and without knowledge of the bacterial cause of infection, they did appreciate the impact of antiseptic agents on reducing infection rates and accelerating healing. The use of alcohol, either the commonly used red wine, white wine, or *aqua vitae* spirits, was frequently recommended for cleaning wounds and soaking bandages and dressings. Vinegar was also frequently used, usually as a vinegar-water mix, 'oxycrate', or *posca* (an ancient Roman water-vinegar drink). Similarly, turpentine ('terebinth') was commonly used in either operative treatment or post-operative wound care.

Concentrated sugars, such as honey or treacle, were also used in dressings to reduce infection, approaches which are still used today, especially in veterinary medicine. The recommendation to treat burns using a poultice of garlic, onions or leeks with salt is also a potentially viable approach to limit infection.[33] These members of the *Allium* family contain organosulphur compounds, such as Allicin, which have antimicrobial properties.[34] Powders, such as chalk, or various mineral clays, or resins, such as 'Dragon's Blood' or mastic gum, were also effective at impeding bacterial growth. Dragon's Blood was a resin from the South American tree, *Croton lechleri*, which had been used as a coagulant in South American traditional medicine for many centuries. Taspine, the active component of Dragon's Blood, has been shown to have anti-inflammatory and anti-viral properties, and promote cell death in cancer tissue.[35]

None of these remedies were understood from a biomedical perspective; but clearly experience, and trial and error showed the practitioners that they worked. These published observations contradict modern assumptions that early modern practitioners were unable to understand the nature of infection until the discovery of the role of bacteria in the nineteenth century. The treatises also demonstrate a good appreciation of the importance of hygiene in surgical practice.

WOUNDS FROM FIREARMS

Surgeons in the British Civil Wars had to deal with a variety of weapon types, but with musketeers typically comprising two thirds or more of infantry units, the most common injury they were likely to encounter would be from gunshot. The projectile shot from a musket was a spherical ball, referred to interchangeably as a ball or bullet (see Figure 3.1).[36] It was typically 15–20mm diameter, weighed around 38–45g and cast in lead. The lead used in seventeenth-century musket balls was softer than modern lead, which is alloyed with a small amount of antimony. The irregular shape of the ball (from casting), its poor fit inside the barrel, and its propulsion by low-quality loose-grain gunpowder, meant the musket ball trajectory was low velocity (400–500 metres per second), with maximum range of up to 180 metres, and moderate-to-poor accuracy.[37] Projectile force lessened with distance, so

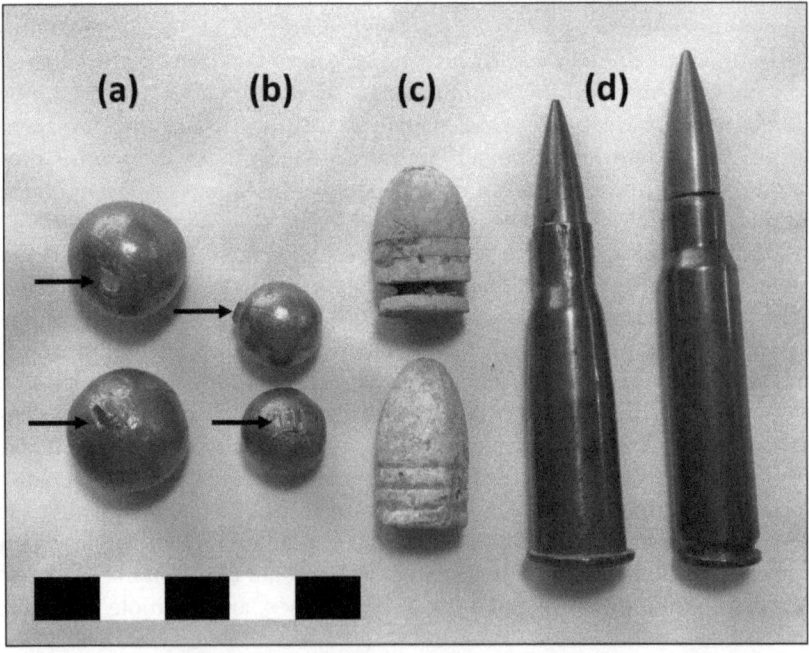

Figure 3.1 Musket/pistol balls. (a) Musket and (b) pistol balls typical of the mid-1600s. Note the visible 'nipple' on the surface (arrows), a relic of the casting process which created an uneven surface to the ball. Comparison with (c) Minié Ball bullets from the American Civil War (1861–65) and (d) two *c.* 7.5 mm calibre rounds from the mid-twentieth century. The scale bar is 5 cm

the effective range was significantly less, possibly as little as 50 metres.[38] A musket ball was expected to be able to penetrate armour, while a pistol ball would be repelled by a metal breastplate or helmet, but would penetrate through clothing.

Modern, high-velocity bullets typically have a small entry wound, and a large exit wound. Surgeons in the seventeenth century recognised the different forms of wound, with the entry wound usually being small, tight and blackish, the exit wound (if one existed at all, as the bullet often did not leave the body), large, ragged and inflamed.[39] The treatment of the exit wound involved debridement and eventual closing of the wound after cleansing. The entry wound was easier to treat, either by cauterisation (using hot metal or oil to close the wound), by suture (stitching), or by a ligature (a bandage or thread tying the wound closed). Paré observed that surgeons around him typically cauterised gunshot wounds using boiling oil of elders, mixed with treacle. However, after running out of this mixture, he resorted to using a non-boiling poultice of egg yolk, oil of roses and turpentine, which resulted in better patient outcomes and is reflected in seventeenth-century writings.[40] Entry wounds could often be mistaken as gangrenous due to the blackish skin around the hole (now termed a 'gunpowder tattoo'), and be erroneously treated as such by inexperienced surgeons, without the wound being investigated for the bullet or other foreign matter taken in with it.[41]

TREATMENT OF SOFT TISSUE DAMAGE FROM GUNSHOT

Musket-shot wounds are complex and variable in their nature, due to the ballistics of the bullet, and this was understood by early modern surgical authors.[42] A travelling bullet causes three potential areas of compression (see Figure 3.2a).[43] Firstly, there is a displacement shockwave ahead of the bullet. Secondly, the bullet tearing through the body will cause direct physical damage (the permanent cavity). Finally, the compression caused by the wake of the bullet, analogous to the wake of a boat through water, will cause damage from temporary pressure on internal tissues (the temporary cavity). The temporary cavity is usually considerably wider than the permanent cavity, though even with a modern high-velocity bullet, rocking or yawing (and in some cases, complete flipping) of the bullet inside the body (see Figure 3.2b) will cause the permanent cavity to widen.[44] Although there have been no published ballistic tests undertaken on seventeenth-century musket balls using seventeenth-century powder mixtures, the internal effect on the body is likely to be broadly similar to a soft-headed bullet (see Figure 3.2c). This bullet flattens and even fragments, and therefore causes a much wider permanent cavity, with a temporary cavity still present. The bullet, if it emerges at all, is likely to be severely misshapen.

The impact of a musket ball on the body was therefore likely to result in deformation of the ball, and some deviation from the direction of travel when

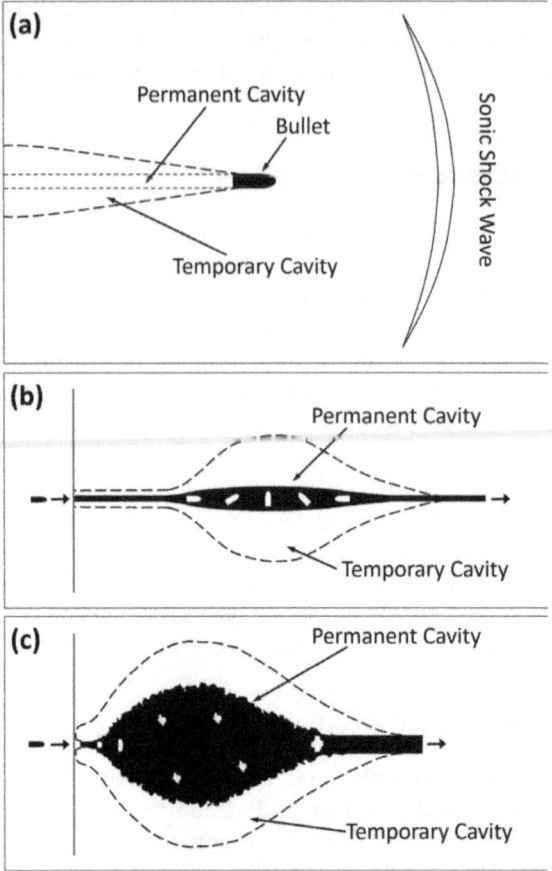

Figure 3.2 Ballistics of modern bullets. (a) Pathway of a bullet, showing the sonic shock wave, permanent and temporary cavities as a bullet passes through the air or a human body. (b) Plotting the permanent (shaded) and temporary (dotted line) cavities in a high velocity (7.62 mm) bullet. The axes represent proportional distances. White bullet shapes demonstrate the yawing and flipping of the bullet. (c) Cavitation from a soft-headed bullet. The bullet deforms and fragments, causing a wider permanent cavity, and a wider exit path

the ball entered the body. As the ball moved between tissues or cavities of differing densities, its pathway would be refracted. This refraction was noted by seventeenth-century surgeons, Wiseman noting that 'It being wonderful to consider how these Shots do twirl about'.[45] There are several accounts of this, such as a soldier who, having been shot in the cheek, had the bullet removed from the back of his neck. Another, shot in the lower leg, had the bullet removed from the thigh above the knee; a third, shot near the breastbone, had the bullet removed from near the spine.[46]

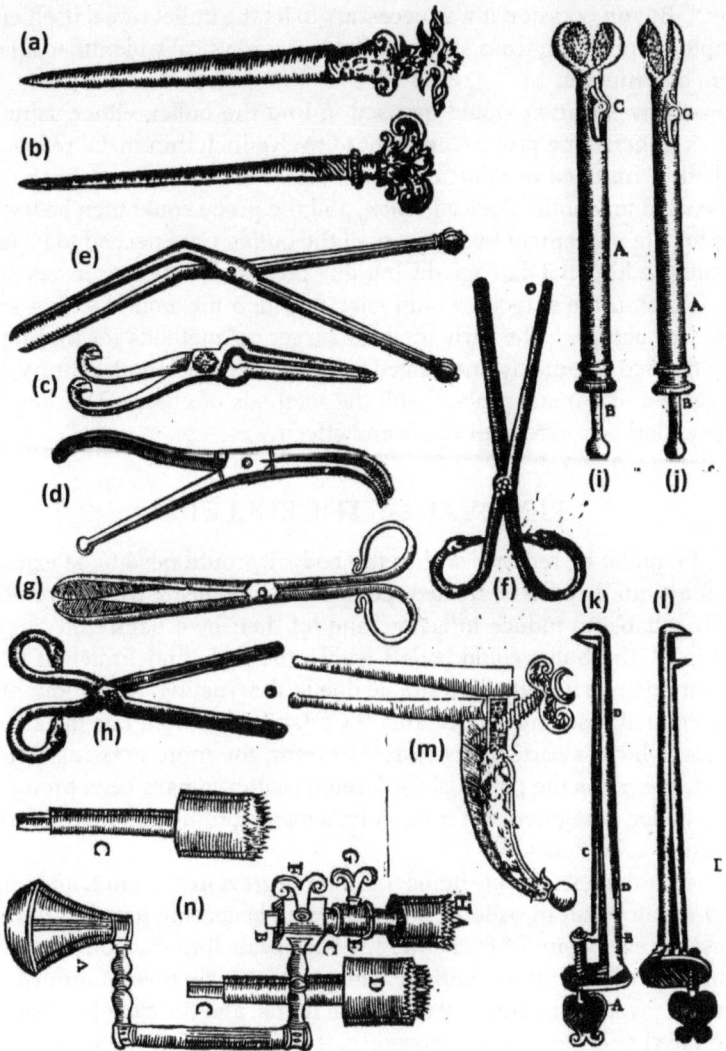

Figure 3.3 Surgical implements. (a, b) Tirefond bullet extractors, (c, d) Crowe's Bill, (e, f) Crane's Bill, (g, h) Drake's Bill, (i) Catch-bullet and (j) Lizard's Mouthe articulated bullet extractors, (k, l) Parrot's Bill, open and closed respectively, (m) Swan's Beake, (n) Trepanning tool showing fittings. Not shown to scale

The erratic path of the ball posed considerable challenges for the surgeon. The bullet was not always straightforward to find. It was advised that the patient should be sat in the same position as when he received the injury, as this gave the surgeon a better chance of locating and accessing the bullet.[47] The symptoms of the patient could also be used as an indicator of the bullet's location.[48] But on occasion it was necessary to let the bullet reveal itself either by symptoms resulting from sepsis, or by being physically identified against the skin, or a muscle.

Internal investigation would be used to find the bullet, either using the surgeon's fingers, or a probe – an eight to twelve-inch thin metal rod, sometimes with a rounded or widened end.[49] The feel of metal touching metal could be used to identify the lead bullet, and the probe could then be used as a guide for the implement used to extract the bullet. Care needed to be taken not to cause additional damage during this process,[50] although it was noted that on occasion the surgeon would have to widen the wound with a knife, to allow free access.[51] The early modern surgeons' methods for finding the bullet remained essentially unchanged until the late nineteenth century, with the finger,[52] and a metal probe,[53] still the methods of choice. This suggests that these methods were both viable and effective.

REMOVAL OF THE BULLET

Should the bullet be retained within the body, it would need to be extracted before the wound could be treated. Lead musket or pistol balls were not in themselves liable to induce infection, and 'of their own nature do carry no Poyson in'.[54] The bullet could be left within the body, indefinitely if necessary,[55] but this was usually undesirable due to the 'rusting' (oxidation) of the metal potentially causing septicaemia.[56] Certainly this would be the case for lead oxide, which is particularly toxic. However, the more pressing concern for the surgeon was the potential for foreign matter to have been brought in with the bullet – fragments of the soldier's own clothing, splinters of wood, hair or other solid items.[57]

The removal of extraneous items was of very great importance, and failure to do so would result in patients failing to heal, becoming feverish, developing sepsis or even dying.[58] Even after the wide-scale introduction of antibiotics in the latter half of the twentieth century, this imperative continued. The importance given to the removal of foreign items, and the clear link between their removal and the patient recovering, is indicative that the surgeons did understand the link between septicaemia/sepsis and contamination of the wound, as shown by Wiseman:

> A person having been shot in the Arm, and the Wound undigested, I being consulted advised the laying open of the Wound, and extraction of the Bullet, Rags, &c. but was over-ruled by others ... Two days after I visited the Patient, and asked the Chirurgeon whether he had laid open the Wound. He replied, there was no need, for he could turn his finger in it, and pull out the Bullet and Rags, if it was necessary. As I was going out of the house, I met the Physician, who inquiring of me the Patient's health, I replied that the Chirurgeon had unwittingly given me the certain sign of his Death ... A day or two after he died, too certainly justifying my Prognostick.[59]

Once it had been located, the soft lead bullet, as well as fragments of bone or splinters of wood, could be removed by a *Terebellum* or Tirefond (see Figure 3.3a and 3.3b), a long hollow tube containing an internal baffle tipped with a sharp screw.[60] There were also other implements for extraction, each a variant on pliers or forceps.[61] The Crowe's Bill (see Figure 3.3c and 3.3d) was a pair of levered pliers, either straight or curved, with short, toothed fronds capable of gripping firmly. The Crane's Bill (see Figure 3.3e and 3.3f) had longer fronds for deeply embedded bullets. The Duck or Drake's Bill (see Figure 3.3g and 3.3h) had tips that were rounded to surround the ball. The 'catch-bullet' (see Figure 3.3i) had capped ends, operated by an internal mechanism. The Parrot's Bill (see Figure 3.3k and 3.3l) had sharpened edges for gripping flat bones, such as skull fragments. Finally, the Swan's Beak (see Figure 3.3m) was used to dilate wounds. Except for becoming more slender and reliable, these implements, as with the probes, remained relatively unchanged for the next two centuries.[62]

Once the bullet had been extracted and the wound confirmed as clean, Wiseman recommended dressing the wound with a clean dressing, soaked in *oleum catellorum* (oil of puppies), as hot as bearable by the patient. *Oleum catellorum* was a recipe gained from Paré,[63] who in turn obtained it from a fellow surgeon, and involves boiling two newborn puppies in lily oil until 'their flesh departed from the bones', along with one pound of earthworms – purified of their stomach contents in white wine – and *aqua vitae*, then strained and mixed with turpentine to make a balm. Wiseman's own summary of the recipe is almost identical to that of Paré, though less detailed.[64] Given that this was a treatment for gunshot wounds, potentially the most common wound type Wiseman would have encountered, it is unlikely that this method was plagiarised and included in the text without being used. Wiseman does not hesitate to challenge the methods of other notable surgeons, and so it is reasonable to conclude that the use of *oleum catellorum* was effective. The biomedical properties of boiled earthworms and puppies are as yet untested by modern science, but are unlikely to be biomedically significant. However, possibly neonates and cleansed earthworms were chosen due to a lack of faecal matter in their intestines, little hair, and high proportion of protein and fat. The balm would be sterilised and kept sterile and malleable through the alcohol and turpentine, properties enhanced by it being applied 'as hot as the Part will bear'.[65] *Oleum catellorum* may have been effective in creating an antibacterial seal to prevent further contamination. However, it is likely that the alcohol and turpentine were the active ingredients, rather than the puppies.

MANAGEMENT OF INFECTION IN WOUNDS

Although, through alcohol, vinegar, heat or poultices, surgeons had methods in place to reduce infection levels, large wounds were prone to developing infection. To address this, instead of being sutured closed, the wound would deliberately be left open,[66] and the lips of the wound kept apart from each other. For this the surgeon would use either tents (rolls of linen pressed into the wound to keep the lips of the cut apart),[67] or setons (thick thread sewn through the wound to aid in drainage, analogous to a modern-day shunt).[68] The tent would typically be made of linen and stiffened with egg white,[69] and then steeped in red wine or oxycrate before inserting into the wound.[70]

The methodology was to keep the wound open and allow it to weep and discharge until it took on the appearance of 'Flesh long hang'd in the Air'.[71] By keeping the wound site open, the surgeon was promoting the accumulation of lymph at the wound site, fortifying the immune system, recruiting white blood cells and limiting bacterial growth.[72] Although the cell biology behind this approach was not known to the seventeenth-century practitioners, they were aware that it was effective. This approach to wound healing, later termed 'delayed primary suture' or 'delayed primary closure' in 1919, or 'healing by second (or third) intention', continued to be used in major conflicts, right up to the modern day.[73] Delayed primary closure is still in use, in civilian surgery, such as for appendicitis and compartment syndrome.[74] The longevity of this approach highlights that the practice used by early modern surgeons was valid, effective and revisited continually over subsequent centuries. Similarly, this approach was a pioneering methodology, as it is absent from medical practice in previous centuries. In the absence of antibiotics, the approach of delayed primary closure by the seventeenth-century surgeon was inventive and effective, and illustrates that these surgeons were undertaking sound, evidence-based medical practice.

TREATMENT OF BLUNT-FORCE TRAUMA DAMAGE FROM PROJECTILES

A musket was a formidable weapon in causing penetrative damage, but the damage caused by blunt force trauma was equally significant. Aside from damage caused using the musket butt as a club in mêlée combat, the musket ball was also capable of causing blunt-force trauma. If a bullet encountered solid bone, then it was possible to cause considerable damage, and either shatter the bone, sever it, or if the strike was a glancing blow, to cause a simple fracture.[75] One of Wiseman's patients had his arm shot off, just above the elbow.[76] Some seventeenth-century military surgeons showed a working knowledge of gun-shot fractures equivalent to the understanding of late nineteenth-century surgeons. When a bone is struck by a bullet of low-medium velocity, it typically receives an X-shaped fracture, the fracture taking the shortest route, combined with the grain of the bone.[77] Wiseman described this appearance, noting that the bone, if not shattered, had the feel of fish scales.[78]

The removal of slivers of bone and extraneous material was the primary concern.[79] Fragmented remnants of bone could cause pressure on nerves, block blood vessels and inhibit healing. Such issues could potentially lead to gangrene, septicaemia, or, at the very least, continued discomfort and increased risk of infection. Where possible the bone would be reset by the application of traction and the manipulation of the bone through the bullet wound until the fracture was aligned.[80] The wound would be splinted, taking care to use wide bandages, so as not to 'restrict the heat' of the wound and cut off circulation.[81] The support of a fracture could be achieved either by splints or by suspending the limb in a sleeve of armour with a long screw along the length of the articulated covering, to enable the limb to be extended.[82] The validity of this method is supported by direct parallels used in later conflicts, such as the 'Thomas splint',[83] used during the First World War, and the Tobruk splint, developed in the Second World War.[84] The latter directly parallels the method Wiseman used to treat patients with multiple fractures of limbs.[85] In Wiseman's approach, pasteboard softened with vinegar could form an indentation of the limb, so the limb could be sandwiched between two sheets and immobilised. For example, a mariner whose arm was completely shattered, to the extent that one could have amputated the arm without a saw, refused to have the arm removed. This would have been normal practice for a multiple-fractured limb, but after eight weeks' immobilisation the arm managed to heal enough to be usable.[86] Wiseman attributed this success to the patient's inactivity during the eight-week treatment; without immobilisation the bones would never have knitted together.

For a fracture caused by a gunshot, the surgeon needed to treat the wound without disturbing the fracture and preventing its healing. The approach suggested by Wiseman to accommodate this was to create a broad bandage of soft linen cloth folded-over three or four times.[87] Three slits were then cut longitudinally towards the middle from either end, leaving an uncut region in the centre. The uncut region was placed under the limb, to support the fracture, then the three strips from either end tied together over an absorptive linen pad over the wound. This could absorb discharges from the wound but be changed regularly by moving the three ties aside. Thus the fracture could be supported and the wound receive ongoing treatment.

For cranial fractures caused by gunshots, the challenge was to raise the skull fragments back into place. The scalp had to be cleansed of blood using red wine or vinegar, and any hair removed from the wound site.[88] The fractures could then be levered upright without the need to remove too many bones. Indeed, Wiseman castigated some of his fellow surgeons for removing too many bones from patients' skulls and keeping them as souvenirs. For depressed fractures of the skull, caused by glancing blows or pressure injuries, in the absence of a penetrative wound, the only approach was to use a trepanning tool (see Figure 3.3n) to cut out a circular disk from the skull, after first paring back the skin of the scalp. Using this hole as an access point, levers could raise skull fragments back into place.[89] The trepanned section could be replaced, or the gap covered using a beaten-out coin. Trepanning appears to have been used for cranial fractures, or to release visible swellings from cranial fluid, and not as a cure for psychiatric disorders or headaches, common in the medieval period.[90]

AMPUTATION

Should a limb prove to be either beyond repair, infected or gangrenous, the surgeon would reluctantly be required to amputate.[91] Wiseman discussed a range of suggested methodologies from noted surgeons and contemporaries in London but his own approach was quite clear.[92] The surgeon should have a well-prepared supply of clean tow (soft linen), bandages, buttons (small, stuffed linen spheres) and an ox bladder to cover the stump. Cooke's advice on amputation suggested similar preparations, including at least two sharp bone saws, so that the operation could be completed rapidly should one break.[93] These items were soaked in oxycrate and left to dry, and buttons also were soaked in wine or oxycrate and dipped in an astringent mix of powders, including mastic and 'Dragon's Blood'.[94] Cooke also noted that some surgeons used red-hot knives and saws. So without understanding the rationale, some seventeenth-century surgeons did seem aware of the benefits of an aseptic environment.

Wiseman's approach was to cut off the blood supply with a strong ligature (a thick strip of linen tied tightly as a tourniquet) to inhibit bleeding and facilitate the post-amputation securing of blood vessels.[95] The ligature applied, the surgeon could then operate without fear of excessive blood loss from the patient. The surgeon's mate would pull the skin and muscle of the healthy part of the limb away from the damaged area, so that when the surgeon cut through the skin and flesh (using a single motion from a curved knife, shaped with the curve on the inside), the musculature was immediately pulled back, exposing the bone underneath, which could then be cut through using a sharpened saw. Speed was of most importance to the procedure, to minimise patient discomfort.[96]

After amputation the severed arteries needed to be sealed. Cooke advised suturing the stump shut with artery ends blocked by linen buttons, or tied with a ligature.[97] Wiseman, emphasising speed, advised the use of an 'actual' (heat-based) cautery to sear the ends of the blood vessels together. Cauterisation of blood vessels was a faster and more secure approach, provided the nerves and bone ends could be avoided, and cauterisation of blood vessels was practiced into the nineteenth century.[98] To seal the stump, the approach then was to pull the skin and muscle back over the bone. The bone had been cut shorter than the musculature to enable the fleshy end of the stump to be sewn shut using two stout stitches at right-angles to each other. The stump was then bound using bandages, and covered with the bladder, each soaked in oxycrate. As a result of the preparations, operation speed and aftercare, the potential for infection of the amputated stump was reduced considerably, although some discharge of pus was expected and encouraged.

The fact that numerous soldiers survived amputations emphasises the potential effectiveness of the procedure, although the propensity for wounded soldiers to be missing parts of limbs suggests that efficacy depended on the severity of the site of the amputation. Subsequent to the seventeenth century, survival rates from amputations were generally low, even well into the twentieth century, and so it was unlikely that survival rates in the seventeenth century were high.

CONCLUSION: HOW EFFECTIVE WAS SEVENTEENTH-CENTURY MILITARY SURGERY?

This chapter has proposed that several of the methods practiced by seventeenth-century military surgeons had biomedical validity, and longevity within the medical professions. Due to the lack of comprehensive medical records from the British Civil Wars, it is impossible to directly evaluate the success rates of surgeons' practice. However, as several chapters within this book attest, it was possible to survive quite severe wounds. The prevalence of severe wounds presented by maimed soldiers seeking military pensions particularly support this view.[99] Hannah Worthen's data on maimed soldiers' reported wounds indicates a prevalence for wounds of the extremities, but also examples of multiple wounds that were survived.[100] Wiseman, Cooke and other authors frequently reported survivors of extreme injuries, and the fact that these are juxtaposed against descriptions of patients who were less fortunate, suggests that these accounts are truthful. Two extreme cases from the civil wars include Colonel William 'Blowface' Forbes of Tolmads, Aberdeenshire, who was stood near to Sir Thomas Fairfax at the siege of Pontefract Castle when a cannon ball passed between them. The force caused by the passing ball knocked Fairfax to the ground and 'spoyled one side of the Colonells face and eyes'.[101] Colonel Forbes survived, despite his injuries, continuing in military service until his death in 1646.[102] While the surgical intervention for Colonel Forbes was not recorded, he was clearly treated successfully, and despite disfiguring injuries was able to continue active duty. Still more extreme were the wounds of John Tinkler of Durham, a gunner at Hartlepool, who survived blinding and the loss of both his arms.[103] Clearly it was possible to survive very significant injuries and medical procedures.

Ian Gentles suggests an estimate of over 90,000, 30,000 and 80–100,000 wounded soldiers in England/Wales, Scotland and Ireland respectively, and suggests the numbers of maimed soldiers in later years to be tens of thousands.[104] It is impossible to know how many of these casualties survived as a result of surgical intervention, or indeed how many casualties died as a result of it, but it was clearly possible to survive a civil-war injury. It should be noted that this chapter focuses on a small number of select surgeons, who were successful or recognised enough to enjoy sufficient patronage to publish. It is likely there were also less-valid practices among unpublished civil-war surgeons, but the consistency of approaches between published authors supports the notion that they were reporting common practices. Based on their published works, it seems that seventeenth-century surgeons were utilising approaches that were valid biomedically, and that they were using an evidence-based approach to their practice, which belies the popular image of dangerously incompetent 'quacks'. Instead it suggests that they were medical pioneers, whose effective methods remained largely unchanged for several generations, and laid the basis for modern surgical practice.

NOTES

1 V. C. McAlister, 'William Harvey, Fabricius ab Acquapendente and the divide between medicine and surgery', *Canadian Journal of Surgery*, 50:1 (2007), 7–8; I. Richards, 'Medicine, religion and the judiciary: a reevaluation of the surgeon's position in the community, 1600–99' (MA dissertation, University of Huddersfield, 2013).

2 I. Mortimer, *The Dying and the Doctors: The Medical Revolution in Seventeenth-Century England* (Woodbridge: Boydell, 2009).

3 S. De Renzi, 'Women and medicine', in P. Elmer (ed.), *The Healing Arts: Death, Disease and Society in Europe, 1500–1800* (Manchester: Manchester University Press, 2004), pp. 196–227; Wyman, 'The surgeoness: the female practitioner of surgery, 1400–1800', *Medical History*, 28:1 (1984), 22–41; Mortimer, *The Dying and the Doctors*, pp. 135–89.

4 Mortimer, *The Dying and the Doctors*, pp. 15–23, 86–90.

5 P. Elmer, 'Medicine, religion and the puritan revolution', in R. French and A. Wear (eds), *The Medical Revolution of the Seventeenth Century* (Cambridge: Cambridge University Press, 1989), pp. 10–45; J. Henry, 'The matter of souls: medical theory and theology in seventeenth-century England', in French and Wear (eds), *The Medical Revolution*, pp. 87–113; P. Elmer, 'Medicine and witchcraft', in B. P. Levack (ed.), *The Oxford Handbook of Witchcraft in Early Modern Europe and Colonial America* (Oxford: Oxford University Press, 2013), pp. 561–74.

6 N. G. Siraisi, *Medieval and Early Modern Medicine: An Introduction to Knowledge and Practice* (Chicago, IL: University of Chicago Press, 1990), p. 183.

7 R. Porter, 'Hospitals and surgery', in R. Porter (ed.), *The Cambridge History of Medicine* (Cambridge: Cambridge University Press, 2006), p. 176. For an extensive review of the progression of medical practice from medieval to early modern periods, see Siraisi, *Medieval and Early Modern Medicine*.

8 G. Guyatt *et al.*, 'Evidence-based medicine: a new approach to teaching the practice of medicine', *Journal of the American Medical Association*, 268:17 (1992), pp. 2420–5.

9 For example, only cursory attention is paid to seventeenth-century surgeons in R. Hollingham, *Blood and Guts: A History of Surgery* (London: Random House, 2008), and M. J. Lewis, *Medicine and Care of the Dying: A Modern History* (Oxford: Oxford University Press, 2007).

10 For example, J. E. McCallum, *Military Medicine: From Ancient Times to the 21st Century* (Santa Barbara, CA: ABC-CLIO, 2008), pp. 291–4; R. A. Gabriel,

Between Flesh and Steel: A History of Military Medicine from the Middle Ages to the War in Afghanistan (Washington DC: Potomac Books, 2013), pp. 65–85.

11 C. Webster, *The Great Instauration: Science, Medicine and Reform 1626–1660* (London: Duckworth, 1975), pp. 252–3; S. De Renzi, 'The sick and their healers', in Elmer (ed.), *The Healing Arts*, pp. 43–9; L. M. Beier, *Sufferers and Healers: The Experience of Illness in Seventeenth-Century England* (London: Routledge, 1987), pp. 51–96; S. M. Rutherford, 'Ground-breaking pioneers or dangerous amateurs? Did early modern surgery have any basis in medical science?', in I. Pells (ed.), *New Approaches to the Military History of the English Civil War* (Solihull: Helion and Company, 2016), pp. 153–85.

12 R. Porter, *The Greatest Benefit to Mankind: A Medical History of Humanity from Antiquity to the Present* (London: Harper, 1997), p. 652.

13 O. P. Grell, 'War, medicine and the military revolution', in Elmer (ed.) *The Healing Arts*, pp. 257–60.

14 For a more extensive account of the early modern military surgeon, see Rutherford, 'Ground-breaking pioneers or dangerous amateurs?'.

15 The London Company of Barber-Surgeons alternated each year between a surgeon and a barber for the Master of the Company: A. Griffin, 'William Clowes (1582–1648)', *ODNB*; McCallum, *Military Medicine*, p. 292.

16 J. O. Robinson, 'The barber-surgeons of London', *Archives of Surgery*, 119:10 (1984), 1171–5.

17 E. Gruber von Arni, *Justice for the Maimed Soldier: Nursing, Medical Care and Welfare for Sick and Wounded Soldiers and their Families during the English Civil Wars and Interregnum, 1642–1660* (Aldershot: Ashgate, 2001), pp. 228–31.

18 Richard Wiseman's surgeon's mate at the battle of Worcester, William Clarke, later became a surgeon based in Bridgnorth: R. Wiseman, *Severall Chirurgical Treatises* (London: Norton and Maycock, 1676), p. 438.

19 S. B. Ghosh, 'Human cadaveric dissection: a historical account from ancient Greece to the modern era', *Anatomy & Cell Biology*, 48:3 (2015), 153–69; Rutherford, 'Ground-breaking pioneers or dangerous amateurs?', p. 160.

20 R. A. Cohen, 'Documents concerning James Cooke, surgeon, of Warwick', *Medical History*, 1:2 (1957), 168–73.

21 *Ibid.*

22 J. Kirkup, 'Richard Wiseman (*bap.* 1620?, *d.* 1676)', *ODNB*.

23 Wiseman left considerable sums to his family in his will (including £2,000 to his son); TNA, PROB 11/352/88, 12 September 1676.

24 The extent to which Wiseman collaborated with his fellow surgeons is discussed in detail in M. McVaugh, 'Richard Wiseman and the medical practitioners of Restoration London', *Journal of the History of Medicine and Allied Sciences*, 62:2 (2007), 125–40.

25 G. Ballingall, *Outlines of Military Surgery* (Edinburgh: A&C Black, 1844), pp. 215–16.

26 P. Hernigou, 'Ambroise Paré's life (1510–1590): part I', *International Orthopaedics*, 37:3 (2013), 543–7; P. Hernigou, 'Ambroise Paré III: Paré's contributions to surgical instruments and surgical instruments at the time of Ambroise Paré', *International Orthopaedics*, 37:10 (2013), 975–80.

27 E. Jones, 'The life and works of *Guilhelmus Fabricius Hildanus* (1560–1634): Part

I', *Medical History*, 4:2 (1960), 112–34; E. W. P. Jones, 'The life and works of *Guilhelmus Fabricius Hildanus* (1560–1634): Part II', *Medical History*, 4:3 (1960), 196–209; J. Scultetus (trans. E. B.), *The Chirurgeons Store-House* (London: J. Starkey, 1674); A. H. Scultetus, J. L. Villavicencio and N. M. Rich, 'The life and work of the German physician Johannes Scultetus (1595–1645)', *Journal of the American College of Surgeons*, 196 (2003), 130–9.

28 W. Fabry (trans. J. Steer), *Gulielm Fabricus Hildamis, His Experiments in Chyrurgerie* (London: Barnard Alsop, 1643).

29 Wiseman, *Severall Chirurgical Treatises*, pp. 445–7.

30 *Ibid.*, pp. 445–6.

31 *Ibid.*, p. 445.

32 It was also known as 'laudable quittor', J. Cooke, *Mellificium Chirurgiae, or the Marrow of Chirurgery Much Enlarged, to which Is Added Anatomy* (London: J. D., 1676), pp. 51, 145.

33 *Ibid.*, pp. 223, 395; A. Paré (trans. W. Hamond), *The Method of Curing Wounds Made by Gun-shot, Also by Arrowes and Darts, with their Accidents* (London: Isaac Iaggard, 1617), pp. 8–9; Wiseman, *Severall Chirurgical Treatises*, p. 442; Wing / B5124, J. Browne, *A Compleat Discourse of Wounds* (London, 1678), p. 95.

34 S. Ankri and D. Mirelman, 'Antimicrobial properties of allicin from garlic', *Microbes and Infection*, 1:2 (1999), 125–9.

35 W. Fayad, M. Fryknäs, S. Brnjic, M. H. Olofsson, R. Larsson, S. Linder, 'Identification of a novel topoisomerase inhibitor effective in cells overexpressing drug efflux transporters', *PLoS ONE*, 4:10 (2009), 7238.

36 V. Eyers, 'Ballistics of matchlock muskets' (MSc dissertation, Cranfield University, 2006), p. 12.

37 *Ibid.*, pp. 29–33. The velocity of bullets from modern rifles is three times faster.

38 *Ibid.*, p. 52.

39 Wiseman, *Severall Chirurgical Treatises*, p. 413.

40 Paré, *The Method of Curing Wounds Made by Gun-shot*, pp. 5–6.

41 M. Tokdemir, H. Kafadar, A. Turkoglu and T. Bork, 'Forensic value of gunpowder tattooing in identification of multiple entrance wounds from one bullet', *Legal Medicine*, 9:3 (2007), 147–50; Wiseman, *Severall Chirurgical Treatises*, p. 408; Browne, *Compleat Discourse*, pp. 100, 102.

42 Wiseman, *Severall Chirurgical Treatises*, p. 411.

43 A. C. Szul (ed.), *Emergency War Surgery: NATO Handbook, US Revision 3* (Washington, DC: United States Government Printing Office, 2004), pp. 1–13.

44 M. L. Fackler, 'Gunshot wound review', *Annals of Emergency Medicine*, 28:2 (1996), 194–203; R. A. Santucci and Y. -J. Chang, 'Ballistics for physicians: myths about wound ballistics and gunshot injuries', *Journal of Urology*, 171:4 (2004), 1408–14.; V. J. M. DiMaio, *Gunshot Wounds: Practical Aspects of Firearms, Ballistics, and Forensic Techniques* (2nd edn, New York: CRC Press, 1999), pp. 51–61.

45 Wiseman, *Severall Chirurgical Treatises*, p. 412.

46 *Ibid.*, p. 413.

47 Browne, *Compleat Discourse*, p. 109.

48 *Ibid.*, p. 412.

49 T. Johnson, *The Workes of that Famous Chirurgion Ambrose Parey* (London: Cotes and Young, 1634), p. 421; Wiseman, *Severall Chirurgical Treatises*, pp. 412, 427.

50 Wiseman, *Severall Chirurgical Treatises*, p. 412.

51 Browne, *Compleat Discourse*, pp. 350–1; Wiseman, *Severall Chirurgical Treatises*, p. 431.

52 T. Chevalier, *A Treatise on Gunshot Wounds: Which Obtained the Premium Given by the Royal College of Surgeons in London for the Year 1803* (London: S. Bagster, 1806), pp. 69–70; S. D. Gross, *A Manual of Military Surgery or Hints on the Emergencies of Field, Camp, and Hospital Practice* (2nd edn, Philadelphia, PA: J. B. Lippincott & Co., 1862), p. 70.

53 F. H. Hamilton, *A Practical Treatise on Military Surgery* (New York: Balliere Brothers, 1861), p. 139; Gross, *A Manual of Military Surgery*, p. 70.

54 Browne, *Compleat Discourse*, p. 100.

55 Browne recounts reading of an individual for whom he had 'extracted a Leaden Bullet, which was received in the Groyn, five years after its reception, in which time it had fallen near the Knee, at which place it was drawn forth', *Ibid.*, pp. 100, 110.

56 Wiseman, *Severall Chirurgical Treatises*, p. 411.

57 *Ibid.*, p. 431.

58 Johnson, *The Workes*, pp. 424–6; Wiseman, *Severall Chirurgical Treatises*, pp. 411–12.

59 Wiseman, *Severall Chirurgical Treatises*, pp. 445–6.

60 Browne, *Compleat Discourse*, pp. 7, 37, 107; Paré, *The Method of Curing Wounds Made by Gun-shot*, p. 52.

61 Johnson, *The Workes*, pp. 421–4; G. Fabritius Hildanus, *Cista Militaris: or A Military Chest* (London: W. Godbid, 1674), pp. 21–8; Browne, *Compleat Discourse*, p. 37.

62 M. Crumplin, *Men of Steel: Surgery in the Napoleonic Wars* (Shrewsbury: Quiller Press, 2007), pp. 188–91; Hamilton, *A Practical Treatise on Military Surgery*, pp. 139–41; Gross, *A Manual of Military Surgery*, pp. 71–3.

63 Paré, *The Method of Curing Wounds Made by Gun-shot*, pp. 6–7.

64 Wiseman, *Severall Chirurgical Treatises*, pp. 414–15.

65 *Ibid.*, p. 415.

66 Cooke, *Mellificium Chirurgiae*, p. 180; Wiseman, *Severall Chirurgical Treatises*, p. 326; G. Keynes (ed.), *The Apologie and Treatise of Ambroise Paré, 1585* (Chicago, IL: University of Chicago Press, 1952), pp. 124–5, 436; Browne, *Compleat Discourse*, pp. 7, 37, 107.

67 W. Clowes, *A Prooved Practise for All Young Chirurgians* (London: T. Cadman, 1588), p. 15; Paré, *The Method of Curing Wounds Made by Gun-shot*, pp. 64–5; Fabritius Hildanus, *Cista Militaris*, p. 29; Cooke, *Mellificium Chirurgiae*, p. 179; Browne, *Compleat Discourse*, p. 108.

68 H. C., *An Explanation of the Fashion and Use of Three and Fifty Instruments of Chirurgery* (London: Sparke, 1631), pp. 52–3.

69 Clowes, *A Prooved Practise*, p. 14; Cooke, *Mellificium Chirurgiae*, pp. 371–2, 456.

70 Wiseman, *Severall Chirurgical Treatises*, p. 437.

71 *Ibid.*, p. 430.

72 J. H. Binns, 'Wound closure by delayed primary techniques', *Journal of the American College of Emergency Physicians*, 4:2 (1975), 133–4.

73 H. H. Hepburn, 'Delayed primary suture of wounds', *British Medical Journal*, 1:3033 (1919), 181–3. Napoleonic period: Chevalier, *A Treatise on Gunshot Wounds*, pp. 125–6; Crumplin, *Men of Steel*, pp. 227–9. The American Civil War: Hamilton, *Practical Treatise on Military Surgery*, pp. 149–52. Crimean War: G. H. B. MacLeod, *Notes in the Surgery of the War in the Crimea: With Remarks on the Treatment of Gunshot Wounds* (London: Churchill, 1858), pp. 322, 352, 392; T. Scotland and S. Heyes, *Wars, Pestilence and the Surgeon's Blade* (Solihull: Helion & Co., 2013), p. 244. First World War: A. J. Hull, *Surgery in War* (London: J. & A. Churchill, 1916), pp. 52–8; T. Scotland and S. Heyes, *War Surgery, 1914–18* (Solihull: Helion & Co., 2012), p. 68. Second World War: W. H. Ogilvie, *Forward Surgery in Modern War* (London: Butterworth, 1944), p. 26. Korean War: T. E. Rasmussen and R. M. Tai, *Rich's Vascular Surgery* (3rd edn, London: Elsevier Life Sciences, 2016), p. 9. Viet Nam War: V. E. Burkhalter, B. Butler, W. Metz and G. Omer, 'Experiences with delayed primary closure of war wounds of the hand in Viet Nam', *Journal of Bone Joint Surgery*, 50A (1968), 945–54. Iraq/Afghanistan Wars: B. E. Leininger, T. E. Rasmussen, D. L. Smith, D. Jenkins and C. Coppola, 'Experience with wound VAC and delayed primary closure of contaminated soft tissue injuries in Iraq', *Journal of Trauma Injury, Infection, and Critical Care*, 61:5 (2006), 1207–11.

74 J. Harrah, R. Gates, J. Carl and J. D. Harrah, 'A simpler, less expensive technique for delayed primary closure of fasciotomies', *American Journal of Surgery*, 180:1 (2000), 55–7. B. Siribumrungwong, K. Srikuea and A. Thakkinstian, 'Comparison of superficial surgical site infection between delayed primary and primary wound closures in ruptured appendicitis', *Asian Journal of Surgery*, 37 (2014), 120–24.

75 Browne, *Compleat Discourse*, p. 101.

76 Wiseman, *Severall Chirurgical Treatises*, p. 423.

77 D. P. Penhallow, *Military Surgery* (London: Oxford University Press, 1916), p. 163.

78 Wiseman, *Severall Chirurgical Treatises*, p. 420.

79 Cooke, *Mellificium Chirurgiae*, p. 198; Wiseman, *Severall Chirurgical Treatises*, pp. 422, 431, 437.

80 Wiseman, *Severall Chirurgical Treatises*, p. 422.

81 *Ibid.*, p. 447.

82 Fabry, *Gulielm Fabricus Hildamis*, pp. 58–64.

83 Penhallow, *Military Surgery*, pp. 171–9.

84 Scotland and Heyes, *War Surgery*, pp. 154–5; Ogilvie, *Forward Surgery*, p. 37.

85 Wiseman, *Severall Chirurgical Treatises*, pp. 425, 428–30.

86 *Ibid.*, pp. 427–30.

87 *Ibid.*, pp. 424–5.

88 *Ibid.*, pp. 384–5.

89 *Ibid.*, pp. 401–4.

90 Cooke, *Mellificium Chirurgiae*, p. 141.

91 Cooke reflected that 'Dismembering is a dreadful Operation; yet necessary, that the dead part may not injure the living, nor procure death. Sphacelus is the

perfect Mortification of any part, invading not only the soft parts, but also the bones.' Cooke, *Mellificium Chirurgiae*, pp. 722–7.

92 Wiseman, *Severall Chirurgical Treatises*, pp. 454–8.
93 Cooke, *Mellificium Chirurgiae*, pp. 724–5.
94 Wiseman, *Severall Chirurgical Treatises*, p. 455.
95 *Ibid.*, p. 457.
96 Wiseman claimed to have performed amputations without needing the patients restrained: *ibid.*, p. 457; Cooke, *Mellificium Chirurgiae*, pp. 723–5.
97 Cooke, *Mellificium Chirurgiae*, p. 725.
98 Crumplin, *Men of Steel*, pp. 186–8.
99 See Chapter 9 of this volume.
100 E. Gruber von Arni and A. Hopper, *'Battle-Scarred': Surgery, Medicine and Military Welfare during the British Civil Wars* (Leicester: University of Leicester, 2016), p. 11.
101 Thomason, E24[23], *Mercurius Civicus*, 9–16 January (London, 1645), p. 790.
102 Gruber von Arni and Hopper, *'Battle-Scarred'*, p. 21.
103 Durham County Record Office, Q/S/OB 5, Quarter Sessions Order Book, 1660–68, fo. 72r (Microfilm M7/2), The petition of John Tinckler of the city of Durham, 3 October 1660.
104 I. Gentles, *The English Revolution and the Wars in the Three Kingdoms, 1638–1652* (Harlow: Pearson Longman, 2007), p. 437.

Chapter 4

'Stout Skippon hath a wound': the medical treatment of Parliament's infantry commander following the battle of Naseby

Ismini Pells

'**S**tout Skippon hath a wound' proclaims Macaulay's poem *Naseby*. It was once claimed that this line was the only reason that anyone had ever heard of Parliament's infantry commander.[1] Regardless of the truth of this claim, the treatment administered to Sergeant-Major-General Philip Skippon following his wounding at the battle of Naseby on 14 June 1645 is one of the best documented examples of the medical care available to a senior officer during the civil wars.[2] Despite the fact that a musket ball had pierced his armour and shot through his body, he refused to leave the field until victory was won. He was treated in nearby Northampton but it was a month before he could be moved back to London and nearly a year before he could return to active service. Such was the importance of Skippon's recovery that medics were sent from London at public expense, prayers were offered up by London's parishes, and newsbooks printed updates on his progress. This generated a wealth of evidence, which together with the numerous eye-witness accounts of the battle, can be used to determine exactly how Skippon came to be wounded, examine the precise nature and seriousness of his wound, and explore the medical care that Parliament provided for his treatment. This evidence demonstrates that the medical care that Skippon received was neither barbaric nor backward but, in fact, representative of significant advances that had been made in medicine as a result of warfare during the early modern period.

However, this chapter will also investigate why Parliament went to such great lengths to keep Skippon alive, and the reasons why parliamentarian writers took such an intense interest in his medical treatment. Both issues were closely connected to the need to overcome residual political opposition to the formation of the New Model Army from within the parliamentarian alliance, and the wider need to secure outright victory over the royalists.

Those in the House of Commons who had supported the New Model experiment were obliged to capitalise upon the victory at Naseby in whatever way they could and Skippon's survival, which was hailed as divine vindication of their cause, provided these men with one such opportunity to do so.

It is well known that the New Model Army, formed as a result of a bitter feud between Oliver Cromwell and the earl of Manchester, had rather inauspicious beginnings. At the passing of the New Model Ordinance on 17 February 1645, Skippon was immediately appointed Sergeant-Major-General of the infantry, under Sir Thomas Fairfax as commander-in-chief.[3] Neither was an apolitical appointment and the two men had caused a storm over the choosing of senior officers for the New Model.[4] Furthermore, the majority of Skippon's infantry was to be recruited from the remnants of the earl of Essex's army but the New Model had a smaller number of regiments, which meant that several officers had to be discharged.[5] Unsurprisingly, this decision was not popular and Parliament had to send Skippon to quell a mutiny in Reading and carry out the tricky task of 'reducement'.[6] While Skippon succeeded in this task 'beyond expectation', the amalgamation had not produced a sufficient number of soldiers and the deficit was made up by conscripts.[7] Given the opposition to the formation of the New Model, it would only have taken a few defeats for the whole project to fall apart. Naseby marked its first real test.

Once battle commenced at Naseby, Skippon's infantry were pushed to the limit. They lay exposed on their left wing, as Prince Rupert's cavalry had shattered the parliamentarian horse under Henry Ireton on that flank, while they also found themselves hard pressed at the front by the royalist infantry under Sir Jacob Astley. This forced Skippon to bring up the reserves.[8] In many ways, as Glenn Foard argued, Skippon's decision to bring up his reserves 'was THE decisive moment of the English Civil War'. If Skippon's reserves had been broken, the battle would have been lost.[9] This is a view shared by Malcolm Wanklyn. He maintained that while it was Cromwell's cavalry on the right wing that decided the battle, it was Skippon's reserves who, by checking the royalist advance and pushing it back, enabled Cromwell to launch his forces in a battle-winning move.[10] It was an overwhelming parliamentarian victory, in which Skippon was credited with a vital role.[11]

However, during the course of the mêlée, as Fairfax reported to the Speaker of the Commons, 'Major General *Skippon* was shot through his Side, but, notwithstanding, he continued in the Field with great Resolution, and when I desired him to go off the Field, he answered, "He would not go so long as a Man would stand", still doing his Office as a valiant and wise Commander'.[12] Skippon seems to have received his wound in the first charge. Contrary to Foard's claim that Skippon was wounded while bringing up the reserves, the politician and diarist Bulstrode Whitelocke, who maintained that his account was as Skippon 'himself related it to me', makes it clear that Skippon 'was sorely wounded in the beginning of the fight'.[13] This version of events is con-firmed by Captain George Bishop, who helped the Major-General from the field. Bishop took him to a nearby house belonging to one Master Stanley in Brixworth (thought to be Wolfage Manor, owned by Ralph Standish),[14] and 'carried him to his Chamber, stript him, and saw his wound drest'.[15] Bishop claimed that 'In the first charge he [Skippon] received his wound ... yet not-withstanding hee kept his Horse, and discharged his place, and would by no meanes be drawn off till the Field was wonne; for the space of two houres and a half'.[16]

Skippon had been shot at close range by one of his own musketeers, who had accidentally fired his weapon while wheeling aside.[17] Due to the close proximity of the perpetrator, the bullet had pierced Skippon's armour (which weighed fifty-eight pounds) and entered on the right side of Skippon's breast, about six inches below the armpit towards the back. It probably hit his scapula, missed the mouth of his stomach and exited, narrowly missing his spine by three to four inches. As Eric Gruber von Arni pointed out, the fact that Skippon remained on the field of battle suggests that the chest cavity was not punctured nor any damage sustained to any vital organ or the spine.[18] However, by 16 June, the newspapers reported that Skippon's wound 'proves worse then we heard'.[19] It emerged that Skippon had fallen into a raging fever and was too ill even to be moved from Stanley's house to Northampton, where he could receive better treatment.[20] By remaining on the battlefield, he had lost much blood, while a large piece of rag from his waistcoat had been taken in through the force of the bullet and lay festering in the wound.[21]

The Commons received news on 20 June that Skippon was dangerously ill and sent him a letter 'to express the great Sense this House has of his many faithful Services, and the Care they have of him'.[22] The Lords did likewise.[23] Furthermore, the Commons sent 'Dr. Clarke a physician to visit him' and ordered Fairfax to require the army surgeons to 'use their best endeavours for his recovery'.[24] This evidence suggests that Clarke was not, as Gruber von Arni has suggested, a surgeon from Wellingborough.[25] A 'Mr Clarke surgeon' was indeed active in Wellingborough with the Naseby casualties but it is unlikely that this was the same individual described as 'Dr' and 'physician' sent from London.[26] It seems that the Commons had, in fact, sent Skippon none other than the man who was elected President of the College of Physicians in 1645. This Dr Clarke has been credited with leading the College through the turbulence of the civil wars and creating a secure institution for the fellows who were at the forefront of the scientific movement in the second half of the seventeenth century. He was a devoutly religious man, who donated any fees earned on the Sabbath to the poor and was an eager signa-tory to the Solemn League and Covenant. Clarke was also, since 1634, one of the two Physicians to St Bartholomew's Hospital. Although Clarke's medical ideas 'broke little new ground', his pre-eminence in the medical world suggests that Parliament were determined that the medical care administered to their wounded general should be nothing short of the best.[27]

Fortunately, Clarke soon reported that Skippon was on the mend and the 'violence of his Feaver asswaged'.[28] Skippon was fit enough to send a short letter of thanks to the Lords from Brixworth on 21 June, though the shakiness of the signature belied his continuing pain and weakness.[29] On 23 June, the same day that the Lords received the letter, the Commons ordered that Dr Meverell and Mr Donne be sent to Skippon, 'being Persons acquainted with the Constitution of his Body; the one having formerly been his Physician, the other his Surgeon'.[30] Othowell Meverell was Clarke's predecessor as President of the College of Physicians. The two men were firm friends as well as professional allies. Meverell had steered the College into the parliamentary camp at the opening of the civil wars. Clarke, who was Treasurer at the time, supported him in this policy and continued it when the two swapped positions in 1645. Meverell's biographer speculated that 'Meverell's and Clarke's friendship and cooperation may have had their origin in their student days together in the intensely puritan atmosphere of Christ's College, Cambridge'. After graduating from Cambridge, Meverell continued his studies in Leiden and subsequently established his practice in London. In testimony to the reputation he had evidently acquired, Meverell was invited by the London Barber-Surgeons' Company to deliver the anatomical lectures at the public dissection held in 1638, since which time he had also been physician to Bethlem Hospital.[31]

George Dunn was an 'approved surgeon' and leading member of the Barber-Surgeons' Company. He sat on the Court of Assistants, acted as an examiner of surgeons and was to be appointed Master in 1646.[32] Like Clarke and Meverell, Dunn displayed godly leanings. For example, in his will, he left provision for a teacher at Christ Hospital to enable the young maidens to learn to read 'that thereby they may the better attaine unto the knowledge of God and understanding of the word' and he funded a minister to preach at St Katherine Creechurch on 5 November each year in commemoration of the 'wonderfull deliverance of the Nation from the hellish Conspiracie of the Gunpowder-Treason'.[33] Dunn also seems to have been a specialist in military medicine. A contemporary recalled that he had become 'acquainted, and into familiarity with Master *George Dunne* Chyrurgion' in 1642 when being treated for cuts and shots.[34] In April 1639, in preparation for Charles I's war against Scotland, Dunn had been tasked with organising the conveyance of surgeons to the army in the north and he was Surgeon at the Savoy, Parliament's permanent military hospital in London, from at least 1648.[35]

Upon arrival in Brixworth, Meverell and Dunn found Skippon 'very weake and much spent'. Yet, they reported in a letter written on 28 June that when they dressed his wound, they had 'found some good digestion coming from his wound, [t]he feaver somewhat abated, but his pains exceeding great'. They also informed the public that they had finally been able to move Skippon to Northampton, their letter implying that he had been moved that day or shortly beforehand. Nevertheless, the medics concluded that 'if it shall please God to recover him, it will be a long time ere he will get strength'.[36]

It is possible to deduce what treatment Dunn may have administered to Skippon through his support for the work of John Woodall. Woodall, who had died in 1643, began his career as a surgeon in Lord Willoughby's regiment in the Normandy campaign against the Catholic League in 1589–90. He then practised throughout Europe, before returning to London and becoming free of the Barber-Surgeons' Company in 1601. He was elected Master of the Company in 1632 and held the post of Surgeon to both the Charterhouse and St Bartholomew's Hospital. In 1613, Woodall was appointed the first Surgeon-General of the East India Company and as a result of this appointment, published in 1617 *The Surgions Mate,* a medical textbook for young sea surgeons. He followed this in 1628 with *Viaticum, the Path-Way to the Surgeons Chest,* which outlined the treatment of gunshot wounds for surgeons who had been sent on Charles I's expedition for the relief of La Rochelle. This short work was incorporated into a revised edition of *The Surgeons Mate* in 1639.[37] This edition was dedicated to the Master and Wardens of the Barber-Surgeons' Company at the time when Dunn was Second Warden.[38] Woodall thanked these men for their 'good likings and well approvings of my former works and editions'.[39] Further evidence of Dunn's 'good likings' of Woodall's work can be found in the two dedicatory poems that Dunn wrote to preface the new edition.[40]

If Dunn followed Woodall's directions in treating Skippon's wound, then he would have been aware that the greatest danger with gunshot wounds was 'putrefaction', that is the wound becoming gangrenous. To prevent this, Woodall recommended an application of Egyptian perfume mixed with wine or spirit of wine, either injected into the wound or applied on lint.[41] The purpose of this alcoholic application was clearly to act as an antiseptic – an interesting procedure in an era predating the discovery of microbiology or a widespread acceptance of germ theory. Next, Woodall directed the surgeon to 'make a very short dressing, and of as gentle medicines as may be'.[42] He favoured a liquid made with tropical tree resin, warmed up and applied with soft lint to the edges of the wound. He then filled the wound with lint and covered it with a *Paracelsus* plaster (made from lead, gum resin and bark), layers of flannel soaked in an alkaline solution mixed with ashes, and soft, warm bandages.[43] Finally, Woodall directed the surgeon to apply a third dressing of warm balm, 'some good emollent [soothing agent]' and 'anodine [painkilling] plaster'.[44]

Woodall's methods, which rested on cleanliness, pain-relief and plasters, appear, as with much of the material in *The Surgeons Mate,* to have been influenced by the principles pioneered by the Swiss physician Paracelsus.[45] Paracelsus was favoured by modernists who questioned the treatments proposed by the ancients that were still widely accepted in the seventeenth century, such as the Greek physician Galen.[46] *The Surgeons Mate* stood the test of time and was long considered a standard work.[47] A copy in the Northampton General Hospital Archives is testimony to its longevity in Northamptonshire. The archive was founded in 1790 as a library of medical works, donated by notable families in the county, as well as surgeons and physicians upon their retirement. *The Surgeons Mate* was one of the first books acquired for this library and annotations throughout this copy show that it was used well into the eighteenth century, before continuing to provide advice for the Northampton hospital staff.[48] Thus, if Dunn did indeed follow Woodall's methods, then the treatment he administered to Skippon was not only the most modern and progressive that was available at the time but also of a standard that set the benchmark in military surgery long after the civil wars.

At some point, Skippon had required surgery to remove the scrap of waist-coat festering in his wound. This must have taken place before Dunn could have got to work with his dressings and probably occurred before his arrival in Northampton, as it is likely that this was linked to the improved state in which Dunn and Meverell found Skippon. The knife for this operation was wielded by Thomas Trapham.[49] Trapham had been Skippon's regimental surgeon since the previous year. A committed parliamentarian, Trapham's estates at Abingdon had suffered great losses due to their close proximity to the royalist headquarters at Oxford.[50] He went on to have a distinguished career, serving as Surgeon-General with the army in Ireland in 1649 and in Scotland in 1650–51, when he also became Cromwell's personal surgeon. He succeeded Dunn as Surgeon to the Savoy upon the latter's death in 1653. However, Trapham is perhaps most famous as the man entrusted with embalming the body of the executed Charles I, when he gained some notoriety for reputedly commenting that he had 'sewn on the goose's head'.[51]

Unfortunately, there is no surviving record of Trapham's operative procedures but Gruber von Arni speculated that it is 'distinctly probable' that Trapham followed the procedures of Ambroise Paré. Paré, a French military surgeon during the sixteenth-century Wars of Religion, had 'revolutionised attitudes towards the treatment of battle casualties'.[52] He is most commonly remembered for his use of ligatures to prevent catastrophic bleeding in place of cauterisation, the method of pressing a red-hot iron on the wound, which often failed.[53] In order to extract foreign bodies from the wound, Paré recommended placing the patient in the same position as he was when he received the shot 'because that the Muscles and other parts being otherwaies situate, may stop and hinder the way'.[54] A 'dilatory' could then be used 'to open and dilate the wounds, to the end that the strange bodyes may the easier bee found and extracted', which could be done using a variety of avian-themed instruments, such as a 'Crowes Bill toothed', 'Cranes bill straight', 'Duckes Bill', 'Parrats Bill' or 'Swans bill'.[55] Paré's methods greatly influenced many contemporary military surgeons and it is known that his procedures were used during the civil wars from the writings of the royalist surgeon Richard Wiseman.[56] Wiseman recalled treating one soldier at Dunbar in 1650 for a wound remarkably similar to that sustained by Skippon.[57] How far this might prove illuminating to Skippon's experience can only be guessed at, but 'As a contemporary, experienced military surgeon, it is therefore reasonable to assume that Thomas Trapham used similar operative techniques to Wiseman'.[58]

As a result of Trapham's surgery and under the careful watch of Meverell and Dunn, Skippon continued to progress. On 28 June, a letter from an unknown correspondent was published in the press, which reported '*Major-Generall* Skippon *recovers (wee hope) of his wound; he is still full of paine, and by a towell fastened to the top of his bed (sitting up in his bed as his usuall manner is) he raiseth, or turnes himselfe ... wee hope the worst is past with him; the Surgeons begin to like his wound better everie day*'.[59] By a week later, readers of *The Kingdomes Weekly Intelligencer* were informed that Skippon was '*much eased of his paine, he riseth every day, falleth to his food, and they hope to bring him to* London *erre it be long on a Horslitter*'.[60] A horse litter was duly hired from one Paul Green and on 15 July, Skippon was carried into London, where 'divers Gentlemen and Citizens of worth rode forth to meet him'.[61] Skippon was left with an eight-inch wound on his left side under the ribs where the bullet had exited and it was not until May 1646, that he returned to active duty at the siege of Oxford.[62] Nevertheless, Skippon had made a miraculous recovery.

The importance of the victory at Naseby had prompted Parliament to ensure that all their wounded received exemplary care, something Skippon played his part in ensuring. Injured soldiers were transported to Northampton, Wellingborough and the surrounding area, where local inhabitants nursed them in their own homes. The most severe cases were sent to London.[63] Forty of the 560 or so casualties brought into Northampton were treated at St John's Hospital in Bridge Street. Throughout the town, treatment was provided by Surgeon-General James Winter with the help of nine other surgeons. To help meet the town's costs in caring for the wounded, Parliament granted £500 on 21 June to Joseph Sergeant, mayor of Northampton, which was followed by a further subsidy of £200.[64] According to Sergeant, in distributing this money he 'acted by the advice of Major General Skippon'.[65] The sophistication of the parliamentarian medical administration following Naseby is particularly apparent when compared to that in place after the battle of Edgehill on 23 October 1642. The sick and wounded were scattered across the countryside, some cared for by local residents, while others struggled to follow the army to Warwick, where, along with Coventry, the most severe cases had been sent. The confused situation of that time is reflected in the hurried and random manner in which the accounts were compiled and there was 'little or no preparation for long term care of the wounded'. The situation improved with the establishment of the Committee for Sick and Maimed Soldiers and the adoption of the Savoy Hospital as a dedicated military facility in November 1642, although Gruber von Arni has argued that it was not until autumn 1644 that tangible improvements began to appear.[66] By the time of Naseby, wounded parliamentarians benefitted from the many lessons in medical administration that had been learnt over the previous three years.

However, Skippon unquestionably benefitted from special treatment. In his letter written from Northampton to the Speaker of the House of Commons, Skippon acknowledged 'the great care and kindnesse of the Honourable House of Commons and your particular favours towards me'.[67] Clarke and Meverell were rewarded by Parliament's Treasurers at War for their efforts and Dunn's expenses were also met out of the public purse.[68] In addition, an apothecary, Henry Potter, was given £7 2s 6d for journeying to Northampton with physic to be administered to Skippon.[69] The Commons granted Skippon himself £200 'as a testimony of their favour' and he and his family were provided with a 'convenient house' for 'their better Accommodation', furnished and rent free, in Long Acre, Westminster, which had been sequestered from the marquess of Worcester.[70]

Why had Parliament gone to such lengths for Skippon? Firstly, most obviously, as a senior officer with thirty years' military experience, an unswerving commitment to their cause and an immense popularity with his men, Skippon was an invaluable asset. Secondly, Parliament naturally could not miss out on the opportunity to dent royalist morale. The parliamentary polemicist John Vicars alleged that after Naseby the King was heard to say 'in a kind of a consolitary way, to himself ... That though he had lost the Victory at Nazeby, yet Skippon was slain'.[71] Unfortunately, it is difficult to corroborate this claim. Vicars was notoriously scathing of the King and his men.[72] That said, Charles had attempted to win Skippon over to his side on more than one occasion, implying that the King respected Skippon's talents.[73] Therefore Parliament's loss of their veteran commander may well have been welcome news to the King's ears. Nevertheless, Skippon's survival only served to make him a high-profile target. Protection measures had to be put in place around Stanley's house in Brixworth after Bishop had taken Skippon there for treatment immediately after the battle. Yet, the 500 men who were allegedly posted there to guard him[74] and two pieces of ordinance were not enough to put off the earl of Northampton, who 'threatned to fetch him from thence'. Parliament could not risk the propaganda coup the royalists might gain from kidnapping Skippon, so moved him to Northampton before he was really fit to travel.[75] The town, which housed one of the most important midland parliamentarian garrisons, was protected on the south and west by the castle and River Nene and surrounded by a curtain wall, which had been strengthened when the fortifications were improved in 1642–43.[76]

Thirdly, and most importantly, Naseby had presented the chance to silence the critics. As the London diarist Thomas Juxon noted: 'There were certainly many that were not very well pleased with this victory. But herein did God vindicate His honour ... This put an honour upon and engage the parliament and kingdom to favour that party who were most active in the service'.[77] The New Model Army had overcome political opposition from within the parliamentarian alliance itself, as well as the royalists, and the Army's supporters were eager to maximise any political capital that could be gained from the battle. While it is difficult to deduce from whom the initiative came for Skippon's medical care, it may well be worth noting that the logistics were entrusted to the Committee for the Army.[78] This seems perfectly reasonable given that the administrative details of military matters were this body's responsibility.[79] However, this committee, which was established in March 1645, was dominated by political 'Independents' who had supported the formation of the New Model and was chaired by Robert Scawen. Scawen had played a vital role in Parliament's military reorganisation over the winter of 1644–45 and he had an input into much of the legislation for paying, recruiting and equipping the New Model.[80] Likewise, it might not be entirely coincidental that Oliver St John and Samuel Browne were the men tasked with thanking Clarke and Meverell for their pains in attending Skippon.[81] St John, together with his cousin and 'close associate' Browne, had been leading supporters of the Self-Denying and New Model Ordinances.[82] As Skippon had been an integral player in the political manoeuvrings surrounding the formation of the New Model, it was natural that the politicians who had supported this venture wished to ensure his survival.

At the same time, it must not be overlooked that it was Anthony Nicoll who was ordered to convey the £200 to Skippon, and Robert Harley who was sent with Oliver St John on 12 July to visit Skippon on behalf of the Commons.[83] Both these men became associated with the political 'Presbyterians', who were to emerge as the New Model's adversaries following the end of the First Civil War in 1646.[84] Skippon was to fall foul of many in the Presbyterian alliance in 1648, when he emerged as a vociferous opponent of their policies during his command in London. Yet, in summer 1645, he still retained the Presbyterians' trust and respect, largely because they regarded his religious views as compatible with their own desire to reorganise the Church of England along Presbyterian lines. This was strongly opposed by many in the Army, who campaigned for more toleration of different views than that allowed in a Presbyterian settlement.[85] Interestingly, it was the clergyman Richard Byfield who denounced toleration, who conceded in his sermon preached before the Commons on their monthly fast held on 25 June that despite the victory at Naseby, 'our estate is very sad', not least because 'our *Skippon* lyes a bleeding'.[86] He took the opportunity to provide a warning against 'Heresies, Blasphemous, Brutish, Atheistical Heresies, Frantique and Fanatique Opinions, Schismes, Proud Divisions upon Divisions' and claimed that 'a Spirit of self-seeking on many in Committees, in City, in the Armies' existed.[87] He therefore urged his listeners to unite in prayer so that the glories of God would become visible.[88]

In fact, what the saga of Skippon's wounding ultimately provided was the opportunity to demonstrate the righteousness of the cause he fought for, behind which all parliamentarians could unite. Skippon was a man with a reputation for godliness, something that he had gone out of his way to promote in the three devotional works he published for his soldiers.[89] Skippon's books made it clear that wounding was an affliction from God. In *The Christian Centurians Observations* (published only days before Naseby), Skippon claimed that 'no bullet can fly, or any other instrument of warre move but according to his especiall disposing, nor doe any hurt to me, but by his expresse commission'.[90] Moreover, Skippon maintained that 'He chastens us for our profit' and *'we shall gaine much good by Affliction particularly, The tryall of our Christian graces'*.[91] Skippon reassured his soldiers that God would 'inable us to beare affliction aright' because afflictions were 'assurance we are Gods children'.[92] Displaying such fortitude in adversity was surely easier said than done. However, while Skippon's 'Christian graces' must have been sorely tested after Naseby, he was no stranger to serious wounding. For example, at the siege of Breda in 1637, while Skippon allegedly held off 200 enemy soldiers with thirty men in 'push of pike', he was shot through the neck and temporarily lost the use of his left arm, although apparently he recovered and carried on fighting.[93] Skippon's past experiences undoubtedly strengthened him to live by his own maxims and he told the Lords that despite being in 'very great Pain' from his Naseby wound, he was 'humbly submitting to the good Pleasure of my God'.[94]

Skippon's attitude was a gift to the newsbooks. It was reported that as Skippon was having his wound dressed, he groaned but 'spake these words (lifting his eyes towards heaven) *Though I groane, I Grumble not*'.[95] A correspondent from Northampton informed readers of *Perfect Passages* that Skippon was *'verie patient, and content with what God will; his discourse is verie sweet and heavenly'*, while Captain Bishop recalled that he had said to Skippon, 'Sir, your wound hath caused a little cloud on this glorious day; hee answered, by no meanes let mine Eclipse its glory, for it is my honour that *I* have received a wound, and it was my God that strengthened mee'.[96] It is hard to believe that the tales of Skippon's saintly patience had not been embroidered with an element of journalistic licence but nevertheless, by holding up Skippon as a paragon of godly virtue, the press implicitly reinforced the worthiness of his cause. Furthermore, in apparently asking for the nation's prayers, Skippon inadvertently issued a political call to arms. According to *Perfect Passages*, 'The prayers of Gods people he [Skippon] desires', while *The Kingdomes Weekly Intelligencer* encouraged the public to 'assist this worthy and ever renowned Patriot with their prayers'.[97] His recovery was duly prayed for in the London parishes.[98] Public prayer is a collective exercise, which brings people together and unites them behind a cause. Thus, the prayers for Skippon's health were intended to increase public backing for the New Model.

Had the capital's prayers fallen on deaf ears, then no doubt the press would have spun a story of martyrdom. As it was, Skippon's recovery represented the ultimate divine vindication of the New Model experiment. For Skippon, just as the Lord wounded, it was 'the Lord that healeth thee'.[99] Moreover, God never did anything without good reason. Skippon noted in *The Christian Centurians Observations* that 'It hath pleased the Lord that I have served many yeers already, and if God spare my life, and please not to work wonderfully for me, am like to serve many yeers more to serve other turnes'.[100] This conveniently pre-existing theme was echoed in the press. *Perfect Passages* expressed the hope that 'the Lord will spare him for further service to his glorie and the good of his Church and people', while *Mercurius Civicus* proclaimed that 'God who delivers from the Gates of Death will upon the prayers of his people yet restore this faithfull and constant souldier of His that hee may live to be serviceable to the publike cause'.[101]

Yet, as Alexandra Walsham reminded us, although Providentialism was a doctrine 'which enjoyed near universal acceptance' in early modern England, 'to insist upon the ubiquity of such convictions is not to ignore their polymorphous and protean qualities'.[102] Skippon's miraculous recovery seems to have become a battlefield over which competing parliamentarian groups fought for ownership. In *England's Worthies*, published in 1647, John Vicars relayed how as Skippon was brought on his horse-litter through Islington back to London in July 1645, a great mastiff ran out of one of the houses and fell furiously upon one of the litter's horses. This made the horse fling about, shaking the litter up and down and Skippon's wounded body inside it. Eventually, a soldier ran the dog through with his sword.[103] For Vicars, Skippon's latest salvation had been ordained by God to show that he had reserved for Skippon 'more glorious worke for the honour of his great Name, and the good of his poore Church'.[104] Vicars was a devout Presbyterian, who emphatically asserted the divine providence of parliamentary achievements.[105] In his *Englands Parliamentary Chronicle* of 1646 he had commended Skippon's conduct at Naseby and claimed that Skippon's wound was 'an *indelible badge of Honour*'.[106]

In that publication, Vicars had also noted that 'Commissary Generall *Ireton* did valiantly also behave himself in this fight'.[107] Ireton too had been severely wounded at Naseby. He was run through the thigh with a pike and struck in the face with a halberd, while his horse had been shot under him.[108] Yet, interestingly, there is no mention of Ireton's valour, or indeed of the Commissary-General at all, in the 1647 publication. Similarly, another Presbyterian polemicist, Josiah Ricraft, also linked Skippon's piety with his recovery from his Naseby wound in *A Survey of Englands Champions*, a collection of biographies of the parliamentarian commanders.[109] This tribute was reprinted in Ricraft's history of the civil war, published in 1649.[110] These works 'were clearly biased' towards the achievements of Presbyterians and, once more, neither Ireton nor his Naseby wounding is afforded any attention.[111]

The comparison with these authors' treatment of Skippon and Ireton is instructive. Ireton emerged in 1647 as a vigorous opponent of the Presbyterians, acting as spokesman for the New Model's rights in the face of Presbyterian pressure for their disbandment and he publicly clashed with the Presbyterian leader Denzil Holles in the Commons.[112] All the immediate accounts of Naseby honoured Ireton's valour and expressed concern for his wounds, though admittedly *The Moderate Intelligencer* reported on 16 June 1645 that Ireton's wound was not as bad as first thought and he was fit enough to return to active service by July.[113] Nevertheless, it was standard fare for the popular press to comment on the heroism of leading commanders. Fairfax developed a reputation that depended upon his ability to lead from the front and inspire his forces with gallantry, which led him to expose himself to extreme danger numerous times throughout his career.[114] Likewise, when Cromwell was wounded in the neck at Marston Moor on 2 July 1644, it only served to embellish his reputation as 'the great agent in this victory' and gave birth to his nickname 'Ironside'.[115] Thus, the silence of the Presbyterian pamphleteers in 1647 on Ireton's wounding at Naseby is deafening. That the portrayal of the parliamentarian commanders had become politicised is perhaps best summed up by the Independent minister and parliamentary chaplain Joshua Sprigg. In *Anglia Rediviva*, an account of the New Model's successes written in 1647, Sprigg provided his own providential interpretation of these victories that was designed to defend the Army's reputation against Presbyterian hostility.[116] Although the seriousness of Skippon's wound meant that Sprigg was unable to avoid singling out Skippon for his 'Spring of Resolution', he added, 'That *I* mention not all those Officers and Souldiers particularly, who behaved themselves so gallantly in this Action, is to avoyd emulation and partiality'.[117]

Naseby was undoubtedly the turning-point in the successful parliamentarian outcome of the First Civil War. Skippon had played an integral part in that victory, commanding his reserves with resolution as discipline disintegrated about him, despite being on the receiving end of 'friendly fire' early in the battle. He had also been instrumental in ensuring that there was a parliamentarian army at Naseby in the first place, in the face of opposition to its formation from within the parliamentarian alliance. The collective sigh of relief with which those who supported the New Model project greeted the news from Naseby is almost palpable. Yet, though they had won some breathing space, their work was not complete. Skippon's condition, though curable, had been made worse by his determination to remain on the field and the infection from foreign bodies in his wound, and there was genuine concern for his life. Although Parliament would have no doubt provided special treatment for any senior commander, the political importance of the victory prompted the New Model's supporters in Parliament to spare no expense in the fight for Skippon's survival. The loss of one of their most trusty and experienced officers, who was respected by parliamentarians of all persuasions and royalists alike, was almost too much to contemplate. Moreover, Skippon's conduct in convalescence provided the perfect material to demonstrate the righteousness of his cause and the means to rally the public behind it. In 1645 his remarkable recovery reflected the divine vindication of the New Model Army and if the story of his providential deliverance was later hijacked by Presbyterian polemicists, that is only tribute to the success with which their parliamentary adversaries had established it. Messrs Clarke, Meverell, Dunn and Trapham had done their work well but it was God who had saved Skippon. Those who had questioned whether Parliament should have pursued the New Model experiment had been answered. But then, as Karl Marx said, 'Medicine heals doubts as well as diseases'.[118]

NOTES

1 Anon., 'A militant saint; Philip Skippon. An account, with excerpts from his devotional manual, Salve for Every Sore, published in 1643', *Transactions of the Congregational Historical Society*, 4 (1909–10), 207.

2 E. Gruber von Arni, *Justice to the Maimed Soldier: Nursing, Medical Care, and Welfare for Sick and Wounded Soldiers and their Families during the English Civil Wars and Interregnum, 1642–1660* (Aldershot: Ashgate, 2001), p. 179.

3 C. H. Firth and R. S. Rait (eds), *Acts and Ordinances of the Interregnum, 1642–1660*, 3 vols (London: HMSO, 1911), I, p. 614.

4 A. Hopper, *'Black Tom': Sir Thomas Fairfax and the English Revolution* (Manchester: Manchester University Press, 2007), pp. 54–62; I. Pells, 'The military career, religious and political thought of Philip Skippon, c. 1598–1660' (PhD dissertation, University of Cambridge, 2014), p. 135; M. Wanklyn, 'Choosing officers for the New Model Army, February to April 1645', *Journal of the Society for Army Historical Research*, 92 (2014), 112, 120–1.

5 *CJ*, IV, p. 76; G. Davies, 'The parliamentary army under the Earl of Essex, 1642–45', *English Historical Review*, 49 (1934), 45–6.

6 *CJ*, IV, p. 81; BL, Thomason E277(8), Anon., *Severall Letters to the Honourable William Lenthall, Esquire, Speaker of the House of Commons* (London, 1645), p. 5.

7 BL, Harleian MS 252, fo. 33, John Rushworth's narrative, 1645; P. Young, *Naseby 1645: The Campaign and the Battle* (London: Century, 1985), p. 182.

8 G. Foard, *Naseby: The Decisive Campaign* (Barnsley: Pen & Sword, 2004), p. 260.

9 *Ibid.*, p. 265.

10 M. Wanklyn, *The Warrior Generals: Winning the British Civil Wars 1642–1652* (New Haven, CT: Yale University Press, 2010), p. 232.

11 BL, Thomason E288(21), Anon., *A Glorious Victory Obtained by Sr. Thomas Fairfax, June, the 14. 1645.* (London, 1645), p. [5]; BL, Thomason E288(25), Anon., *A Relation of the Victory Obtained by Sr. Thomas Fairfax, Generall of the Parliaments Forces, over the Enemies Forces, neer Harborough, on Saturday, June, 14. 1645* (London, 1645), pp. 3–4; BL, Thomason E288(38), G. Bishop, *A More Particular and Exact Relation of the Victory Obtained by the Parliaments Forces under the Command of Sir Thomas Fairfax* (London, 1645), pp. 1–2.

12 LJ, VII, p. 433.

13 Foard, Naseby, p. 264; B. Whitelocke, Memorials of the English Affairs, 4 vols (Oxford: Oxford University Press, 1853), I, p. 448.

14 Northampton General Hospital Archives, 'Email communication from Brixworth History Society' (9 August 2012). I am extremely grateful to Martin Marix Evans for bringing this unique archive to my attention and for the help and assistance of Sue Longworth and her volunteers, and the curator, Dr Andrew Williams.

15 BL, Thomason E288(38), Bishop, More Particular and Exact Relation, p. 3; BL, Thomason E289(10), Mercurius Civicus, no. 109, 18–25 June (London, 1645), p. 970; BL, Thomason E290(16), The Kingdomes Weekly Intelligencer, no. 106, 24 June–1 July (London, 1645), p. 847.

16 BL, Thomason E288(38), Bishop, More Particular and Exact Relation, p. 3.

17 BL, Thomason E290(16), The Kingdomes Weekly Intelligencer, p. 847.

18 Evaluation of Skippon's wound from Gruber von Arni, Justice to the Maimed Soldier, p. 179, based on the description in BL, Thomason E290(16), The Kingdomes Weekly Intelligencer, p. 847.

19 BL, Thomason E288(37), The Moderate Intelligencer, no. 16, 12–19 June (London, 1645), p. 126.

20 BL, Thomason E289(10), Mercurius Civicus, p. 970; BL, Thomason E290(5), The Scotish Dove, no. 88, 20–27 June (London, 1645), p. 696.

21 BL, Thomason E290(16), The Kingdomes Weekly Intelligencer, p. 847; Wing / V304, J. Vicars, England's Worthies (London, 1647), p. 57.

22 CJ, IV, p. 180.

23 LJ, VII, p. 441.

24 Whitelocke, Memorials, I, p. 452; CJ, IV, p. 180.

25 Gruber von Arni, Justice to the Maimed Soldier, p. 179.

26 TNA, SP 28/173/I, fo. 22a, money paid for the wounded men at Northampton from 14 June 1645; TNA, SP 28/31, fo. 504, payment to Dr John Clarke, 11 July 1645.

27 W. Birken, 'Clarke, John (1582?–1653)', ODNB.

28 BL, Thomason E290(5), The Scotish Dove, p. 696.

29 Beinecke Rare Book and Manuscript Library, Osborn Collection, FB 67/17, Philip Skippon to Lord Grey, 21 June 1645.

30 CJ, IV, p. 183.

31 N. Moore, 'Meverell, Othowell (1586x8–1648)', rev. W. Birken, ODNB; Guildhall Library, MS 5257/5, Barber-Surgeons' Company Court Minute Book, 1621–51, fo. 232.

32 Guildhall Library, MS 5257/5, Barber-Surgeons' Company Court Minute Book, 1621–51, fos. 167, 253 and 372–3.

33 TNA, PROB 11/221/36, Will of George Dunn, 3 March 1652.

34 Wing (2nd edn) / J47, W. J., A Collection of Seven and Fifty Approved Receipts Good Against the Plague (London, 1665), p. [i].

35 Guildhall Library, MS 5257/5, Barber-Surgeons' Company Court Minute Book, 1621–51, fo. 260; CSPD 1648–49, pp. 323, 341; Gruber von Arni, Justice to the Maimed Soldier, p. 179.

36 BL, Thomason E290(16), The Kingdomes Weekly Intelligencer, p. 847.

37 J. H. Appleby, 'Woodall, John (1570–1643)', *ODNB*; STC (2nd edn) / 25963, J. Woodall, *The Surgeons Mate* (London, 1639), pp. [v]–[vi].

38 *Ibid.* p. [iii].

39 *Ibid.*, p. [iv].

40 *Ibid.*, pp. [v]–[vi].

41 *Ibid.*, p. 96.

42 *Ibid.*, p. 96.

43 *Ibid.*, p. 97.

44 *Ibid.*, p. 97.

45 Appleby, 'Woodall, John'.

46 Gruber von Arni, *Justice to the Maimed Soldier*, p. 145.

47 Appleby, 'Woodall, John'.

48 Northampton General Hospital Archives, STC (2nd edn) / 25963, Woodall, *The Surgeons Mate*, pp. [i], 85 and 275v.

49 Wing / V304, Vicars, *England's Worthies*, pp. 57–8; Gruber von Arni, *Justice to the Maimed Soldier*, p. 250.

50 Historical Manuscripts Commission, *Thirteenth Report, Appendix, Part 1*, 10 vols (London: Eyre and Spottiswoode, 1891–1931), I, p. 187; *CJ*, III, p. 658; *CSPD 1644–45*, p. 25.

51 Gruber von Arni, *Justice to the Maimed Soldier*, p. 250.

52 *Ibid.*, p. 185.

53 *Ibid.*

54 A. Paré (trans. W. Hamond), *The Method of Curing Wounds Made by Gun-shot, Also by Arrowes and Darts, with their Accidents* (London: Isaac Iaggard, 1617), p. 43.

55 *Ibid.*, pp. 44–51.

56 Gruber von Arni, *Justice to the Maimed Soldier*, p. 185.

57 R. Wiseman, *Severall Chirurgicall Treatises* (London, 1676), p. 411.

58 Gruber von Arni, *Justice to the Maimed Soldier*, p. 185.

59 BL, Thomason E262(19), *Perfect Passages of Each Dayes Proceedings in Parliament*, no. 37, 2–9 July (London, 1645), p. 292.

60 BL, Thomason E292(15), *The Kingdomes Weekly Intelligencer*, no. 107, 1–8 July (London, 1645), p. 855.

61 TNA, SP 28/173/I, fo. 20a, Money paid for the sick and wounded men that came into Northampton from 14 June 1645; BL, Thomason E262(26), *A Perfect Diurnall of Some Passages in Parliament*, no. 103, 14–21 July (London, 1645), p. 818; BL, Thomason E293(7), *Mercurius Civicus*, no. 112, 10–17 (London, 1645), p. 998.

62 Wing / V304, Vicars, *England's Worthies*, p. 55; Wing / S5070, J. Sprigg, *Anglia Rediviva* (London, 1647), p. 248.

63 Gruber von Arni, *Justice to the Maimed Soldier*, pp. 55–6.

64 *Ibid.*, p. 55.

65 *Ibid.*, pp. 57, 180.

66 *Ibid.*, pp. 43–5, 55. Surgeon-General James Winter is misnamed here as Daniel Winter – see TNA, SP 28/30 fos. 460, 502, 517 and 518, payments to James Winter, June 1645.

67 BL Thomason, E292(21), *The Moderate Intelligencer*, no. 19, 3–10 July (London, 1645), p. 152.

68 TNA, SP 28/31, fo. 504, payment to Dr John Clarke, 11 July 1645; TNA, SP 28/31, fo. 505, payment to Dr Othowell Meverell, 9 July 1645; TNA, SP 28/31 fo. 454, payment to George Dunn, 12 August 1645.

69 TNA, SP 28/31, fo. 506, payment to Henry Potter, 9 July 1645.

70 Whitelocke, *Memorials*, I, p. 456; *CJ*, IV, pp. 190, 206, 225; M. A. E. Green (ed.), *Calendar of the Proceedings of the Committee for Advance of Money, 1642–1656*, 3 vols (London, Eyre and Spottiswoode: 1888), I, p. 47.

71 Wing / V304, Vicars, *England's Worthies*, p. 56.

72 J. Gasper, 'Vicars, John (1580–1652)', *ODNB*.

73 BL, Additional MS 34,253, fo. 13, summons to Captain Skippon to attend the King at York, 17 May 1642; BL, Thomason E256(3), *A Perfect Diurnall of Some Passages in Parliament*, no. 59, 9–16 September (London, 1644), p. 468.

74 This seems an improbably high number of troops and I have found no evidence to corroborate this figure.

75 BL, Thomason E289(10), *Mercurius Civicus*, p. 970; BL, Thomason E290(16), *The Kingdomes Weekly Intelligencer*, p. 847.

76 W. Page (ed.), *A History of the County of Northampton: Volume 3* (London: University of London/Institute of Historical Research, 1970), p. 12; M. Marix Evans, P. Evans and M. Westaway, *Naseby: June 1645* (Barnsley: Leo Cooper, 2002), p. 45.

77 K. Lindley and D. Scott (eds), *The Journal of Thomas Juxon, 1644–47* (Camden Society, 5th series, 13, 1999), p. 80.

78 *CJ*, IV, pp. 180, 183, 190.

79 M. Kishlansky, *The Rise of the New Model Army* (Cambridge: Cambridge University Press, 1979), p. 23.

80 D. Scott, 'Scawen, Robert (*bap.* 1602, *d.* 1670)', *ODNB*.

81 *CJ*, IV, p. 190.

82 W. Palmer, 'St John, Oliver (*c.*1598–1673)', *ODNB*.

83 *CJ*, IV, pp. 190, 206.

84 J. Eales, 'Harley, Sir Robert (*bap.* 1579, *d.* 1656)', *ODNB*.

85 Pells, 'Military career, religious and political thought of Philip Skippon', pp. 133–69.

86 J. Gurney, 'Byfield, Richard (*bap.* 1598, *d.* 1664)', *ODNB*; BL, Thomason E289(12), R. Byfield, *Zion's Answers to the Nations Ambassadors* (London, 1645), pp. 15–16.

87 *Ibid.*, p. 15.

88 *Ibid.*, p. 16.

89 E. Hyde, earl of Clarendon, *The History of the Rebellion and Civil Wars in England Begun in the Year 1641*, ed. W. Dunn Macray, 6 vols (Oxford: Clarendon Press, 1888), I, p. 509.

90 Wing / S3951, P. Skippon, *A Salve for Every Sore* (London, 1643), p. 63; Wing / S3950, P. Skippon, *The Christian Centurians Observations, Advices, and Resolutions* (London, 1645), p. 318. *The Christian Centurians Observations* was entered in the Stationers' Register on 31 May 1645 – see G. E. Briscoe Eyre, *A Transcript of the Registers of the Worshipful Company of Stationers; From 1640 to 1708 A. D.* (London: Privately Printed, 1913), I, p. 172.

91 Wing / S3951, Skippon, *Salve for Every Sore*, p. 104.
92 *Ibid.*, pp. 102, 104.
93 STC (2nd edn) / 13265, H. Hexham, *A True and Briefe Relation of the Famous Seige of Breda* (Delft, 1637), pp. 23–4.
94 *LJ*, VII, p. 450.
95 BL, Thomason E262(10), *Perfect Occurrences of Parliament*, no. 25, 13–20 June (London, 1645), p. [4].
96 BL, Thomason E262(19), *Perfect Passages of Each Dayes Proceedings in Parliament*, p. 292; BL, Thomason E288(38), Bishop, *More Particular and Exact Relation*, p. 3.
97 BL, Thomason E262(19), *Perfect Passages of Each Dayes Proceedings in Parliament*, p. 292; BL, Thomason E290(16), *The Kingdomes Weekly Intelligencer*, p. 848.
98 BL, Thomason E289(10), *Mercurius Civicus*, p. 970; Wing / V304, Vicars, *England's Worthies*, p. 57.
99 Wing / S3951, Skippon, *Salve for Every Sore*, p. 128.
100 Wing / S3950, Skippon, *Christian Centurians Observations*, p. 18.
101 BL, Thomason E262(19), *Perfect Passages of Each Dayes Proceedings in Parliament*, p. 292; BL, Thomason E289(10), *Mercurius Civicus*, p. 970.
102 A. Walsham, *Providence in Early Modern England* (Oxford: Oxford University Press, 1999), pp. 2–3.
103 Wing / V304, Vicars, *England's Worthies*, pp. 56–7.
104 *Ibid.*, pp. 56, 58.
105 Gasper, 'Vicars, John', *ODNB*.
106 BL, Thomason E348(1), J. Vicars, *Magnalia Dei Anglicana. Or, Englands Parliamentary Chronicle* (London, 1646), p. 162.
107 *Ibid.*, p. 162.
108 I. J. Gentles, 'Ireton, Henry (*bap.* 1611, *d.* 1651)', *ODNB*.
109 Wing / R1436, J. Ricraft, *A Survey of Englands Champions and Truths Faithfull Patriots* (London, 1647), p. 55.
110 Wing / 399:08, J. Ricraft, *The Civill Warres of England* (London, 1646), p. 81.
111 J. T. Peacey, 'Ricraft, Josiah (*d.* 1688)', *ODNB*.
112 Gentles, 'Ireton, Henry', *ODNB*.
113 *LJ*, VII, p. 433; BL, Thomason E288(25), Anon., *A Relation of the Victory*, p. 3; BL, Thomason E288(38), Bishop, *More Particular and Exact Relation*, p. 2; BL, Thomason E288(28), Gentleman in Northampton, *A More Exact and Perfect Relation of the Great Victory* (London: 1645), p. 6; BL, Thomason E288(37), *The Moderate Intelligencer*, p. 126; D. Farr, *Henry Ireton and the English Revolution* (Woodbridge: The Boydell Press, 2006), p. 51.
114 Hopper, *'Black Tom'*, pp. 177–9.
115 BL, Thomason E2(14), L. Watson, *A More Exact Relation of the Late Battell Neer York* (London, 1644), p. 7; J. Morrill, 'Cromwell, Oliver (1599–1658)', *ODNB*.
116 I. J. Gentles, 'Sprigg, Joshua (*bap.* 1618, *d.* 1684)', *ODNB*.
117 Sprigg, *Anglia Rediviva*, p. 44.
118 P. McDonald, *Oxford Dictionary of Medical Quotations* (Oxford: Oxford University Press, 2004), p. 66.

Chapter 5

'Dead Hogges, Dogges, Cats and well flayed Carryon Horses': royalist hospital provision during the First Civil War

Eric Gruber von Arni

An army without good hospitals perishes easily, it being impossible that combat actions and sickness will not fill them often and all too abundantly.[1]

This chapter will examine the attitudes and actions adopted by the King and his Council of War towards maintaining the health and welfare needs of their troops in Oxford.[2] Unfortunately, whereas the comprehensive hospital records of their opponents survive in some quantity, those of the royalist army are hard to find. Despite a centralised command structure vested in the Council of War, which, under the King's personal direction, exercised a feudalistic attitude towards servants, a lackadaisical approach to administration compounded by the wholesale destruction of documents when the royalist cause collapsed in 1646 has resulted in the survival of very few references to medical and nursing care in the royalist camp. The King's autocratic command structure assumed that regimental commanders would adopt a responsible approach towards the sick and wounded of their individual commands and paid only lip service to formulating a centrally coordinated casualty care policy. Naturally, in practice standards varied according to the capabilities and commitment of each regimental commander. Although the widows and orphans of a few royalist officers who died in service were granted sums of money to tide them over their immediate loss, the relatives of dead soldiers were rarely mentioned until a flood of petitions to county Quarter Sessions was generated many years later in the immediate post-Restoration period.

Oxford was the centre of the royalist war effort from October 1642 until June 1646. A deep division existed between town and gown in a city governed by wealthy merchants and craftsmen with widespread commercial interests, particularly in the Cotswold wool trade. These city fathers were wary of the

King's taxation of their business interests and were heavily sympathetic towards Parliament. In addition, north Oxfordshire contained a high proportion of Puritan inhabitants who distrusted their monarch's version of the Anglican faith.[3] Conversely, the university, conscious of its reliance upon the monarchy for the retention of the high status and many privileges enjoyed by its colleges (including exemption from various taxes and the right to return its own representatives to Parliament) naturally sided with the King's party.[4]

A rapidly-growing city population had encouraged the erection of much poor-quality housing. Town regulations prohibited thatched roofs but continual complaints claimed that many thatched cottages remained. By 1642, the total population of Oxford had reached approximately 10,000, to which a further 3,000 were added during the following winter.[5] Following the first major pitched battle, at Edgehill in Warwickshire on 23 October 1642, royalist casualties left behind by their army found little sympathy among the predominantly parliamentarian sympathisers of the surrounding villages. Little evidence survives related to the circumstances of their evacuation. While a few casualties were cared for locally, most were transported to Oxford in wagons and deposited in various churches, almshouses, hostelries and private houses. The city's parish officers found themselves obliged to provide the arrivals with succour and sustenance. The churchwardens of St Aldate's paid for thirty-one shrouds for the burial of wounded soldiers who had died in that parish subsequent to returning from Edgehill and a further £2 8s 4d was spent on food for casualties accommodated in local almshouses.[6] As a result of the widespread public revulsion following the uncontrolled behaviour of Prince Rupert's men during the storming of Brentford, and the subsequent rebuff that the King suffered at Turnham Green, Charles retired to Oxford to establish his headquarters where it remained for the next three and a half years.

The royal army and the King's entourage filled every available nook and cranny. The King's court, officers and members of the government, as well as their servants, dependants, soldiers, families and a variety of refugees from surrounding areas, all sought accommodation. The court's arrival caused intense overcrowding, grossly insanitary conditions and a huge increase in the number of horses and other animals brought into the city. Both human and animal waste was carelessly disposed of in cesspits, dunghills or open drains running through the middle of the streets providing an ideal breeding ground for all types of communicable diseases from which the army inevitably began to suffer. In March 1643 the city council appointed two men in each parish as street cleaners but this proved totally inadequate and, at the height of an uncomfortable and noisome summer, the King personally ordered the council to take further action. The council's hired wagons subsequently removed twenty-nine cartloads of rubbish followed, four months later, by a further twenty-six loads.[7]

The housing shortage was aggravated by the destruction of all cottages and the flooding in pastures lying within three miles of the city to prevent their use by the enemy. Finding sufficient accommodation for the army was extremely difficult. Some of the lower royal servants lived in St Ebbe's and ordinary soldiers were billeted in St Michael's, St Martin's and St Mary Magdalen parishes. Some 4,000 cavalry were billeted in churches and houses in Abingdon, all of which required constant cleaning.[8] By January 1644, in Oxford's St Aldate's parish alone, each of the seventy-four recorded households contained an average of more than five unwelcome strangers.[9] More than one churchwarden paid bribes to encourage them to move out of the town into the surrounding countryside.[10] To add insult to injury, on 16 November 1642 the council imposed a permanent weekly tax of £12 to be collected from city parishioners to cover the ever-mounting costs of the royalist war effort – including casualty care – and this was not the end of it. On 30 December a levy of £150 was demanded and, in April 1643, the King enforced a 'loan' of £2,000.[11]

Food shortages, supply problems and overcrowding were not the only factors which contributed to a higher national incidence of sickness and morbidity. When the King retired from Turnham Green to Oxford he left a strong garrison in Reading, a town that had endured a particularly high incidence of plague throughout the preceding four decades. The new arrivals were not spared from the infection and, following the town's surrender to the earl of Essex's army on 27 April 1643, some 1,200 royalist soldiers withdrew towards Oxford carrying the plague with them.[12] The infection spread rapidly and the Council of War addressed the situation by publishing formal arrangements for the long-term care of soldiers incapacitated by injury or sickness.[13]

A military hospital was established in the surviving portion of the former St Mary's College which stood in New Inn Hall Street, now known as Frewen Hall. On 2 May 1643 it was announced that every wounded officer and soldier would be rewarded with a pension, or be admitted into such hospitals and almshouses as lay within the King's area of control, or receive an annuity from their home county as specified by the old Elizabethan Poor Laws.[14]

Regimental commanders were required to submit the names of worthy candidates for pensions to the Secretary of State for consideration, while, in the counties loyal to the King, JPs were instructed to raise the necessary funds through weekly levies 'for the relief of such poor soldiers as have either lost their limbs or disabled their bodies in His Majesty's most just defensive wars, so as the said soldiers may reap the fruits of their good deservings'.[15] Although the proclamation avoided specifying the amount of relief each wounded soldier should receive, it soon became obvious that the royal treasury could not possibly cope with the predicted financial burden and, five days later, the proposals were effectively consigned to oblivion when the royalist newsletter *Mercurius Aulicus* announced that they related 'only to the future and not likely to yield help and comfort ... for the present'.[16] On the same day, a third call for parish donations was made in the churches and chapels of

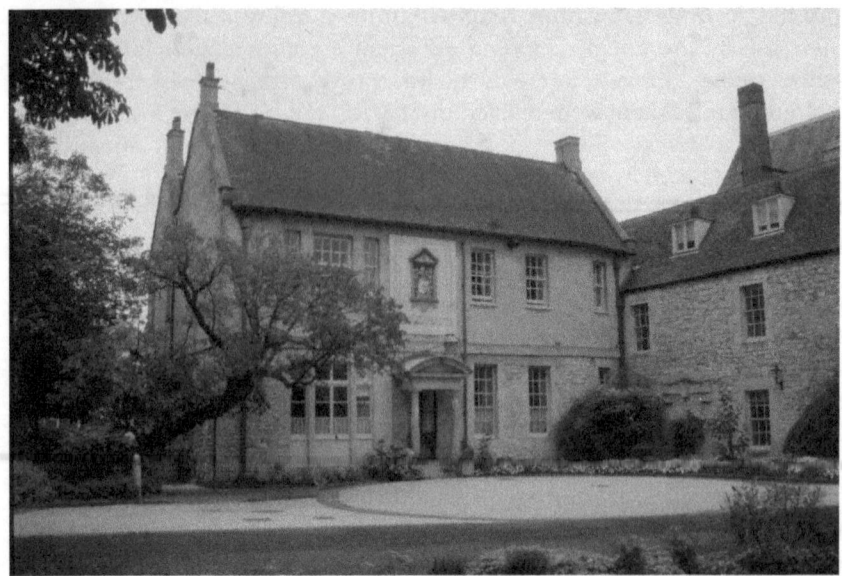

Figure 5.1 Frewen Hall, Oxford

the university and city. Reportedly, the King contributed 'in a very bountiful manner' and the court followed his example. Leonard Bowman, a city alderman, was appointed Treasurer for Sick and Wounded Soldiers and charged, in consultation with the medical staff, with allocating the proceeds, primarily for the purchase of food.[17]

Churches continued to be used to accommodate soldiers. In 1644, St Michael's fed wounded soldiers billeted there and the following year further expense was entailed in cleaning the church with pitch, resin, frankincense and other fumigants when the soldiers were moved into a small chapel in the church's grounds that was converted for semi-permanent use as a sick berth. Subsequently, on five separate occasions, several bodies of soldiers who had died there were transferred from the old chapel to St Mary Magdalen's for burial. In 1645 a parishioner, Goodman Compton, received a shilling for going about the latter parish gathering rags for use as bandages and dressings.[18] St Martin's also recorded several payments for the carriage of sick soldiers to alternative parishes or to the hospital in New Inn Hall Street.

On 2 May 1643 the royalist army, which had been feverishly constructing an outer defence for the city, marched out of Oxford into an entrenched and fortified camp or 'leaguer' on Culham Hill, south-east of Abingdon, the perceived direction of the approach of parliamentary forces from Reading.[19] The Culham leaguer was maintained throughout May and into June, continually being enlarged with earthworks, trackways and deep trenches until at least 700 defensive positions had been constructed.[20] Eventually almost 20,000 soldiers were stationed on the hill, some accompanied by their families.[21] Only 500 tents were provided, supplies were infrequent and, inevitably, poor sanitation, overcrowding, lack of food and suspect water brought disease. In addition, the hill's proximity to the River Thames was a mixed blessing as, in order to survive, soldiers, who normally drank water only as a last resort, were 'constrained to drink water, and to rob, pillage and plunder all the country thereabouts'.[22] A graphic contemporary description of the river's contents was conveyed in the words of John Taylor, assistant water-bailiff at Oxford, from which the heading for this chapter is drawn:

> I was commanded with the Water Baylie
> To see the River clensed, both night and dayly
> Dead Hogges, Dogges, Cats and well flayed Carryon Horses,
> Their noysom Corpses soyld the water courses;
> Both swines and stable dunge, Beasts guts and Garbage,
> Street durt, with Gardners weeds and Rotten Herbage.
> And from these Waters filthy puterfaction,
> Our meat and drink were made, which bred Infection.[23]

Given that Culham was downstream from Oxford, the effects were soon evident. The parish records of St Helen's, Abingdon recorded a total of 184 burials during the summer of 1643, of which more than a third (sixty-six) were those of soldiers.[24] In late May sixteen irate and influential royalist commanders presented a nine-point petition to the King's Council of War. In addition to measures aimed at preserving the army's fighting strength, this influential lobby requested a supply of shoes and stockings, better food supplies, regimental wagons for use as ambulances, the establishment of a medical facility in a village near the leaguer and the presence of both a physician and an apothecary. On 1 June 1643 the Council of War responded by appointing one of the King's physicians, Dr Francis Goddard, and an apothecary, Thomas Clarges. Goddard, conscious of his duty to advise on such matters, pressed for the removal of the sick to a healthier location.[25] An emergency hospital was established in the local manor at Nuneham Balding (now Nuneham Courtney and Marsh Baldon), which lay some five miles to the south of the city, not far from the Culham leaguer.[26] As a result the situation slowly began to improve.

On the same day as Goddard's appointment was promulgated, emergency warrants were issued to the sheriffs of Oxfordshire and Berkshire requiring them to order local inhabitants to collect and deliver sixty flock beds, with sheets and other necessaries, 'to either Nuneham or such other place near the leaguer as the Commissary for the Sick should appoint, for use by the sick soldiers of the Army'.[27] On 2 June 1643 the Paymaster-General was instructed to release the back-pay owed to sick soldiers to Goddard for his use in providing the patients with adequate food and treatment.[28] The expected bedding was slow to arrive and when Goddard wrote a letter of complaint to the Council of War, he took the opportunity to attach a list of amended and additional requirements. The house at Nuneham was inadequate and he requested sufficient space to contain beds for all the sick.[29] He also suggested that the clergy of nearby parishes should appeal to their congregations for old linen and clothes so that his patients could receive clean garments while their own were laundered. However, the situation deteriorated further and, on 5 June, parliamentarian spies reported that the enemy on Culham Hill were short of food and drink, that discipline and morale were poor, that desertions were frequent and that a very dangerous sickness had spread among them.

On 8 June the headquarters of the parliamentary army was established at Thame, eight miles east of Oxford and, as a result of the altered threat, the Culham leaguer was abandoned. The troops moved to Bullington Green (Horspath Common) between Oxford and Wheatley, but, by this time exposure and disease had seriously depleted the King's forces among whom over 3,000 men were now 'so sick and weak that, if they were put to march, it is thought half of them were scarce able to march away'.[30]

In response to Goddard's previous plea for additional space, the facility at Nuneham was also vacated and transferred to the village of Sunningwell, a short distance north of Abingdon, where a semi-permanent hospital for the Abingdon garrison was opened at the manor house of the Baskerville family in the adjacent hamlet of Bayworth, described by the contemporaneous writer Anthony Wood as 'private and lone – a romancy place'.[31]

The King was also requested to issue a warrant to the sheriffs of Oxfordshire and Berkshire reiterating the demand for straw beds, redirecting their delivery to Sunningwell. Goddard also asked for the appointment of a senior officer to supervise the issue of sick soldiers' pay and authority for the Wagon-Master-General, who, as Commissary-General for Victuals, was also responsible for the adequate supply and transportation of rations and necessaries for the sick, to commandeer wagons and boats for their carriage.[32] The physician's requirements ended with a complaint that his salary payments were irregular and, because his military duties had forced him to neglect 'all his (private) practice for the furtherance of his Majesty's service', he was suffering financial embarrassment. In response Matthew Bradley, the Paymaster-General, was instructed to provide regular salary payments to both Goddard and Clarges.[33]

The employment of a number of local civilian surgeons was approved but it was made clear that funding for this would have to be made through regimental commanders who were required to 'take care of the hurt soldiers in their own Regiment that they be provided for accordingly', and to 'recommend ... to the Council of War ... the means how the surgeons attending be rewarded for their pains and charges in their cures'.[34] In other words, the King was transferring the financial burden of paying for such care away from himself onto individual commanders. Subsequent orders from the Council of War appear to have been drafted verbatim from Goddard's

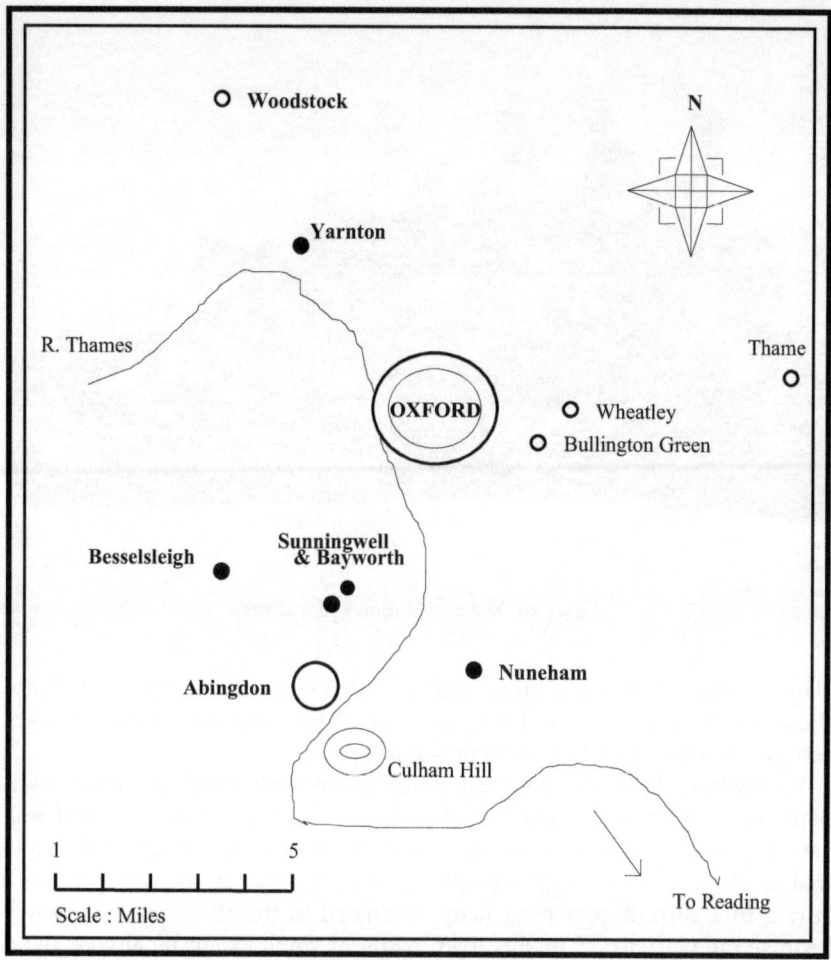

Figure 5.2 Sketch map showing locations of royalist military hospitals in the Oxford area, 1643–45

list, including opening a third hospital at Yarnton Manor, some four miles north-west of the city.

Yarnton Manor lay in a small, quiet village lying on the trackway along which local farmers had traditionally herded their stock into Oxford market. It was specifically designated as a medical, or isolation hospital to supplement the existing facilities at New Inn Hall Street and at Sunningwell. The village was probably chosen because of its relative isolation and distance from the city, as, while wounded patients requiring surgery continued to be treated in the city and at Sunningwell, henceforth infectious cases were sent to Yarnton. Unfortunately, the military presence initiated an outbreak of

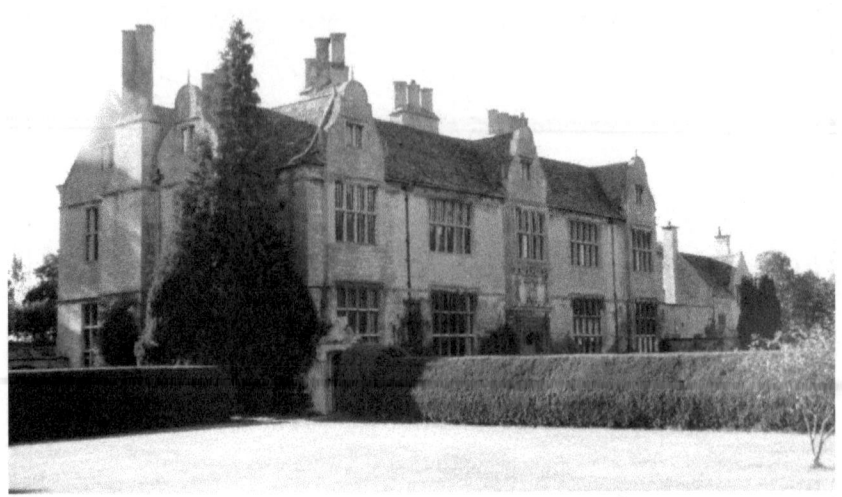

Figure 5.3 Yarnton Manor, Oxfordshire

plague in the village that is graphically recorded in the parish registers. These show that between May and August 1643, there were twenty-four military and twenty-six civilian burials in the churchyard.[35]

Meanwhile, the city's death toll continued at such a high level that additional burial plots were required. The final resting place for the dead was determined by status as regulations were promulgated specifying that any soldier who died in the city 'who [was] not of that quality as to [be] fit to be buried in a shroud, that their body be carried to the churchyard at Osney because the churchyard in this town being of small extent be already overfull'.[36] Military funeral services were conducted by regimental chaplains who were also responsible for ensuring that an appropriate number of the dead man's comrades accompanied the body to the graveside.[37]

Despite the opening of a third hospital, the provision of adequate quantities of beds and bedding continued to pose problems. Even though Oxfordshire had been ordered to supply 300 beds, still more were required and, on 7 July 1643, an additional warrant was issued to the sheriffs of Gloucestershire and Berkshire extending the demand for beds and fresh straw to the inhabitants of the villages bordering Oxfordshire.[38]

Unfortunately the hospitals' capacity is unknown and, although regulations for the twelve women employed as nurses among the three hospitals stipulate that they were 'to act as nurses for the soldiers, to attend them and perform those offices which are necessary', regrettably no further documentary evidence relating to their work survives.[39]

Table 5.1 Staff establishments and pay in Oxford's military hospitals, 1643

Appointment	Daily pay rate
Two female nurses	8d
Three overseers	6d
The commissary, John Bissell	5d
The physician's servant	2s 6d
The apothecary's servant	2s 0d

Source: BL, Harleian MS 6,804, fo. 121; BL, Harleian MS 6,852, fo. 181

Although William Barlow and Elizabeth Matthews, two employees at Yarnton hospital, found the time to marry in the manor chapel, the intense work in the three hospitals took its toll on everyone caring for the sick. All three senior hospital officers, Bowman the Treasurer for Sick and Wounded Soldiers, Clarges the apothecary and Dr Goddard, reported their exhaustion and overwork. Bowman complained that his burden was excessive and he was subsequently authorised to appoint two or three assistants 'to overlook the poor soldiers every day and to supply their necessities ... that they [the patients] may be provided for that they perish not'.[40] On 14 July 1643, Clarges found it necessary to write to Edward Walker, Secretary to the King's Council of War, complaining sarcastically that he was overworked and had 'by some subtle Philosophy, become a Doctor of Physick, two apothecaries, three overseers and twelve attendants'.[41] With the war producing a continual flow of wounded men in addition to the victims of disease, Clarges and Goddard both pressed for implementation of earlier requests for surgical assistance 'which some course must speedily obtain for we ... bury more toes and fingers [unnecessarily] than we do men'.[42] Eventually a surgeon and two mates were added to the hospital establishment. Goddard also pleaded for two personal assistants, 'because the number of the sick are beyond all expectation and too many for the care of one man', both to be Bachelors of Physick at the university, although this last request seems to have fallen on deaf ears as nothing further was heard of the matter.[43]

By mid-June 1643 the significantly-increasing costs of providing the troops with medical care began to worry the King and his Council. Dr Bayley, the Dean of Salisbury, and William Gerrard were appointed to form a committee to investigate and supervise the accounts of the treasurer, physician and apothecary who presented their records for audit on 23 June. Bowman had received money from the various church collections, Goddard had finally been paid £100 in arrears from the Paymaster-General, though Clarges had purchased his stock of medicines, at a cost of £50, for which he had not been remunerated. Amazingly, the audit committee determined that the medical financial situation was not unreasonable and recommended that Goddard be provided with the wherewithal to maintain a constant cash float for hospital staff salaries. The debt related to Clarges and his stores was referred to the Council of War for repayment.[44] On 17 July 1643, John Bissell was appointed Commissary for the Sick, to whom the Paymaster-General was instructed to pay the wages of soldiers in hospital. Bissell was then charged with passing this money on to individual patients according to a prescribed scale, having made various deductions to offset the cost of care.[45] While a patient in the hospital, each soldier would be entitled to be paid 3s a week of which 2s was given to the soldier. The remainder was retained by Bissell to fund the cost of medicines and the pay of doctors providing care.

Funding for the provisioning of the sick and wounded of the army was authorised at the rate of £10 weekly for food for 100 men and £5 weekly for their medicines and treatment. With Parliament controlling the national treasury, Charles I was perpetually struggling to prosecute the war while paying and sustaining his troops and maintaining his household expenses. The unfortunate population living within the areas controlled by the royalist army provided the only readily available source of revenue and sustenance, the villagers living in the marginal territories between the opposing factions being particularly oppressed by frequent taxation and pillage by both armies.

Meanwhile, Sir Samuel Luke's parliamentarian spies continued to report the spread of infection in the royalist ranks throughout the summer months and his papers provide a running commentary on the sufferings of the royalist forces, not only in the city but also in the garrisons of outlying villages.[46] On 16 June 1643 some 300 sick soldiers were taken in wagons from Gosford Bridge to Woodstock, which was garrisoned by the Lord General's regiment. Such a move would seem to infer the presence of either a treatment facility or convalescent camp, but, unfortunately, this cannot be confirmed.[47] By 22 June disease had struck the King's army in Headington and also forced the withdrawal of all royalist troops from the area between Chiselhampton and Abingdon, including any remaining on Culham Hill.[48] By 10 July 1643 the deaths in Oxford garrison from sickness numbered forty a week besides those from other causes. At Radley, of the forty-two burials recorded during 1643 in the parish, twenty were in July and, of these, thirteen were for military personnel.[49] The enormous difficulties experienced in providing care for the Oxford army's sick were aggravated further on 12 July when thirty cartloads of injured soldiers from Prince Maurice's army arrived in the city following their evacuation from the field of Lansdown. On 29 July, a letter directed to the Paymaster-General informed him that 469 soldiers had now recovered, were fit to march and ordered him to supply their relevant regimental commanders with a week's pay to cover the soldiers' transport costs.[50]

Following his capture of Bristol on 26 July 1643, the King besieged Gloucester, but, by 6 September, with Essex and his relieving force approaching Cheltenham, the journey to Oxford over the Cotswolds had become too risky for royalist sick and wounded and some 400 were dispatched by boats down the River Severn from Berkeley to Bristol.[51] Within days, with Essex having broken Gloucester's siege, a further 300 royalist casualties were transferred in forty carts from Sudeley Castle to Cirencester where local overcrowding forced the onward transfer of five cartloads to Oxford. Three days later more followed them on horseback.[52]

In August a new danger was added to this sorry predicament when a particularly virulent form of typhus, called 'the new disease' or 'morbus campestris' in contemporary records, presented itself causing many deaths in Oxford and surrounding villages such as Wheatley, a town of some ninety-two cottages. There, the annual average of twenty-one burials during the decade 1632–42 rose to fifty-two civilians in 1643 and seventy-three in 1644.[53]

By November 1643 the royalist garrisons in Abingdon and Wallingford had been reduced to below 800 by disease and, on 14 December 1643, Oxford's overcrowding was exacerbated by further arrivals from Bristol and Winchester, the latter having escaped from the fall of Alton to Sir William Waller on 13 December.[54] Garrisons lying at a greater distance from Oxford were forced to make their own local arrangements for casualty care. Insidiously, typhus spread westwards along the major highways, assisted by the frequent movement of troops, following the royalist army into the West Country.

In late September 1643, Oxford's housing difficulties became even worse when approximately 1,000 casualties arrived following the first battle of Newbury (20 September), a number of whom were captured parliamentarian wounded. The King decreed that these parliamentarians should receive the same treatment as his own casualties:

> Though they be rebels and deserve the punishment of traitors, yet out of our tender compassion upon them, as being our subjects, our will and pleasure is that you carefully provide for their recovery, as well as for those of our own army.[55]

Newbury's mayor, to whom the order was sent, was charged with collecting and transporting the wounded as well as supervising burial of the dead. On 7 November 1643, despite the continuing high number of patients, both sick and wounded, the Council of War surprisingly decided, on the grounds that they were under-employed, to dispense with the services of two surgeon's mates and the apothecary's mate, a saving of 7s a day. They also decided that the cost of caring for sick and wounded soldiers in outlying garrisons would henceforth be funded out of the county contributions or local taxes.[56]

Lack of pay had reduced the morale of medical staff drastically, particularly among the long-serving regimental surgeons of the King's 'old regiments'. Seven regimental surgeons, namely Stephen Fawcett, Henry Johnson, Humphrey Paynton, John Robinson, James Rammage, Nicholas Thompson and John Thornhill, had not been paid for months when they congregated in Oxford to petition the King for their arrears. In response, on 24 November 1643, Ashburnham, the Treasurer at War, was ordered to provide them with £20 each on account.[57]

All of these measures were, undoubtedly, a reflection of the King's desperately deteriorating financial situation. With bad beer, poor food and a shortage of fuel for fires, life in Oxford during the ensuing winter became particularly uncomfortable for the population and soldiers alike. However, the incidence of disease eventually diminished and the number of hospital in-patients fell accordingly. By March 1644, with the pace of work at Yarnton significantly reduced, Sir William Spencer agitated for the return of his property. The Council of War agreed, and, on 16 March 1644, ordered Clarges and Bissell to transfer all the resident patients to Besselsleigh, the requisitioned house of parliamentarian William Lenthall, Speaker of the House of Commons, situated on the main road from Oxford to Faringdon.[58]

The hospital remained at Besselsleigh for a mere eleven weeks as nearby Abingdon was abandoned by the royalists on 25 May 1644 and was occupied by the enemy the following day. By 30 May Oxford was almost surrounded by parliamentary forces. Clarges was ordered to move his practice into the city and to continue caring for 'the soldiers of Our Army as are now there or shall be brought thither diseased or wounded' under the directions of Dr Samuel Turner, the King's personal physician and Physician-General. Thenceforth, until Oxford's surrender in 1646, the hospital in New Inn Hall Street provided the royal army's only static medical facility with other temporary houses being requisitioned as necessary.[59]

During the night of 4 June 1644, fearing capture by the combined armies of the earl of Essex and of Sir William Waller, the King made a daring escape from Oxford. Waller attempted to follow the King, but Essex abandoned the pursuit and led his army into the West Country. On 20 June, the King sent his army's sick into Oxford and ordered his Wagon-Master and Commissary-General of Victuals, Captain Henry Stevens, who was continually hard pressed to maintain supplies of cereals and other food items, to issue two quarts of wheat and two quarts of malt to Commissary Bissell for consumption by the sick soldiers, most likely for baking bread and brewing beer. Two weeks earlier he had been ordered to take special care that each soldier received a daily issue of one pound bread and half a pound cheese, and it is difficult otherwise to see how the wheat and malt were intended to alleviate the condition of the sick. Contemporary brewing methods suggest that the allowance issued to Bissell represented the meagre equivalent of a week's supply of bread and ale for about twenty sick soldiers.[60]

The same day, acting on the advice of Dr Goddard, the Council of War ordered Stevens to consult with Commissary Bissell before additional quarters for the sick and wounded were requisitioned in outlying towns and villages. With the closure of Yarnton and Sunningwell, the care of the sick had become fragmented and scattered, causing difficulties and duplication of work, confusion over numbers and unnecessary expense. Almost inevitably, the summer of 1644 brought a resurgence of the plague and, on 6 August

1644, sixteen cartloads of sick soldiers were carried from Abingdon into Oxford with many more being left behind.[61]

In an attempt to limit the spread of infection, the Council dictated that only one, or at most two, houses in any town or village should be used for medical purposes. Unfortunately, the resultant widespread dispersal of patients through several villages aided the spread of infection rather than containing it. On 10 June 1644, a report by *Mercurius Aulicus* (that the King's intention of the previous year, to provide for the hurt and maimed soldiers in charitable institutions, had been frustrated because many of the nominated hospitals and almshouses had fallen under the control of parliamentarian forces) provides us with a clue to defining the royalist approach to casualty care. The King's response was a direct reflection of pre-war society's approach to community benevolence, which separated itinerants and the impotent poor from society, keeping them out of sight and out of mind. Pre-war society had fulfilled its obligations to the needy by establishing charitable almshouses, endowed by wealthy members of the community, where they could be maintained as a permanent charitable charge and living proof of the donor's generosity. Naturally, this system failed to solve the root cause of the problem and was in direct contrast to Parliament's war-time response, which accepted full, centralised responsibility for those killed or incapacitated in its service.[62]

Nevertheless, minor administrative re-structuring brought some practical benefits to the sick and wounded. The Treasurer for the Sick Soldiers, Leonard Bowman, was now appointed 'Governor of the Sick and Wounded'. He assumed responsibility for ensuring 'the present comfort and relief of such wounded soldiers as were under care in and about the City of Oxford' and, in addition to receiving monies raised for their relief, he became accountable for these funds and for paying the surgeons, nurses and other attendants. He was also expected to notify Oxford's governor when soldiers became fit to return to their regiments or, should the soldier be deemed unfit for further service, to inform the Justice of the King's Bench. In response, the justices were to make suitable recommendations to the appropriate county treasurers for the award of annual pensions according to individual merits and necessities.[63] However, as the following example shows, royal patronage frequently circumvented these arrangements and specific warrants continued to be issued by the Council of War for cases that attracted the King's interest:

> Whereas we have been informed that our right dear nephew Prince Rupert did lately order the sum of £150 to be paid unto the officers of Sir William Russell's Regiment of Foot out of the Contribution of the County whereof £30 as yet unpaid was the proportion due unto Lt. Colonel Davis, slain lately in our service. Our will and pleasure therefore is and we hereby do require and authorise you out of such Contribution money as you have or shall speedily receive that you pay unto Thomasina Davis, widow of the said Lt. Colonel, the said full sum of £30 and for your so doing this shall be your warrant.[64]

The prevailing cramped and insanitary conditions affected all levels of society. The King's court in Christ Church had become the hub of the royalist war effort. Courtiers, staff and visitors thronged the halls, rooms and stairs, and, at times, especially after victories, captured enemy standards were draped over the main staircase adding to the overall clutter. During her time in Oxford the Queen established herself at Merton College while Princes Rupert and Maurice took over the house of the Town Clerk. In St Aldates, three earls, three barons and several baronets and knights took up residence alongside the King's surgeon, apothecary, barber, tailor and seamstress.[65] A herd of cattle was maintained in the quadrangle of Christ Church as well as a forge. Naturally, with such over-crowded conditions, the court was by no means immune from infection. Among the members of the Royal Household, ninety-five died during the years 1642–46, including the King's Comptroller, the Keeper of the Great Seal and two Yeomen of the Wardrobe. On 7 August 1643 even the Queen was reported to be very sick and one of her attendant ladies, suffering from the plague, expired in a room adjacent to the Queen's bedchamber.[66] A graphic description of the situation that met those who accompanied the court to Oxford was left by Lady Fanshawe who commented:

> From as good a house as any gentleman of England had, we came to a baker's house in an obscure street, and from rooms well-furnished, to lie in a very bad bed in a garret, to one dish of meat, and that not the best ordered, no money, for we were as poor as Job, no clothes more than a man or two brought in their clothes bags: we had perpetual discourse of losing and gaining towns and men; at the windows the sad spectacle of war, sometimes plague, sometimes sickness of other kinds by reason of so many people being packed together.[67]

The morale of Oxford's population must have reached its nadir when, on Sunday 6 October 1644, the most devastating fire of the civil-war years broke out there. The conflagration was reported variously as having been started either by a soldier carelessly roasting a stolen pig or by deliberate action – three men suspected of involvement were reputedly tortured afterwards. The wind blew strongly from the north so that the fire, which started in the central area, spread rapidly to the south of the city where it burned for ten to fifteen hours. A total of 300–350 houses in all were lost, representing between a quarter and one third of the city.[68] As a result of the overcrowding, those made homeless by the fire, including many solders, could not be rehoused and faced the oncoming winter without a roof over their heads.[69]

Battle casualties continued to flow into the city. Three weeks after the great fire, on 27 October 1644, wounded soldiers struggled into a devastated Oxford following the second battle of Newbury. Although royalist losses in that battle were less than those of their enemy – they claimed 529 soldiers and 59 officers hurt against 1,000 – it was impossible, in the circumstances, to provide shelter and food in the city. Many were diverted to Bristol or to

Marlborough, where, for two weeks after the battle, the King's Council of War met and where, on 13 November 1644, Humphrey Paynter, Paymaster-General, received instructions to purchase whatever medicines as were required by the army's physicians and surgeons using money gained from local taxation.[70] As the weeks passed the severe winter of 1644–45 increased the hardships suffered in Oxford where the bitter cold was accompanied by increased shortages of fuel for warmth and cooking.

Finally, on 7 May 1645, the King departed Oxford at the head of his army and embarked on a campaign which, in the words of his astrologer, was to be 'the battle of all for all'.[71] His departure was followed by an attempt to surround Oxford by the New Model Army under Fairfax, but this was abandoned in early June following vigorous royalist counter-raids. Eventually, although the King captured Leicester, his total defeat by Fairfax at Naseby on 14 June 1645, where 1,000 of his troops were killed and some 5,000 captured, was the beginning of the end for his cause.[72] The royalist wounded struggled off the field and attempted to find succour in Leicester. For a further four months, during which his remaining forces experienced a series of crushing losses at Langport, Bristol, Rowton Heath and in Scotland, the King covered some 1,200 miles in his attempts to recoup support and reform his army, exhausting his few remaining troops in the process. He returned to Oxford during the following October but the weather during the coming winter was even worse than that of the previous year.

On 27 April 1646, leaving his son the duke of York behind, the King embarked on a final attempt to determine his own future and secretly left the city in a bid to seek an arrangement with the Scots army. The garrisons around Oxford capitulated one by one but the city held out until 24 June 1646, when, after delivering himself to the Scots at Southwell on 5 May, the King ordered the Oxford garrison to surrender. With the end of the siege food supplies could once again reach the city, and, on 6 May 1646, the main provision store was opened to feed 4,700 people daily.[73]

The logistical, medical and environmental problems that faced Charles I's army throughout its occupation of Oxford were horrendous. Little is known about the recruitment of physicians and surgeons for the royalist cause but, in the absence of an inherited infrastructure or ready-made hospitals such as those that Parliament had enjoyed in London, coupled with a loss of backing by the College of Physicians (who favoured Parliament), and with poor administrative support, a shortage of medical staff and gross overcrowding, the care and welfare of the King's sick and wounded troops compared badly with Parliament's achievements. Theoretically the faculty of medicine at the university should have been in a position to influence the provision of physicians but there is no evidence to indicate that this happened.[74] Widows and children appear to have been disregarded altogether and referred to their home parishes for support, in line with the Elizabethan vagrancy laws. These same parishes were themselves bowing under the weight of punitive taxation and the cost of 'free quartering', which left little or nothing for charitable causes.[75] However, notwithstanding the disadvantages they experienced, it is hard not to draw the conclusion that the royal army failed to attach the same high priority to the care of its sick and wounded as that adopted by Parliament to its soldiers.

NOTES

1 Marquis de Feuquières in L. André, *Michel Le Tellier et l'Organisation de l'Armée Monarchique* (Paris: Felix Alcan, 1906), pp. 475–6.

2 The nature, membership and function of the King's Council of War has been discussed at length in I. Roy, 'The royalist Council of War, 1642–6', *Bulletin of the Institute for Historical Research*, 35 (1962), 150–68.

3 L. Rice-Oxley, *Oxford Renowned* (Oxford, 1925), p. 96; D. Eddershaw and E. Roberts, *The Civil War in Oxfordshire* (Stroud: Sutton, 1995), pp. 1–50.

4 I. Roy, 'The city of Oxford, 1640–1660', in R. C. Richardson (ed.), *Town and Countryside in the English Revolution* (Manchester: Manchester University Press, 1992), pp. 130–68.

5 Bodl., MS 28,289, fo. 17. Return of the Names of the Inhabitants and Lodgers within each several parish [aged] from 16 to 60, 7 June 1643. This document was compiled to identify those available to participate in a work force employed in constructing new city defences.

6 OHC, Ref. Mss., D. D. Par. Oxford, St Aldate's parish churchwardens' accounts.

7 Eddershaw and Roberts, *The Civil War in Oxfordshire*, pp. 59–60.

8 A. Clark (ed.), *The Life and Times of Anthony Wood, Antiquary, of Oxford, 1632–1695, Described by Himself*, 5 vols (Oxford, 1891–1900), I, p. 68.

9 BL, Harleian MS 2,125, fo. 66, 134v; S. Porter, 'The Oxford fire of 1644', *Oxoniensis*, 44 (1984), 289–300.

10 *CSPD 1644*, p. 10; OHC, Ref. Nos. Par. D. D. Mss: Oxford, Churchwardens' accounts for St Aldate's and St Michael's parishes.

11 M. G. Hobson and Rev. H. E. Salter (eds), *Oxford Council Acts, 1626–65* (Oxford Historical Society, 95, 1933), pp. 369–71.

12 OHC, Churchwardens' accounts for St Mary's parish. In 1639, in Reading's St Mary's parish alone, there was recorded a total of eighty-three deaths, of which twenty-one were attributed to plague or fevers. A further two plague victims were buried in that parish during the following year.

13 BL, Thomason E102(1), *Mercurius Aulicus*, 18th week (Oxford, 1643), p. 224.

14 The hospital buildings, now part of Brasenose College, were later renamed 'Frewen Hall'. BL, Thomason E103(10), *Mercurius Aulicus*, 19th week (Oxford, 1643), p. 235.

15 *Mercurius Aulicus*, 2 May 1643, OHC, OXFO 072, Microfiche 94/857.

16 Ibid.

17 I. G. Philip (ed.), *Journal of Sir Samuel Luke*, 3 vols (Oxford, 1947–53), I, p. 72.

18 OHC, Parish records for St Michael's and St Mary Magdalen.

19 Council to Heydon, 2 May 1643: TNA, WO55/459, fo. 117.

20 Philip (ed.), *Journal*, I, p. 24.

21 Ibid.
22 BL, Thomason E102(1), Mercurius Aulicus; Philip (ed.), Journal, I, pp. 24, 72.
23 Quoted by I. G. Philip, 'River navigation at Oxford during the civil war and Commonwealth', Oxoniensis, 2 (1937), 156.
24 St Helen's, Abingdon parish register 1640–78 (not deposited).
25 BL, Harleian MS 6,852, fo. 74; BL Harleian MS 6,804, fo. 204; K. Park, 'Medicine and society in medieval Europe, 500–1500', in A. Wear (ed.), Medicine in Society: Historical Essays (Cambridge: Cambridge University Press, 1992), pp. 86–7.
26 M. D. Lobel (ed.), A History of the County of Oxford: Vol. 5, Bullingdon Hundred (London: Oxford University Press, 1957), pp. 234–45.
27 BL, Harleian MS 6,852, fos. 72–3.
28 Ibid., fo. 74.
29 BL, Harleian MS 6,804, fo. 204.
30 Clark (ed.), The Life and Times of Anthony Wood, I, p. 100; Philip (ed.), Journal, II, pp. 90–102.
31 Clark (ed.), The Life and Times of Anthony Wood, I, p. 270.
32 BL, Harleian MS 6,804, fo. 204.
33 Council of State to Matthew Bradley, 2 June 1643: BL, Harleian MS 6,852, fo. 74.
34 BL, Harleian MS 6,852, fo. 181.
35 OHC, Mss, D. D. Yarnton parish register, 1629–1721.
36 Ibid.
37 See M. Griffin, Regulating Religion and Morality in the King's Armies, 1639–1646 (Leiden: Brill, 2004).
38 BL, Harleian MS 6,804, fo. 115.
39 Ibid.
40 BL, Harleian MS 6,842, fo. 203.
41 Ibid.
42 OHC, Mss, D. D. Yarnton, fo. 203.
43 BL, Harleian MS 6,804, fo. 204.
44 Ibid., fo. 202.
45 John Bissell was probably a Worcester man who was paid 5s a day for his services: M. Toynbee (ed.), The Papers of Captain Henry Stevens, Waggon-Master-General to King Charles I (Oxfordshire Record Society, 42, 1961), pp. 54–5.
46 Philip (ed.), Journal, II, pp. 114–5.
47 Ibid.
48 Philip (ed.), Journal, I, pp. 26–140, and II, pp 146–53.
49 W. Bradbrooke, 'The Church during the Commonwealth in the Abingdon Deanery', Berkshire Archaeological Journal, 37 (1934), 19–32.
50 Council of War to Matthew Bradley, 29 July 1643: BL, Harleian MS 6,852, fo. 163.
51 The River Severn was one of the King's main communication routes at this time.
52 W. O. Hassell, 'Typhus in Oxfordshire Billets, 1643–44', Journal of the Royal Army Medical Corps, 101 (1955), 244–5.
53 Ibid.
54 S. R. Gardiner, History of the Great Civil War, 4 vols (London: Longmans, 1886–93), I, p. 254.
55 BL, Thomason E69(18), Mercurius Aulicus, 38th week (Oxford, 1643), p. 531.
56 Council of War to the constable and churchwardens of Barrington and Rissington,

13 November 1643: BL, Harleian MS 6,852, fo. 225; Council of War to Surgeon Humphrey Paynton, 13 November 1644: BL, Harleian MS 6,802, fo. 293.

57 Council to John Ashburnham, Treasurer at War, 7 November 1643: BL, Harleian MS 6,852, fo. 210; Council of War to Ashburnham, 27 November 1643: BL, Harleian MS 6,851, fos. 229–30.

58 BL, Harleian MS 6,852, fo. 41; BL Harleian MS 6,804, fos. 92, 124; Toynbee (ed.), *The Papers of Capt. Henry Stevens*, p. 35; BL, Harleian MS 6,804, fos. 92, 124; *CSPD 1644–45*, pp. 204–5; M. D. Lobel (ed.), *A History of the County of Oxford: Lewknor and Pyrton Hundreds* (London: Oxford University Press, 1964), VIII, p. 209.

59 BL, Harleian MS 6,802, fo. 198.

60 H. Hall and F. J. Nicholas (eds), 'Select tracts and table books relating to English weights and measures, 1100–1742', *Camden Miscellany XV* (Camden Society, 3rd series, 41, 1929), p. 8; M. Prestwich, 'Victualling estimates for English garrisons in Scotland during the early fourteenth century', *The English Historical Review*, 82 (1967), 536–8; Toynbee (ed.), *The Papers of Capt. Henry Stevens*, p. 28.

61 WRO, R. O. 265/2, Naworth (ed.) (*Dugdale*) (n.d.) 'Transcription of Ms. Note by Sir William Dugdale in his Diary of 1644, A New Almanack and Prognosticator for the year of our Lord 1644'; BL, Harleian MS 6,851, fo. 163.

62 W. K. Jordan, *The Charities of Rural England, 1480–1660* (London: Allen & Unwin, 1961), pp. 33–4.

63 BL, Thomason E53(5), *Mercurius Aulicus*, 24th week (Oxford, 1644), pp. 1021–2.

64 Council of War to Sir Barnaby Scudamore, Constable and Governor of Hereford, 30 June 1645: BL, Harleian MS 6,852, fo. 268.

65 A. Crossley and C. R. Elrington (eds), *History of the County of Oxford: Vol. 4, The City of Oxford* (London: Oxford University Press, 1979), p. 69.

66 Philip (ed.), *Journal*, II, p. 130.

67 A. Fanshawe, *The Memoirs of Ann, Lady Fanshawe, Wife of the Right Honble. Sir Richard Fanshawe, Bart., 1600–72* (London, 1907), pp. 24–5.

68 *CSPD 1644–45*, pp. 16, 46.

69 Porter, 'The Oxford fire of 1644', 289–300; Toynbee (ed.), *Papers of Capt. Henry Stevens*, p. 25.

70 Council to Paynter, 13 November 1644: BL, Harleian MS 6,802, fo. 293. BL, Harleian MS 6,804, fo. 92; W. Money, *The First and Second Battles of Newbury and the Siege of Donnington Castle during the Civil War, 1643–6* (2nd edn, London: Simpkin, Marshall, 1884), *passim*.

71 C. Carlton, *Charles I: The Personal Monarch* (London: Routledge & Kegan Paul, 1983), p. 285.

72 I am grateful to David Appleby for drawing my attention to BL, Thomason E288(46), *The True Informer*, 21 June (London, 1645), p. 70 – wrongly paginated as p. 61 and *The True Informer*, p. 67.

73 WRO, R. O., 265/2; Naworth (*Dugdale*).

74 N. Tyacke, *The History of the University of Oxford, Volume 4: Seventeenth-Century Oxford* (Oxford: Clarendon Press, 1997), pp. 707–9.

75 The nationwide decline in charitable donations during the civil-war years has been eloquently described in W. K. Jordan, *The Charities of London, 1480–1660* (London: Allen & Unwin, 1960), p. 25, and Jordan, *The Charities of Rural England*, p. 26.

Chapter 6

Gerard's *Herball* and the treatment of war-wounds and contagion during the English Civil War

Richard Jones

On 14 September 1644, Lieutenant-Colonel Thomas Johnson, a royalist field officer at Basing House, sustained a gunshot to his shoulder while coming to the aid of Captain Fletcher's musketeers. Charged with protecting carts bringing provisions from the town to the besieged garrison, Fletcher's men had been routed by a parliamentarian force of mounted and foot soldiers. Johnson's rearguard action was a success: sixteen parliamentarians were killed, eleven taken prisoner, and their defensive emplacement destroyed. For Johnson himself, however, the outcome of this skirmish proved fatal. A fortnight later he died of fever brought on by his wounds. Thomas Johnson was no ordinary man. According to the marquis of Winchester's diary, his death prompted: 'Funerall teares, being no lesse eminent in the Garrison for his valour and conduct, as a Souldier, then famous through the kingdom for his excellancy as an Herbarist, and Physician.'[1] The marquis did not exaggerate: Johnson was the pre-eminent apothecary/herbalist of his age.

During the late 1620s Johnson had undertaken extensive field visits to collect plant specimens in Kent and on Hampstead Heath. His findings were published together as *Iter plantarum investigationis ... in agrum cantianum* and *Ericetum Hamstedianum* in 1629.[2] Further tours to the Bath region and North Wales resulted respectively in *Mercurius botanicus* in 1634,[3] and his last book *Mercurii botanici pars altera* in 1641.[4] But his contemporary renown was based not on his own original research but on his enlarged and heavily amended edition of John Gerard's *Herball*. This was first published in 1633 and was so well received that by 1636 it had gone into a second edition.[5] On the eve of the civil wars, Johnson's 'Gerard' was unquestionably the most comprehensive and most up-to-date medical manual available in the English language, and Johnson himself, as a Doctor of Physic, a most extraordinary asset for the royalist cause.

John Gerard's *Herball, or, Generall Historie of Plantes* had first been published in 1597.[6] In reality the work was simply a re-arranged English translation
of Dutch scholar Rembert Dodoen's highly popular *Stirpium historiae pemptades sex sive libri XXX* of 1583.[7] Gerard had not initially been commissioned by
the publisher John Norton to undertake the translation. This had been a task
given to Robert Priest of the London College of Physicians. But Priest died
before its completion and Norton asked Gerard to finish the work. Gerard,
however, sought to obscure the book's derivative origins. He would claim in
his preface to the *Herball* that Priest's translation had perished along with
its author and that he had instead written an entirely new book. Distancing
himself both from Dodoen's original and Priest's efforts, Gerard also failed
to acknowledge material that he had borrowed and incorporated from his
celebrated Flemish botanist friend Matthias de l'Obel.

Gerard's disingenuity did not go unnoticed. After errors were identified
in the final draft text and some of the 1,800 accompanying woodcuts, most
taken from Jacobus Theodorus' *Eicones plantarum* published only a few years
earlier in Frankfurt,[8] were shown to have been assigned to the wrong plants,
the publishers asked l'Obel to check and ensure the book's accuracy. L'Obel
identified over a thousand errors, but Gerard had him dismissed and the
herbal was published uncorrected.[9] Recognising the borrowings Gerard had
made, l'Obel would later accuse Gerard of plagiarism.[10] Gerard's work was
thus tainted by controversy from the outset, at least within late sixteenth-
century scholarly circles. The social elites, by contrast, who were unconcerned
by issues of authorship, and unaware of the *Herball*'s inaccuracies, reacted
warmly to its publication, delighting in its scope, content and preservation.

Gerard's *Herball* as it soon came to be known – a clear reflection of the
success of Gerard's efforts in promoting himself as its true author – would
become the most popular herbal of the seventeenth-century well-to-do. More
specifically, Johnson's edition of the *Herball* became an essential reference
work in many aristocratic and gentry households, as well as among some
professional classes.[11] The *Herball* was depicted, for instance, among other
titles in the first panel of the triptych attributed to the Dutch painter Jan van
Belcamp chronicling the life and erudition of Lady Anne Clifford, widow of
the earl of Dorset.[12] On her death in 1647, Dame Margaret Heath, widow
of Charles I's Attorney-General Sir Robert Heath, possessed two copies of
Gerard's *Herball*.[13] The commonplace books of Elizabeth Freke, a relative
of Nicolas Culpeper, the other great herbalist of the seventeenth century,
contain several remedies taken from Gerard, suggesting that she was familiar with the work.[14] Symptomatic of their popularity and also their intrinsic
value, editions of Gerard's *Herball* appeared in book sales towards the end
of the century as family libraries were auctioned off.[15] A copy of Johnson's
enlarged 1636 edition was sold for £2 16s by Nathaniel Ranew on 2 December
1678; and the auctioneer Millington singled out another, describing it as
'judiciously coloured, a book very rare and not easily to be parallel'd', in his

catalogue of over 8,000 books prepared in advance of a sale held at Brydge's Coffee House, opposite the Royal Exchange, on 16 June 1684.[16]

Johnson's 'Gerard' became the foremost English work on botany and herbal medicine across the seventeenth century, rivalled only by the publication of Nicolas Culpeper's *Complete Herbal and English Physician* in 1653.[17] There can be little doubt that for those charged during the civil wars with treating soldiers and civilians, Johnson's 'Gerard' was essential reading and much consulted. Yet how it was used, by whom, and in what contexts largely evades the view of the historian, perhaps because consulting this work was so commonplace that it was deemed unworthy of contemporary report.

Placed centre stage here is a single copy of Johnson's extended Gerard's *Herball*. The work is heavily annotated throughout. Most of these annotations take the form of stylized hands known as manicules, a graphic device commonly used by early modern book readers to identify key sections of text.[18] These manicules, and other marginal writings found in the volume, are characteristic of the seventeenth century. In what follows, the early ownership of this *Herball* is reconstructed from the internal evidence found in the book itself. The *Herball* is shown to have been in the possession of a Nottinghamshire gentry family, active in the royalist cause throughout the First Civil War. Analysis of the annotated sections of the *Herball* suggests that it was consulted specifically for the treatment of ailments and conditions commonly associated with siege warfare. Since the location of the family seat can now be identified, a context for the annotation of the herbal is proposed. Through these interpretative stages, it is suggested that this herbal offers a unique perspective on the care of the war-wounded and diseased during the civil wars.

THE *HERBALL* AND ITS SEVENTEENTH-CENTURY PROVENANCE

The copy of Johnson's 'Gerard' that is the subject of this study is in good but imperfect condition. It has lost its decorative frontispiece and the indices that it originally carried are incomplete. Several pages show signs of foxing, possible water damage, and a few insect holes but nothing that challenges the legibility of the text. At some point it has been sensitively rebound in full calf with six raised bands. This was probably the occasion when some of the pages were slightly trimmed and tidied up. The gilt-lettered spine label reads 'Gerard's Herbal 1633' but this is in error, probably caused by the earlier loss of the dated frontispiece. The volume carries several pagination errors that are sufficiently diagnostic to be absolutely certain that this is the second edition of Johnson's amended text published in 1636. Its recent provenance can only be traced back to c.1959.[19]

The volume carries a number of handwritten signatures and names (Figure 6.1). At the base of the title page there is a heavy inscription in a crude gothic

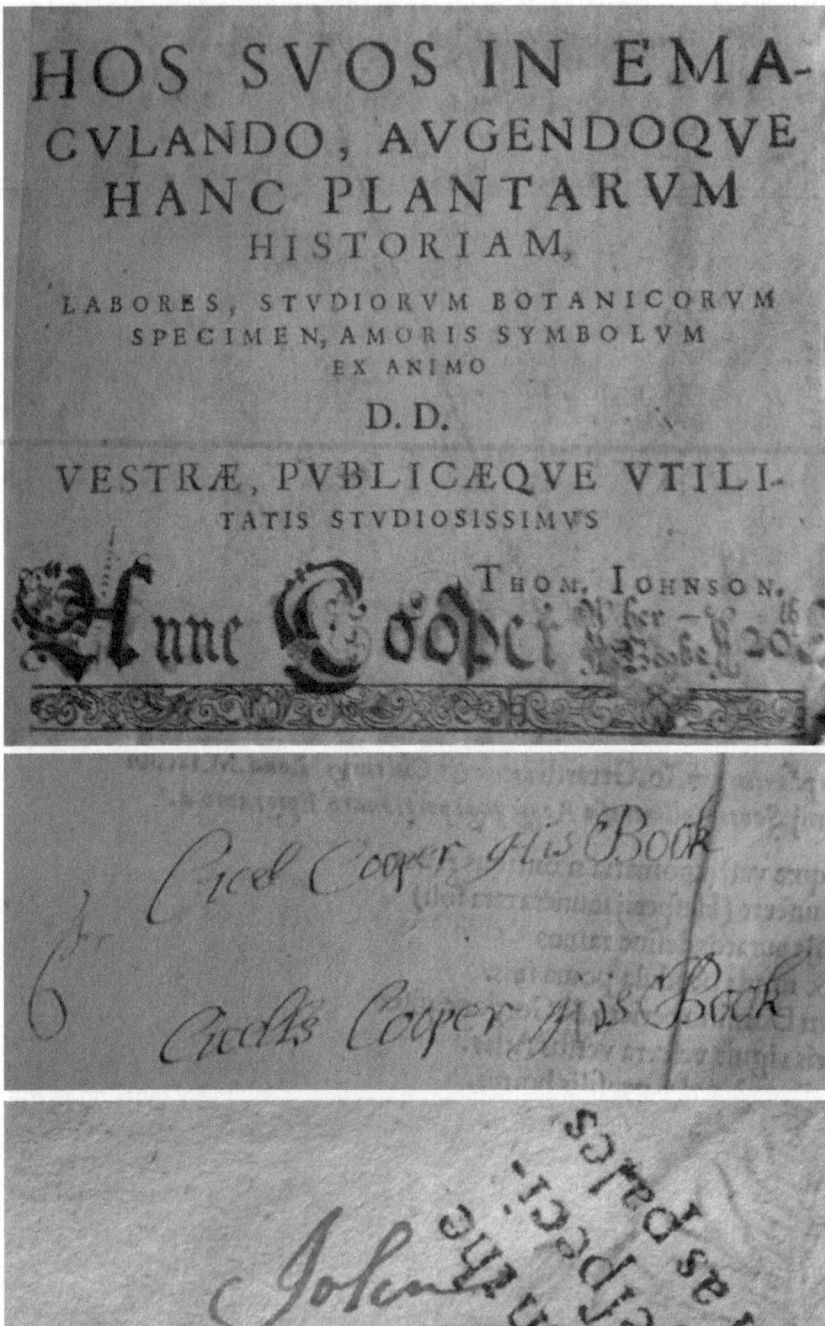

Figure 6.1 Cooper inscriptions found in the *Herball*

script. Unfortunately truncated through trimming, it reads 'Anne Cooper her Booke 20th ...'.[20] The prominent positioning of this inscription and its formal style is highly suggestive of the fact that Anne must have been an early, if not the original, owner. A much smaller inscription in a contemporary seventeenth-century hand, appearing at the top of page one, reads 'Madame Cooper'.[21] It is tempting, but perhaps unwise, to assume that this too refers to Anne; as might the many scribbled initial 'A's which feature in the margins throughout the volume. That this copy of the *Herball* was owned by a woman should come as no surprise. Female ownership of such books was common in the seventeenth century, stemming from the central role that women played as principal household carers. In fact, many surviving copies of this herbal carry female inscriptions.[22]

At the end of Gerard's original preface, two other names appear in this particular copy. These are less formal, but again written in a seventeenth-century hand, perhaps the same hand seen in the 'Madame Cooper' inscription. The inscription reads: 'Cicel Cooper His Book', and set on the line below, 'Cicells Cooper His Book'. Despite the duplication of the name, and the fact that both names are written in the same hand, inscriptions of this kind generally signal a change in ownership and thus point to a Cooper family containing not one but two Cecils. Other names written in the margins appear elsewhere in the book. There are two intriguing *bas-de-page* inscriptions in the same hand, one reading 'Col Thomas', the other 'The place Thos';[23] while the name 'Johnes' recurs in several places together with several initial 'J's.[24]

Cooper is a common surname, but armed with this collection of Christian names, the book can be confidently connected to the Cooper family of Thurgarton in Nottinghamshire. The family's association with the village began in the aftermath of the Dissolution with Henry VIII's grant of the Augustinian Priory of Thurgarton to William Cooper.[25] By the early seventeenth century, the estate had passed, not entirely smoothly, through three generations to Roger Cooper. It was this Roger who was in possession of Thurgarton at the start of the First Civil War. The Nottinghamshire antiquarian Thoroton provides a family tree but this is not without its problems. From it we know that Roger had three sons, Cecil (hereafter Cecil I, probably born in the mid-1620s), John and Roger, as well as one daughter, Anne. John would die in 1672, while Cecil I died three years later in 1675.[26] Cecil I married late to Sarah, daughter of Sir John Hotham, in January 1669. Their union produced a son named Cecil (Cecil II) recorded as being aged four in 1673.[27] It was this Cecil who married Ann Midlemore (baptised 1668), daughter of William Savile of Newton, Lincolnshire in Winkburn church on 6 December 1692.[28] Here then is a Cooper family with multiple generations of Cecils who became head of the household, with siblings christened John and Anne.

On the balance of the evidence, we might propose the book's seventeenth-century provenance: in the possession of Anne, sister of Cecil I, eldest son of Roger Cooper, before passing to her brother at some time (perhaps on her death), thence to his son Cecil II, and which at various times may have been available to Cecil I and Anne's brother John. The most likely date that the book left the possession of the Cooper family is 1677. In March that year Sarah Cooper consented to the Samine and Cooper Bill, allowing trustees to sell lands for payment of debts on behalf of her infant son Cecil.[29] The library catalogue of nearby Southwell Minster coterminously records the donation of the Thurgarton Priory Cartulary and a copy of Sir Walter Raleigh's *History of the World*.[30] Both the manuscript and the book contain the inscription 'The gift of Cecil Cooper Esq'. This feels like the dispersal of the Cooper family library, the reasons for which may be found in the Coopers' debt accrued as a consequence of their involvement in the civil wars.

THE COOPERS OF THURGARTON AND THE CIVIL WARS

In December 1642, Sir Roger Cooper declared for the King.[31] From that moment the fortunes of the family would be closely linked to the successes and failures of the royalist cause. From 1642 to 1644 Roger acted as one of five Commissioners of Array for Nottinghamshire, serving at Newark where the commission was based, but also holding privy sessions at Thurgarton.[32] He fortified his house and garrisoned it with forty men. In December 1644, musketeers under his command ambushed a troop of parliamentary horse on their way to Newark, killing one Captain Heywood. What followed was reported in Lucy Hutchinson's biography of her husband, Colonel John Hutchinson, then governor of Nottingham:

> Hereupon Coll. Thornhagh sent to the governor, and desir'd to borrow some foote to take the house. The governor accordingly lent him three companies who tooke the house, and Sr. Roger Cooper and his brother, and forty men, in it, who were sent prisoners to Nottingham, where, although Sr. Roger Cooper was in greate dread to be put into the governor's hands, whom he had provok'd before upon a private occasion, yet he receiv'd such a civill treatment from him, that he seem'd much moov'd and melted with it. The foote had done all the service, and run all the hazard, in taking the house, yet the booty was all given to the horse.[33]

Ransacked, Thurgarton was sequestered as a consequence of Sir Roger's delinquency. In June 1646 Sir Roger appeared before the Committee for Compounding and in May 1647 before the Committee for the Advancement of Money seeking the restoration of his estate.[34] His fine of £2,256 was accepted by the House of Commons in March 1648 whereupon he was granted pardon and his estate returned. This was confirmed by the House of Lords just over a month later.[35] Raising the fine had come at a cost, however. Sir Roger was forced to sell property in the nearby parishes of Fiskerton, Morton and Bleasby, including Ashwell Hall to Dr Huntingdon Plumtree, a Nottingham physician and member of the parliamentarian county commit-

tee.[36] These sales raised £2,250. But this was not the end of Sir Roger's financial problems, nor their only cause. He was obliged via Articles of Agreement
to pay £1,117 2s to those who had lent money 'for the Use of the Garrison of
Newark' at the end of 1647.[37] Clearly he and his son Cecil I had to resort to
loans: they were both bound to John Hacker of nearby Flintham for repayment of £1,200 in 1648, a sum probably borrowed to cover the additional
demands made by Parliament for the final restoration of the estate.[38] In 1651
this additional fine was reduced to £270, but not before Sir Roger had mortgaged the estate at £2,000 in 1650. He would die in debt six years later.[39]

Cecil I appears to have been an apprentice in Lichfield before the civil
wars and, if Griffith Higg's account of the events of 1643 is accurate, was
involved in the royalist siege of the cathedral close that April.[40] Certainly
he was later listed as a Major of Horse in Colonel Hervey Bagot's regiment
garrisoned in the city.[41] Higg viewed Cecil as 'a man of supreme endeavour
and possessed of great experience in military matters', although nothing is
known about where this might have been gained. Four years later, in July
1648, Cecil I, now a lieutenant-colonel, and his brother John, a captain, were
both taken prisoner at Willoughby-on-the-Wolds but appear to have been at
liberty by the early 1650s.[42] The two brothers next emerge as ringleaders of
the failed Nottinghamshire royalist uprising of March 1655. According to
later testimony, much of the planning for the uprising had taken place at
Thurgarton.[43] Cecil I and John's nocturnal assembly at Rufford in Sherwood
Forest attracted upwards of 300 men. But the conspirators were betrayed and
were forced to abandon their arms and flee. Cecil was arrested and sent to
gaol in Nottingham, later being allowed to leave the country.[44] John escaped,
probably joining other royalist sympathisers in the Low Countries.[45]

John was still abroad in 1658 when his wife, Jane, wrote to Richard
Cromwell, the new Lord Protector, asking for permission for him to return.[46]
Cecil I probably returned that year. He was bound to Sir Thomas Hatton of
Long Stanton, Cambridgeshire for a colossal £10,000,[47] a symptom of the
continuing financial straits that the Cooper family found themselves in, and
the reason, perhaps, why twenty years later his son Cecil II was forced to
disperse their library and with it the family *Herball*.[48] John returned with the
King in 1660. Immediately, the two brothers were rewarded for their loyalty.
Cecil I was named as a Knight of the Royal Oak, although the Order was never
initiated, the Thurgarton estate being valued at £1,000 per annum.[49] John
was appointed Carver to his Majesty.[50] It was on the orders of Cecil I, issued
in the wider context of disarming former parliamentarians, that Governor
Hutchinson's house in Owthorpe was plundered, perhaps in revenge for the
ransacking of the Coopers' Thurgarton home sixteen years previously, even
if Cooper would later be ordered to return what he had taken.[51] Thereafter
the brothers returned to the usual civilian duties of the county gentry: Cecil
I served as a magistrate between 1660 and 1674 and was Deputy Lieutenant
of Nottinghamshire;[52] John acted as Receiver General of the Royal Aid and

Additional Supply, and Collector of Hearth Taxes.[53] Thurgarton, however, was leased out to William Leeke of Wymeswold in 1669.[54]

THE *HERBALL'S* ANNOTATIONS

The Coopers' *Herball* contains 244 marginal annotations in the form of stylised hands known as manicules (Figure 6.2). Establishing how and why they were being used requires an understanding of the internal arrangement of the *Herball* itself. Gerard dedicated a separate chapter to each plant in the

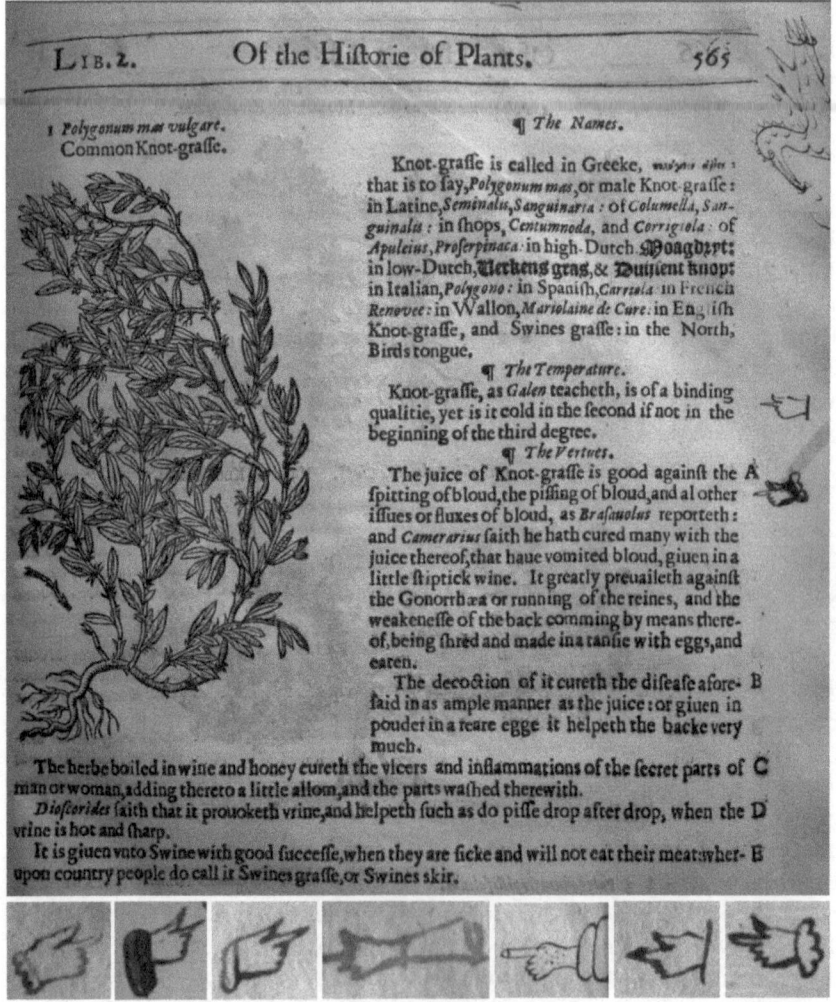

Figure 6.2 Medical conditions identified by the marginal annotations in the *Herball*

Herball, his text often accompanied by a woodcut image. These chapters were then subdivided following a standardised form. Each entry begins with 'The Kindes', a short description of subspecies or, if the plant lacked varieties, with a section called 'The Description' defining the physical attributes of the plant. Where the plant grew and under what conditions were dealt with in 'The Place' and its seasonal flowering or fruiting laid out under 'The Time'. The next section, 'The Names' dealt with the etymology of the name, and its Latin and 'vulgar' variants. There then followed two medico-philosophical sections: first a short section on 'The Temperatures' that dealt with the elemental and humoral qualities of the plant (hot, cold, wet, moist); and finally a section, often the longest of all, on 'The Vertues', that outlined the ailments and conditions the plant was most effective in treating.

177 plant and tree species are singled out by the manicules in the *Herball*. Most relate to plants commonly found in the English countryside; but exotics are also identified such as the Frankincense and the Balsam Tree.[55] Both were available to English apothecaries from the early seventeenth century as a consequence of increased overseas trade, and may here indicate that the annotator was expecting not simply to collect medicinal plants in the field, but also to purchase some.[56] In some instances several individual hands are used to indicate multiple sections of text under a single plant heading. Three hands, for instance, isolate passages in the chapters on Yarrow or Nose-Bleed (*Achillea millefolium*) and Land Plantain (*Plantago major*) respectively.[57] The greater majority of the manicules point to text in the final section on the plants' virtues. This, above everything, indicates that the annotator's purpose was medicinal not botanical. Such an impression is strengthened by the significant number of other manicules which point to 'The Temperature' of plants, since the elemental qualities of plants formed the basis of all early modern medicine. Thus the annotator was clearly interested in the fact that Knot-grasses (*Polygonum aviculare*) were 'cold in the second degree and dry in the third, astringent and making thicke'; and that 'Wortle berries [*Vaccinium uliginosum*] are cold and dry, hauing withall a certain thinnesse of parts and substance, with certaine binding quality joyned'.[58] That the annotator had some *a priori* knowledge of the properties of plants is indicated by their correction of the qualities of the Bastard Floure de Luce (*Iris palustris*).[59] The text, which erroneously stated the plant to be 'cold and dry in the third degree', has been underlined by the annotator and against which 'hot & dry' has been written in the margin.

In the case of those manicules directing attention to the temperature of plants, the shortness of the original text leaves little doubt that this was the information intended to be noted. But the same does not hold true for many of the manicules pointing to parts of the 'Vertues' section where Gerard's verbosity introduces considerable uncertainty. Two examples might stand as illustration. The paragraph highlighted by the manicule used in the entry for Rhubarb (*Rheum rhabarbarum*) reads:

Rhubarb is commended by Dioscorides against windinesse, weaknesse of the stomack and all griefes thereof, Convulsions, diseases of the Spleen, liuer, and Kidnies, gripings, and inward gnawings of the guts, infirmities of the bladder and chest, swellings about the heart, diseases in the matrix [womb], pain in the huckle bones [hip bone or astragalus], spitting of bloud, shortnesse of breath, yexing [belching], or the hicket [hiccupping], the bloudy flux [dysentery], the laske [diarrhoea] proceeding of raw humors, fits in the agues [fevers], and against the bitings of venomous beasts.[60]

That for Herb Twopence (*Lysimachia nummularia*): 'The juice drunke in wine is good for the bloudy flix and all other issues of bloud in man or woman; the weaknesses and loosnesse of the belly and laske, it helpeth those that vomit bloud, & the whites [non-venereal vaginal discharge] in such as haue them.'[61] The range of ailments and conditions listed here thus makes it impossible to isolate the precise medical issue or issues that the annotator had mind to identify. Indeed, in the case of Herb Twopence, even the gender of the potential patient is thrown into doubt.

Elsewhere, however, there is less ambiguity. Again two examples might stand as archetypes. Of the Daffodil (*Narcissus*), the manicule isolates the following section: 'Galen saith, That the roots of Narcissus haue such wonderfull qualities in drying, that they confound and glew together very great wounds, yea and such gashes or cuts as happen about the veins, sinues, and tendons. They haue also a certaine clensing and attracting facultie.'[62] That for tobacco (*Nicotiana tabacum*):

I doe make hereof an excellent Balme to cure deep wounds and punctures made by some narrow sharpe point of weapon. Which Balsame doth bring vp the flesh from the bottome verie speedily, and also heale simple cuts in the flesh according to the first intention, that is, to glew or soder the lips of the wound together, not procuring matter or corruption to it, as is commonly seene in the healing of wounds.[63]

A degree of clarity emerges if all ailments mentioned in sections of the text identified by manicules are tabulated in a bar chart (Figure 6.3). The largest number (n=68) point to paragraphs including references to wound healing. Bloody flux and spitting blood (n=48 and n=46 respectively) together with bleeding (n=28) also stand out; and to a slightly lesser extent ulcers and the laske (n=23 and n=22 respectively). Women's courses (n=16) form a minor spike but in Gerard's text these are almost always mentioned alongside other issues of blood. Everyday ailments such as eye complaints (n=4), coughing (n=4) and flatulence (n=2) feature far less prominently even than pissing blood (n=9) and dysentery (n=8).

What is clear, however, is that the annotator had not systematically trawled the *Herball* for all references to particular conditions. The original index notes eighty relevant entries for the 'bloody flux', for instance, yet only forty-eight are highlighted; seventy-three cures for the 'laske' are itemised, yet only twenty-two are identified by manicules;[64] dysentery is indexed twelve times

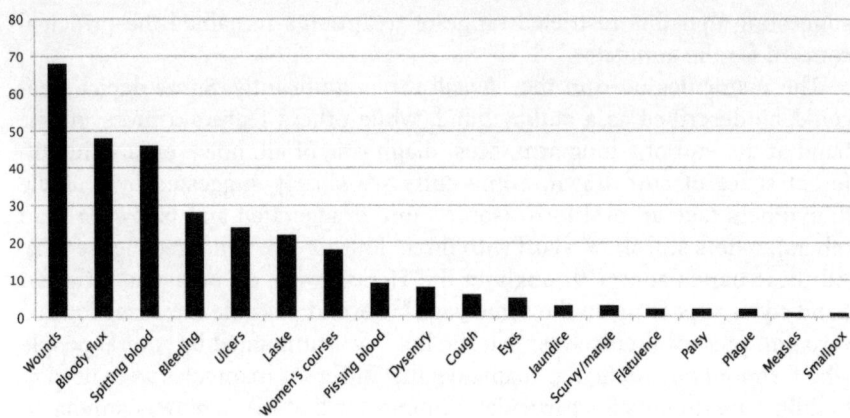

Figure 6.3 Examples of manicules and their use in highlighting sections of text

but only eight are picked up by the annotator. The annotations thus appear rather *ad hoc* and certainly do not appear to have been generated simply by consulting the index.[65] The greatest degree of consistency shown by the annotator relates to their selection of plants said to be cold and dry nature. Beyond those already mentioned, the annotator notes Hawke-Weed (*Hieracium*),[66] Water-Docke (*Rumex hydrolapathum*),[67] Bistort or Snake-Weed (*Persicaria bistorta*),[68] Water and Land Plantaine (*Plantago*),[69] Ribwort (*Plantago lanceolate*),[70] Sea Buck-Horne (*Hippophae*) and Bucke-Horne Plantaines or Harts-Horne (*Plantago lanceolate*),[71] Rampions or Wild Bell-Floures (*Campanula rapunculus*),[72] Willow-Herbe or Loose-Strife (*Epilobium*),[73] Cranes Bill (*Pelargonium*),[74] Pulse,[75] Cloud-Berry (*Rubus chamaemorus*),[76] and tellingly the Medlar Tree (*Mespilus germanica*) which flourishes in Nottinghamshire.[77]

The annotator's interest in cold and dry plants appears to be revealed in four instances. Of Wild Horehound (*Marrubium vulgare*), the text reads: 'This is of singular vse (as most of the herbes of this kinde are) to keep wounds from inflammation and speedily to heale them up, as also to say all fluxes and defluctions, hauing a drying and moderate astrictive faculty.'[78] Of Silver Knapweed (*Centaurea*): 'The seeds and leaues are astringent, wherof the decoction of them is cast up in Dysenteries and into purulent eares, and the leaues applud in manner of a pultis are good to hinder the blacknesse of the eyes occasioned by a blow, and to stop the flowing of bloud.'[79] Of Holly Roses or Cistus: 'the leaues and the first buds being beaten do only dry and bind, in such sort as they may close up ulcers, and joine together green wounds'.[80] And of Goat's Thorn (*Astragalus gummifer*): 'it doth consolidate or glew together sinues that be cut: but the root boiled in wine haue that facultie specially, being given to those that haue any griefe or hurt in the sinues'.[81] In short, then, cold and dry plants were most useful to treat the kinds of ailments otherwise picked out by the majority of other manicules, further suggesting that this restricted range of treatments remained the principal concern for the annotator.

The manicules used in the *Herball* vary significantly. Some depict what could be described as a stubby hand, while others feature a more gracile hand at the end of a long arm. Most diagnostic of all, however, are the different styles of cuff drawn. Some cuffs are simply suggested by a single line; others take an oval form (some more exaggerated and billowing than others); others still show a cuff with three, four, or five frills (see Figure 6.2). All these hands appear throughout the *Herball* with, on occasion, different hand styles appearing on the same page.[82] Several possible scenarios for this variation present themselves: that the book was annotated by several people who favoured one particular manicule; that different manicules were used to highlight treatments for particular ailments; or that the book was annotated on several occasions by the same individual who used different manicules on each occasion. It is ultimately impossible to be certain which, if any, of these scenarios accounts for what is found in this *Herball*. But it is possible to rule some out. There is no consistency, for instance, in the use of manicules used to highlight text containing references to certain ailments. Menstruation, for example, is picked out by the long-armed, oval-cuffed, and frilly-cuffed hands.[83] The same is true for references to spitting blood, which are isolated by an even greater range of manicules.[84] Explored from the other side, it is clear that no correlation can be discerned between a use of a particular manicule and a certain ailment: issues referred to in the extended texts identified by the long-armed manicule include drowsiness, eye problems, bleeding, inflammation, gall stones, watery humors, the bloody flux, spitting blood, ulcers, wounds, dysentery, ruptures and bad stomachs.[85] On the balance of the evidence, one annotator using different manicules haphazardly, seems most likely.

PLACING THE *HERBALL* AND THE ANNOTATION MOMENT

Wounds, bloody flux, spitting blood, bleeding, ulcers and laske stand out in the annotated sections of the *Herball*. To a lesser, but perhaps no less significant, extent so do pissing blood and dysentery. Individually, none of these medical matters would merit comment. Each might result from quotidian activities, poor food hygiene or everyday contagion. Found together, however, they appear to point in a very specific direction.

Retrospective diagnoses should be avoided, but the likely modern medical afflictions which the symptoms highlighted in the *Herball* suggest, and the conditions under which these are most likely to occur, might be suggested. Bloody flux is a form of bacillary dysentery whose transmission is feco-oral. Laske appears in two forms: red laske, a 'stomach affliction involving diarrhea with mucus and blood in stools'; and white laske which equates to 'lientery, diarrhea with undigested passage of food in feces'.[86] Together with those generic entries for dysentery found in the *Herball*, sixty-eight manicules point to these related conditions. Dysentery in all these forms presents in those affected as a high fever with intestinal haemorrhaging and diarrhoea. The disease most commonly originates in places where large groups of people live close together in poor sanitation. These are the very same conditions, exacerbated by malnutrition, in which tuberculosis, one physical symptom of which is spitting blood (forty-six manicules), together with scrofula and smallpox which both manifest as skin ulcers (twenty-two manicules), are able to spread easily.[87] This is true also for typhus, spread from person to person by body lice, ticks, mites and fleas, and which results in headaches, fever, rashes, nausea and vomiting, abdominal pain, diarrhoea, joint and muscle pain and coughing. Tellingly, a further symptom of typhus is the passing of urinary blood.

When combined with the annotator's interest in healing wounds, all internal evidence from the *Herball* points to the book being used to treat the war-wounded and those suffering from the deprivations of living in cramped and unhygienic surroundings. Diseases and contagions of the kind identified were omnipresent threats for both civilians and soldiers throughout the civil wars.[88] The great killers of the age were plague, typhus and tuberculosis.[89] Towns where garrisons swelled the usual number of inhabitants and who stabled their horses within their confines, provided the perfect conditions in which epidemics might spread quickly, and to deadly effect. Plague affected Oxford throughout the 1640s, Banbury in 1644, Bristol in 1645 and Newark in 1646.[90] Typhus epidemics are recorded at Oxford and Reading in 1643, and Tiverton in 1644, where burial registers mention the 'sweating sickness' as cause of death.[91] The plight of these places was worsened when subjected to siege for prolonged periods. The sordid conditions in which besieging forces or armies on the move were forced to live meant that they too were not immune from the same contagions: typhus, dubbed 'camp fever' by contemporaries, was a particular threat to the soldiery during the winter months.[92]

Given the *Herball*'s provenance – in the possession of a staunchly royalist family, whose house was garrisoned for the royalist cause during the early 1640s – the circumstantial evidence strongly indicates that its annotation was occasioned by the plight of the townspeople and garrison of nearby Newark. From January 1643 through to May 1646 the town was permanently garrisoned, doubling and on occasion tripling the number of people in the town. Overcrowding was intensified by the clearance of properties around the defences, forcing more people to live or to be billeted in fewer properties; while the stabling of horses caused sanitary problems for the town's authorities.[93] The population fell prey to typhus across 1642–46, attested by the rising number of adult burials recorded during the winter months in the registers of St Mary's.[94] The epidemic reached its peak during the period October 1644–February 1645 but was a constant presence. Against this backdrop of disease, the town was besieged on three occasions. If the first siege of Newark was short-lived (27–28 February 1643), the second (29 February–21 March 1644) and third (26 November 1645–8 May 1646) sieges were longer and drawn out. Contemporary descriptions make clear the devastation of the parliamentarian bombardment and the damage to life and property during both sieges. They also make clear the violence of the skirmishes that took place beyond Newark's defences as the royalists sought to break these sieges, and as the parliamentarians sought to tighten their grip around the town in 1645.[95]

The impact of these sieges was felt throughout the surrounding country-side. From the constables' accounts for the village of Upton, six miles from Newark and five miles by the same road from Thurgarton House, it is clear that significant numbers of injured soldiers on both sides of the conflict were moving up and down the road to Nottingham during 1644. In that year these accounts record six separate payments to sick soldiers totalling 2s 10d and nine entries for payments made to lame soldiers amounting to 2s 7d. Precise dates for these payments are not provided but they do offer other details: 4d was given to 'a lame Souldier which came from Winfeld Manner [Wingfield Manor, Derbyshire]' and 6d was given to 'a Sicke Souldier which had been prisoner at Bouser [Bolsover, Derbyshire]'. The majority who received payments appear to have passed quickly through the village. But others stopped to convalesce: 10d, for example, was 'Payed for a Souldier which did lie Sicke at Kerkes [Kirk's Inn] for his lodging & meat & drinke', while 4d was accounted 'For Sacke for a trooper which did lye Sicke at John Kitchin his house'. Tellingly, one of the last entries for the year notes 4d 'Given to a lame Souldier which came from Newarke'.[96]

There is one further reason to suspect that the *Herball* was annotated in this year too. Pointing in this direction is the annotator's lack of inter-est in the treatment of plague. Plague was brought to Newark from Bristol by Prince Rupert's troops in advance of the third siege. In the spring and summer months of 1646, following the end of the siege, the disease was spread with devastating effect to neighbouring villages by the newly liberated townsfolk.[97] It seems implausible, had the *Herball* been annotated during or following this siege, that plague treatments would have been ignored.

CONCLUSION

In contrast to the early years of the civil war, when Sir Roger Cooper was active in Newark as a Commissioner of Array, and their house served as a royalist garrison, the Coopers largely disappear from view in Thurgarton in the years following the ransacking of the house in December 1644. The wording of the pardon issued in 1648 indicates that Sir Roger and his sons were forced to quit their estate after its sequestration.[98] It may be that the family was forced to take up temporary residence in Newark. Sir Roger was certainly in the town on its surrender in 1646.[99]

The precise circumstances that prompted the annotation of the Coopers' *Herball* can never be known. But it is suggested here, based on the internal evidence from the *Herball* itself, and from what is known about the Cooper family's wartime activities, that its annotation was most likely occasioned by the second siege of Newark in 1644 and was done at their family home in Thurgarton. If this was indeed the case, then the book provides a unique insight into how those caught up in the siege were treated for the wounds they had received and the diseases they had contracted. It opens up the possibility that Thurgarton House briefly served as a royalist hospital as well as garrison; just as Yarnton Manor, four miles from Oxford, was requisitioned for similar purposes between 1643 and 1645.[100] And it suggests that as well as typhus, whose effects can be traced with some certainty through the burial registers of Newark, and plague (about which the historical sources have so much to say), dysentery was an ever-present and grave issue faced by the people and garrison of Newark. The *Herball*, it would seem, stands as a witness to the fact that during the second siege, the town was ravaged from within by a suite of contagious diseases, not just typhus, and from without by parliamentarian bombardment. To paraphrase the witness to the third siege, Newark in 1644 appears to have been more miserable, more stinking and more infected than historians have hitherto estimated.[101]

NOTES

1 *A Description of the Siege of Basing Castle Kept by the Lord Marquisse of Winchester* (Oxford, Leonard Lichfield, 1644; reprinted Newbury: Walter James Buckley, 1880), p. 16.

2 T. Johnson, *Iter plantarum investigationis ergo susceptum a decem socijs, in agrum cantianum, anno. Dom. 1629. Iulii. 13. Ericetum Hamstedianum sive Plantarum ibi crescentium observatio habita, anno eodem I. Augusti* (London, 1629). His Kentish study would be updated and enlarged three years later: T. Johnson, *Descriptio itineris plantarum investigationis ergô suscepti, in agrum cantianum anno Dom. 1632 Et enumeratio plantarum in Ericeto Hampstediano locisq[ue] vicinis crescentium* (London, 1632).

3 T. Johnson, *Mercurius botanicus. Sive Plantarum gratiâ suscepti itineris, anno M. DC.XXXIV. descriptio Cum earum nominibus Latinis, & Anglicis, &c. Huic accessit de thermis Bathonicis tractatus* (London, 1634).

4 C. J. King, 'Thomas Johnson', *ODNB*.

5 J. Gerard, *The Herball, or, Generall Historie of Plantes. Gathered by Iohn Gerarde of London Master in Chirurgerie Very Much Enlarged and Amended by Thomas Iohnson Citizen and Apothecarye of London* (London: Adam Islip, Joice Norton and Richard Whitakers, 1633, 2nd edn, 1636).

6 J. Gerard, *The Herball, or, Generall Historie of Plantes. Gathered by Iohn Gerarde of London Master in Chirurgerie* (London: Iohn Norton, 1597).

7 R. Dodonaei, *Stirpium historiae pemptades sex sive libri XXX* (Antwerp: Christophori Plantini, 1583). This work was an extended Latin version of Dodoen's earlier *Crujde Boeck, in den welcken die gheheele historie, dat es tgheslacht, tfatsoen, naem, natuere, cracht ende werckinghe van den Cruyden* (Antwerp: Jan van der Loe, 1554). Gerard was responsible for some additions: notably the potato and sunflowers, North American plants that Gerard had had imported and which he then cultivated in his own London garden.

8 Tabernaemontanus, Jacobus Theodorus, *Eicones plantarum* (Frankfurt: Nicolaus Bassaeus, 1590).

9 L. Knight, *Of Books and Botany in Early Modern England: Sixteenth-Century Plants and Print Culture* (Farnham: Ashgate, 2009), pp. 69–110; M. Willes, *The Making of the English Gardener: Plants, Books and Inspiration, 1550–1660* (New Haven, CT and London: Yale University Press, 2011), pp. 91, 113.

10 F. J. Anderson, *The Herbal of John Gerard: An Illustrated History of the Herbals* (New York: Columbia University Press, 1977), pp. 218–26; A. Arber, 'Gerard', in W. T. Stearn (ed.), *Herbals. Their Origins and Evolution: A Chapter in the History of Botany* (Cambridge: Cambridge University Press, 1938, 3rd edn, 1988), pp. 129–32.

11 J. T. Cliffe, *The World of the Country House in Seventeenth-Century England* (New Haven, CT and London: Yale University Press, 1999), p. 167. One copy of the 1636 edition, recently put up for sale by Bonhams of London, carries a handwritten inscription: 'Jeffrey Thomas at the Wheat Sheaf in Common [Covent] Garden in York Street Mercer. Precium 4s besides the cover. Bought of [sic] William Adderton Stationer at the 3 Golden birds in Duck-Laine.' The bookseller, William Adderton, was active at his shop, the 'Three Golden Falcons' between 1628–71, suggesting that this unbound copy was thus bought as new by Thomas around the time of its release: H. R. Plomer, *A Dictionary of Booksellers and Printers Who Were at Work in England, Scotland and Ireland from 1641 to 1667* (London: Blades, East and Blades, 1907), p. 1.

12 G. Parry, 'The great picture of Lady Anne Clifford', in D. Howarth (ed.), *Art and Patronage in the Caroline Courts* (Cambridge: Cambridge University Press, 1993), pp. 202–19; G. Parry, *The Seventeenth Century: The Intellectual and Cultural Context of English Literature 1603–1700* (London: Routledge, 2013), p. 80; N. Wheale, *Writing and Society: Literacy, Print and Politics in Britain, 1590–1660* (London: Routledge, 1999), p. 127. The triptych is dated to 1646.

13 Willes, *The Making of the English Gardener*, p. 235.

14 R. A. Anselment (ed.), *The Remembrances of Elizabeth Freke 1671–1714* (Camden Society, 5th series, 18, 2001); E. Leong, '"Herbals she peruseth": reading medicine in early modern England', *Renaissance Studies*, 28:4 (2014), 556–78.

15 The costs of publication meant that the herbal only went into three editions. As Leong, 'Herbals' noted, by the end of the century these were sought after items.

16 J. Lawler, *Book Auctions in Seventeenth-Century England (1676–1700)* (London: Elliot Stock, 1898), pp. 69, 125.

17 N. Culpeper, *Culpeper's Complete Herbal and English Physician* (London: J. Gleave and Son, 1653).

18 W. H. Sherman, *Used Books: Marking Readers in Renaissance England*

(Philadelphia, PA: University of Pennsylvania Press, 2008), chapter 2, 'Towards a history of the manicule', pp. 25–52.

19 The book is currently in private hands, part of the library of Professor Michael and Dr Elizabeth Jones.

20 CH, title page.

21 CH, p. 1.

22 R. Laroche, *Medical Authority and Englishwomen's Herbal Texts, 1550–1650* (Farnham: Ashgate, 2009). At the time of writing, a copy of the 1636 edition was being offered for sale on the internet by Horden House Rare Books (Potts Point, New South Wales, Australia) described as carrying a '17th-century signature of Elizabeth Taylor of Wimbish Hall [Essex].'

23 CH, pp. 330, 332. It is common in the volume for the annotator to pick phrases from the page to repeat. This appears to be the case here: 'The Place', noting where plants might be found and under what conditions they grow best, is a standard subheading in each description of each plant. The clearest example is a rendering of 'Ducks meat' found at CH, p. 829.

24 CH, pp. 133, 639, 794, 838, 923.

25 14 and 16 June 1538: *Letters and Papers, Foreign and Domestic, Henry VIII, vol. 13, part I, Jan–July 1538* (London: HMSO, 1892), pp. 439, 442.

26 Cecil I's gravestone survives in Thurgarton parish church recording his death on 9 December 1675. In 1677, Thomas Shipman (1632–80) dedicated, presumably as a posthumous tribute, a poem entitled 'The Badge of Good-Fellowship' and subtitled 'Vpon Scarlet-Faces, Rosie-Cheeks, and Ruby Noses' to his friend Cecil Cooper (T. Shipman, *Carolina, or; Loyal Poems* (London: Samuel Heyrick, 1683), pp. 171–3). With thanks to Ellis Morgan for bringing this poem to my attention.

27 Parliamentary Archives, HL/PO/JO/10/1/367: 8 March 1677 and *CJ*, IX, pp. 420, 423, 432, 436, 453, 457.

28 Nottinghamshire Parish Registers: Marriages at Winkburn 1553 to 1773: www.nottshistory.org.uk/winkburn/parishregisters/registers3a.html (accessed 27 November 2016).

29 Parliamentary Archives, HL/PO/JO/10/1/367: 8 March 1677 and *CJ*, IX, pp. 420, 423, 432, 436, 453, 457.

30 T. Foulds (ed.), *The Thurgarton Cartulary* (Stamford: Paul Watkins, 1994), p. cxcvi.

31 Roger had been knighted on 16 August 1624 at Derby: J. Nichols, *The Progresses, Processions, and Magnificent Festivities of King James the First*, 4 vols (London: J. B. Nichols, 1828), IV, p. 995.

32 M. Bennett, 'The Nottinghamshire Justices and the social order, 1604–1652', *The Nottinghamshire Historian*, 47 (1991), 7–15; M. Bennett, 'The royalist war effort in the North Midlands, 1642–1646' (PhD thesis, University of Loughborough, 1986).

33 L. Hutchinson, *Memoirs of the Life of Colonel Hutchinson* (London: Longman, Hurst, Rees, and Orme, 1806), p. 240.

34 'Cases before the Committee: June 1646', in M. A. E. Green (ed.), *Calendar of the Committee for Compounding (Domestic), 1643–1660*, 5 vols (London, 1890), II, pp. 1324–5; 'Cases brought before the committee: May 1647', in M. A. E. Green

(ed.), *Calendar of the Committee for the Advance of Money (Domestic), 1642–1656*, 3 vols (London, 1888), II, pp. 805–6.

35 March 1648: CJ, V, p. 9; 15 April 1648: LJ, X, pp. 199–200.

36 NAO, DD 2B 2/17–51.

37 NAO, D 48.74/32. 29 December 1647: '"A partickler of the publicke debts at Newarke": A Schedule or Particuliar of all such knowne Debts entered into by the Parties hereafter named for the Use of the Garrison of Newark and now agreed to bee payd by those said partyes according to certain Articles of Agreement made amongst them'.

38 NAO, CA 3422, p. 17: 17 March 1648.

39 Bennett, 'Royalist war effort', p. 279.

40 N. Ellis and I. Atherton, 'Griffith Higg's account of the sieges of and iconoclasm at Lichfield Cathedral in 1643', *Midland History*, 34:2 (2009), 233–45 at 244, 69n; P. R. Newman, *Royalist Officers in England and Wales, 1642–1660* (New York: Garland Publishing, 1981), p. 85.

41 Bennett, 'Royalist war effort', p. 345.

42 E. W. Hensman, 'The East Midlands and the Second Civil War, May to July, 1648', *Transactions of the Royal Historical Society*, 6 (1923), 126–59 at 154.

43 'The examination of George Clayton, March 13, 1654', in T. Birch (ed.), *A Collection of the State Papers of John Thurloe Esq*, 7 vols (London: Thomas Woodward, 1742), III, pp. 228–9; 'The examination of John Baggelow servant to Mr. John Cooper, of Thurgaston, taken the 14th day of March, 1654. before col. Berry and captain Needham', in Birch (ed.), *A Collection of the State Papers of John Thurloe*, III, pp. 241–2.

44 J. Hunter, *Familiae Minorum Gentium* (Publications of the Harleian Society, 40, 1896), p. 1230.

45 A. C. Wood, *Nottinghamshire in the Civil War* (Oxford: Clarendon Press, 1937, reprinted 1971), p. 169; Birch (ed.), *A Collection of the State Papers of John Thurloe*, III, pp. 261–76, and IV, pp. 474–88.

46 NAO, CA 3431 f19v: Statute Merchant Bond registered at Nottingham, 18 February 1658 to be repaid 20 April.

47 www.historicalresources.myzen.co.uk/BONDS/statutes2.html (accessed 26 November 2016), CA3431, fo. 19v. (18 February 1658). It was also recorded that in 1652 Cecil Cooper was bound to Henry Gilbert of Lockoe and Gilbert Ward of Tickhill, Derbyshire for £3,000: NAO, CA3426, p. 15 (4 March 1652).

48 These facts support the observations of antiquarian Robert Thoroton, a contemporary of Cecil Cooper, on the family fortunes: 'Sir Roger Cooper, a worthy honest gentleman, whose fidelity and constancy to the royalist interest weakened his fortunes, so that Cecill Cooper, esquire, his son, will have too hard a task to make his house and demesnes intirely his own': J. Thoresby, *Thoroton's History of Nottinghamshire*, 3 vols (Nottingham, 1796), III, p. 59.

49 J. Burke, *A Geneaological and Heraldic History of the Commoners of Great Britain* (London: Henry Colburn, 1835), I, pp. 688–94 at p. 691.

50 'A proclamation of both houses of parliament for proclayming of his Majesty King of England, Scotland, France, & Ireland, Defender of the Faith etc.', in Sir Edward Walker, *A Circumstantial Account of the Preparations for the Coronation of his Majesty King Charles the Second* (London: T. Baker, 1820), p. 13.

51 Hutchinson, *Memoirs*, pp. 385–6.
52 *Ibid.*, p. 440.
53 *Calendar of Treasury Books*, Volume 2, 1667–68; *Calendar of Treasury Books*, Volume 3, 1669–72.
54 Derbyshire Record Office, D231M/E5187.
55 CH, pp. 1426, 1529. On the Balsam Tree, Gerard can be found at his withering best. The annotator notes, indeed was perhaps amused by, the following section: 'The marvellous effects it [the Balsam Tree] worketh in new and green wounds, were here too long to set down, and also superfluous; concerning the skilful Surgeon, whom it most concernes, knoweth the use thereof; and as for the beggarly Quakesaluers, Runnagates, and knavish Mountibankes, we are not willing to instruct them in things so far above their reach, capacities, and worthinesse.'
56 P. Wallis, 'Exotic drugs and English medicine: England's drug trade, *c.*1550– *c.*1800', *LSE Working Papers*, No. 143/10 (2010).
57 CH, pp. 1073–4.
58 CH, pp. 568, 1419.
59 CH, p. 51.
60 CH, p. 395.
61 CH, p. 631.
62 CH, p. 132.
63 CH, p. 360.
64 The annotator, for instance, does not pick up references to Laske under the entries for Sea Rush Grasses, Barley and Darnell to take examples from the first hundred pages of the *Herball*.
65 Since, in its current state, the book does not include 'The table, wherein is contained the Nature, Vertue, and Dangers of all the Herbes, Trees and Plantes, of which are spoken in this present Herball', that lists their value against particular ailments, this may suggest that the Coopers' herbal never had such an index. This would not be that unusual since the herbal could be bought loose leaved. When issued in 1633, Johnson's first edition of Gerard sold at 48s bound and 42s 6d unbound: A Sim, *The Tudor Housewife* (Stroud: The History Press, 2006), p. 96.
66 CH, p. 300.
67 CH, p. 391
68 CH, p. 400.
69 CH, pp. 418, 421.
70 CH, p. 422.
71 CH, p. 428.
72 CH, p. 456
73 CH, p. 480.
74 CH, p. 936.
75 CH, p. 1210.
76 CH, p. 1420.
77 CH, p. 1455.
78 CH, p. 697.
79 CH, p. 732.
80 CH, p. 1281.

81 CH, p. 1330.

82 Variations on the frilly-cuffed hand, for instance, appear on CH, pp. 3, 18, 67, 72, 52, 279, 285, 430, 541, 565, 632, 633, 681, 715, 811, 842, 856, 884, 901, 1012, 1073, 1078, 1097, 1128, 1150, 1202, 1263, 1281, 1303, 1325, 1326, 1330, 1341, 1367, 1379, 1420, 1431, 1432, 1451, 1455, 1471, 1475, 1499, 1524 and 1529.

83 CH, pp. 355, 413, 419 and 1116 (long-armed); pp. 895, 949, 1072, 1325, 1328, 1373, 1452 and 1564 (oval-cuffed); pp. 1475, 1499 and 1524 (frilly-cuffed).

84 CH, *passim*.

85 E.g. CH, pp. 355, 370, 407, 413, 419, 421, 425, 480, 1046, 1047, 1116, and 1518.

86 J. Norri, *Dictionary of Medical Vocabulary in English, 1375–1550: Body Parts, Sicknesses, Instruments and Medicinal Preparations* (London: Routledge, 2016), p. 584.

87 Tuberculosis or White Plague is thought to have accounted for 20 per cent of deaths in England and Wales c.1650: R. J. Dubos and J. Dubos, *The White Plague: Tuberculosis, Man and Society* (Boston, MA: Little, Brown & Co., 1952), p. 8.

88 B. Donagan, 'The casualties of war: treatment of the dead and wounded in the English Civil War', in I. Gentles, J. Morrill and B. Worden (eds), *Soldiers, Writers and Statesmen of the English Revolution* (Cambridge: Cambridge University Press, 1998), pp. 114–32, at p. 121.

89 It has been estimated that 20 per cent of deaths in London during the seventeenth century can be attributed to tuberculosis.

90 J. A. Dils, 'Epidemics, mortality and the Civil War in Berkshire, 1642–46', *Southern History*, 11 (1989), 40–52; I. Roy, 'The English Civil War and English society', *War and Society: A Yearbook of Military History*, 1 (1975), pp. 24–43.

91 This is challenged by Shrewsbury who believes this to have been an outbreak of bubonic plague: J. F. D. Shrewsbury, *A History of Bubonic Plague in the British Isles* (Cambridge: Cambridge University Press, 1970, reprinted 2005), p. 407.

92 Typhus was otherwise described in contemporary sources as 'spotted fever'. Donagan suggests that the 'New disease' that spread through Fairfax's army in 1645 and the 'ordinary raging disease' that affected Maurice's army may also have been typhus: Donagan, 'The casualties of war', p. 121.

93 S. B. Jennings, *'These Uncertaine Tymes': Newark and the Civilian Experience of the Civil Wars, 1640–1660* (Nottingham: Nottinghamshire County Council, 2009), p. 45.

94 S. B. Jennings, '"A miserable, stinking, infected town": pestilence, plague and death in a Civil War garrison, Newark 1640–1649', *Midland History*, 28 (2003), 51–70.

95 BL, Thomason E39(8), *A Brief Relation of the Siege of Newark*, 26 March (London, 1644); *A Copie of Colonell Rossiter's Letter to the Lords and Commons. Commissioners at Lincoln* (5 March, 1645); Jennings, *'These Uncertaine Tymes'*.

96 M. Bennett (ed.), *A Nottinghamshire Village in War and Peace: The Accounts of the Constables of Upton 1640–1666* (Thoroton Society Record Series, 39, 1995), pp. 13–23.

97 S. B. Jennings, 'The anatomy of a Civil War plague in a rural parish: East Stoke, Nottinghamshire, 1646', *Midland History*, 40:2 (2015), 201–19.

98 March 1648: *CJ*, V, p. 9; 15 April 1648: *LJ*, X, pp. 199–200.

99 'Cases before the Committee: June 1646', in Green (ed.), *Calendar of the Committee for Compounding*, II, pp. 1324–5.

100 M. Toynbee (ed.), *The Papers of Captain Henry Stevens, Waggon-Master-General to King Charles I* (Oxfordshire Record Society, 42, 1961), p. 19.

101 T. Bailey, *Annals of Nottinghamshire: History of the County of Nottingham including the Borough*, 4 vols (Nottingham: Simpkin, Marshall and Co., 1853), II, p. 763.

Part III

The hidden human costs

Chapter 7

The third army: wandering soldiers and the negotiation of parliamentary authority, 1642–51

David J. Appleby

Harassed officials struggling to cope with the burdens of civil war might well have empathised with the old German proverb which states that 'war leaves a country with three armies: one of cripples, one of mourners, and one of thieves'.[1] The wars in Charles I's three kingdoms devoured some 540,000 human beings and spat out many more half-chewed.[2] Thousands of civilian refugees, maimed soldiers and war widows trod the roads of England and Wales. Churchwardens routinely provided financial assistance to facilitate their onward journey. At the same time, parish officials had to deal with a more menacing figure: the so-called 'wandering soldier'. These individuals could be disbanded veterans or escaped prisoners-of-war, but were very often deserters. Wandering soldiers were unsupervised, generally able-bodied, and very often armed. Whether such men posed a genuine threat to local communities will be considered below, but it is clear that there were a great many of them, and that they presented the authorities with serious problems.

   C. H. Firth's ground-breaking *Cromwell's Army* (1902) encouraged historians to consider the social world of early modern soldiers, and their relations with civilian communities.[3] Remarkably, it was not until 1991 that the issues of demobilisation and desertion were considered in any depth, with Ronan Bennett's essay on policing in civil-war Yorkshire, and the invidious effects of unsupervised soldiery.[4] In 1992 Ian Gentles dispelled the myth of the New Model's efficiency by emphasising the strategic implications of its high desertion rates. More recently, Barbara Donagan has offered a series of valuable insights into the nature of desertion.[5] It is still the case, however, that far more is known about wandering soldiers of other periods. Philip Thomas, Gervase Phillips and Linda Salamon have explored the world of Elizabethan deserters and veterans, while John Childs has highlighted links between demobilisation and crime in the later seventeenth century. Desertion in the eighteenth century has been covered by scholars such as Neal Garnham and Thomas Agostini.[6]

A student of the civil wars will rarely find such detailed sources as those utilised by Garnham and Agostini, and the difficulties of seeking to liberate marginalised groups from the condescension of posterity are well known. However, the fact that we now know that early modern vagrants did not wander aimlessly, and that crowds were not mindless mobs shows what can be achieved if individuals, events and mentalities are placed within their proper historical context, and subjected to structured analysis.[7] Peter Burke and John Walter, influenced by social anthropologists such as Clifford Geertz and James C. Scott, have demonstrated the efficacy of constructing narratives that operate 'on several levels and within various time spans'.[8] The intention here is to demonstrate that the issues surrounding wandering soldiers were complex and mutable, and should be placed within wider historiographical debates concerning the negotiation of authority in early modern England.

Desertion was so endemic to early modern armies that Gentles has described recruitment as akin to ladling water into a leaky bucket.[9] Mounted troops were less likely to desert than foot soldiers, for the simple reason that most horsemen were volunteers. Cavalry troopers tended to come from the respectable middling sort, and, being more literate than the average soldier, were more cognisant of the cause they served. On the rare occasions when cavalry or dragoons had to be conscripted, the authorities tried to select well-affected individuals of good character; after all it was unwise to conscript an unreliable man only to provide him with a horse on which to escape.[10] Naturally, there were occasions when cavalry commanders discovered knaves in their unit. Two such men were admitted into the troop of Oliver Cromwell junior but, finding less opportunity for plundering than they anticipated, they deserted, taking their horses and weapons with them. Cromwell described them as 'dishonorers of God's cause, and high displeasers of my father, my selfe and the whole regiment'.[11] These tended to be isolated incidents, however, unlike the infantry, who deserted in droves. Most foot soldiers were conscripts, and even volunteers were rarely as eager as propagandists pretended. Volunteers for Parliament's field army in 1642 were privately described as 'runaway cowards', one official declaring that he had 'never seen such indisposition in men to the service in my life'.[12] It is telling that the first assignment given to dragoons raised in Essex in 1643 was to herd hundreds of their impressed fellow countrymen north to the Eastern Association army.[13]

Parliament's shift in emphasis from a regionalised war effort to a national one over the winter of 1644–45 exacerbated the problem. As money was diverted from regional armies to finance the New Model Army, cash-strapped local commanders struggled to retain their men.[14] The foot regiments of the New Model itself, although initially well funded, were heavily dependent on conscription and even more prone to mass desertion. Thousands of conscripts did not even reach the front. Colonel John Venn reported to Parliament in April 1646 that the negligence of the Lincolnshire county committee had resulted in the escape of almost half of their latest crop of conscripts. Several hundred men had scattered before it had been possible to organise their conveyance.[15] By this time it was considered advisable to provide at least one guard for every two impressed men.[16] The royalist high command was similarly plagued by 'enlistment desertion': in April 1644 the earl of Forth sent two officers to Abingdon to collect 834 Berkshire conscripts, only to learn that 713 had already disappeared. Fifty-one more would abscond over the next two days.[17]

Venn suggested that the Lincolnshire incident was indicative of a deeper problem, declaring that:

> most [counties] press the scum of all their inhabitants, the king's soldiers [i.e. prisoners-of-war], men taken out of prison, tinkers, pedlars and vagrants that have no dwelling, and such of whom no account can be given. It is no marvel if such run away.[18]

Venn's jaundiced analysis is at odds with desertion patterns in other periods. Most enlistment deserters from Count Mansfeld's expedition in 1624 had been artisans and husbandmen rather than vagrants, many indignant at being forced to leave their families on parish charity.[19] Garnham and Agostini have observed a similar demographic among eighteenth-century deserters.[20] Venn's comments might even be questioned with respect to enlistment desertion in his own time; by 1646, having drained their respective catchment areas of marginalised males, both sides had begun to conscript breadwinners and householders. If these family men could give their guards the slip while still reasonably close to home, they had a reasonable chance of melting back into their native communities. County justices had proved remarkably sympathetic to such men in 1624, allowing them to return to their civilian occupations 'as soon as it could be done discreetly'.[21] Magistrates were even more circumspect during the civil wars, as leniency could easily be interpreted as disaffection, but many empathised with local complaints that conscription was causing depopulation and economic depression.[22]

Conductors (officers commanding conscript columns) knew that stopping to search for absconders only gave the other conscripts an opportunity to escape. They therefore hurried to deliver their remaining charges as quickly as possible. Months might elapse before the new recruits saw combat. This, and the fact that few could fully appreciate the horrors that awaited them, may explain why fear was low on the list of reasons to desert. Indeed, one contemporary argued that English soldiers in Ireland were more likely to desert if *not* engaged in fighting.[23] Major-General Richard Browne did not list fear as a factor in January 1645 when attempting to explain to his superiors why his army had become so depleted. Instead he pleaded that the soldiers 'for want of pay, desert us daily, their duty is hard, their quarters very strait, victuals very scant, and no money sent to us'.[24] This reflects Gervase Markham's description of a soldier's life as one of 'sicknesse, mortality, slaughter, ill diet and lodging, hunger, cold and surfeits'.[25] There were regular complaints that men were inadequately clothed. In the winter of 1643 an Eastern Association officer observed that 'the winter is already come, and our lying in the field hath lost us more men than have been taken away either by the sword or bullet'.[26] Such privations were exacerbated by boredom and brutal discipline, leaving little reason to wonder why men continued to desert long after they had joined their regiments.

Early modern military regulations invariably prescribed the death penalty for any soldier who strayed more than one mile from his army without licence.[27] In actuality officers tended to exercise discretion when dealing with men who fled from the fight, and they were tacitly supported by generals who appreciated that they could do little more than execute a token handful of reprobates. Those who turned tail in the heat of battle risked being beaten or shot if caught in the act, but if they returned within a few hours there was a good chance that nothing more would be said. Commanders frequently allowed enemy troops to escape rather than risk their own men's lives trying to apprehend them. Captain Edward Kightley confided to his cousin that when he had encountered a large body of royalist deserters fleeing the battlefield at Edgehill in October 1642 he had 'let them passe, disarming them, and giving the spoile to my Troopers'.[28] Although there were several occasions on which hundreds of captives changed sides after their army had been defeated, many officers chose not to recruit enemy deserters, and generally turned them loose rather than waste resources keeping them prisoner. When a Cavalier commander wrote to Thomas Bulstrode, parliamentarian governor of Aylesbury to protest that he had let royalist deserters go free, Bulstrode replied testily that 'this garrison is not suffered to be a receptacle for your fugitives'.[29]

Stragglers fell into a slightly more serious category than battlefield runaways. These were men who went absent without leave while the army was on the move, but who might return after a few days. It was common practice to redistribute stragglers' pay and food around the rest of the unit, in the expectation that they would eventually return. Edward Kightley was typical in this respect:

> I stop their pay, some of them for two dayes, some three dayes, and some four dayes, which time they were gone from me, and give their pay to the rest of the souldiers ...[30]

This had the effect of punishing the delinquent while at the same time rewarding the rest for their fidelity. More serious punishments awaited turncoats and permanent deserters – providing they could be caught. Early modern armies had a rudimentary policing system headed by a provost-marshal-general, but if deserters managed to put a few miles between themselves and their army they were unlikely to be pursued. Regimental provost-marshals ranked below lieutenants and quartermasters, despite having more duties. Naturally they were responsible for subduing and detaining offenders, but were also expected to patrol the camp, supervise the disposal of garbage and human excrement, collect and distribute captured booty, keep camp followers in order, monitor victuallers' goods and prices, and assist regimental quartermasters and wagon-masters with billeting and transportation. Seventeenth-century military theorists presumed that regimental provosts would be watchful for stragglers, but said nothing about pursuing deserters once they had escaped.[31] Some commanders were more energetic than others: Lord John Byron diverted men from frontline duties in order to hunt down deserters, while the earl of Manchester detailed officers to retrieve men who absented themselves from his Eastern Association army.[32] For the most part, however, the manuals reinforce the impression given by contemporary legislation, that it was the civilian authorities' responsibility to detect, detain and return deserters to the military for punishment. Before considering how local officials coped with this burden it is necessary to appreciate the size and nature of the problem.

It is difficult to quantify the effect wandering soldiers had on civilian communities, but as there were significant numbers involved they must have had a significant impact. Part of the solution may lie in aligning entries in parish and county records with military events. There are, for example, well-documented instances of peaceful demobilisation: thousands of royalist troops were released into the community after the general capitulation of 1646. Royalist garrisons negotiated honourable terms and marched out in good order, but, having nowhere to go, they dispersed almost immediately. The soldiers of the Lichfield garrison were instructed to go home or stay with friends, on condition that they lived peaceably thereafter.[33] Thousands of parliamentarians were discharged in 1647, 1651 and 1654. Although these troops were released in an orderly manner, many retained their weapons, and several appear to have caused as much trouble as deserters.

Desertion was disorderly by definition, particularly when it involved large numbers. Gentles calculates that fully 4,000 soldiers of the New Model deserted following Parliament's victory at Naseby on 14 June 1645.[34] Communities in the south Midlands and East Anglia did not simply have to contend with these men, however. According to *The True Informer*, 4,508 captured royalist soldiers were herded into Northampton the day after the battle.[35] A number subsequently agreed to serve in Parliament's forces in Ireland. The remainder were to be set free, provided they could convince their captors that they would never again take arms against Parliament. Those unable or unwilling to do this were to be transported to Barbados.[36] Around 1,500 prisoners were missing by the time the convoy marched through London on 21 June. Those who had accepted Parliament's terms may already have been detached, but there are indications that many prisoners had escaped during the march, in an incident near Barnet.[37] By any calculation therefore, thousands of unsupervised able-bodied ex-soldiers were circulating around southern and eastern parishes from June 1645 onwards – a sizeable addition to those who had deserted royalist, parliamentarian and Scottish armies over the preceding years.

Many of these wandering soldiers were harmless, and simply intended to return home. As has already been noted, both sides quickly became so desperate for recruits that they were forced to pluck men from the heart of the community, as well as vagrants and ne'er-do-wells. When respectable men deserted they often sought to legitimise their behaviour by emphasising the need to contribute to the wellbeing of their local community, such as helping with the harvest. Essex volunteers had deserted *en masse* in 1642 when they learned that their officers were to be replaced by strangers, and their companies assimilated into Parliament's main field army. Having enlisted on the assumption that they would only be expected to defend their own county, the men had no scruples about quitting Parliament's cause and heading home.[38] The pull of localism was also evident in concerns that the enforced absence of breadwinners would cause financial difficulties for their families. Local leaders took steps to alleviate individual cases of hardship, but these were not sufficient to prevent further desertion.[39] A soldier's plea to Sussex justices in 1645 that he had gone home to care for his aged mother had been heard before by magistrates elsewhere.[40] Families were forced to beg for charity when men had seized the opportunity to desert their wife and children as well as the army.[41] The desire to keep families off parish poor relief provided a powerful incentive for justices to respond slowly to pressure from higher authority to track down 'respectable' deserters.

The vast majority of pressed men came from the margins of society, however. In the Suffolk parish of Cratfield, for example, only two out of thirteen men taken for soldiers were ratepayers.[42] Throughout the conflict petty constables invariably sought to meet their quotas by following Sir Robert Cotton's dictum that 'men of lesse livelihood were the best spared'.[43] This encouraged civilians to assume that armies consisted principally of itinerant lowlife and the scum of the parish. As a result, even honest men returning home from the wars could find themselves shunned by their erstwhile friends and neighbours.[44] Communities were snobbish about soldiers and at the same time intensely scared of them. 'The rugged Souldier that from War returns', Thomas Otway later wrote, 'still with heat of former Action burns'.[45] Lurid popular literature and increasing numbers of horrifically maimed veterans passing through their parishes left civilians with a vivid impression of the savagery of war.[46] Sergeant Henry Foster wrote of his first experience of action that 'it were somewhat dreadful when men's bowels and brains flew in our faces', but he also noted how quickly he and others became desensitised to the horrors of the battlefield.[47] Modern studies have found that some combatants come to derive intense gratification from killing – psychopathic behaviour which can be linked with other wartime activities such as rape and vandalism, and which is very often an attempt to compensate for feelings of powerlessness and inadequacy.[48] There is mounting evidence that many others displayed signs of post-traumatic stress disorder. Entries in Quarter Sessions order books and other documents suggest that county officials were generally sympathetic to mentally disturbed veterans and their families, even in cases where the individual posed a danger to themselves or others.[49] However, it was one thing for a justice to deal with unpredictable veterans in the safe environment of the Quarter Sessions; it was quite another to be a parish official patrolling a lonely road, with orders to challenge passing strangers. Constables and churchwardens who confronted wandering soldiers were well aware that they were taking a serious risk. Magistrates' reports in earlier decades (particularly those in the vicinity of traditional embarkation centres such as Chester, Harwich and Portsmouth) had repeatedly linked unsupervised soldiers with robbery, rape and homicide.[50] Historians have been too eager to dismiss these allegations as mere rhetoric, for, as Ronan Bennett has shown, wandering soldiers were guilty of very serious crimes in civil-war Yorkshire, including several murders. Among the victims was a petty constable, stabbed to death by a gang of soldiers while attempting to detain one of their comrades.[51]

As has been suggested earlier, marginalised males may actually have found army life less miserable than their previous existence – at least until disease, starvation and slaughter became too much to bear, or when the acquisition of plunder (as at Naseby) gave them something to live for. When men such as these deserted they became wandering soldiers in the truest sense of the term. 'Home' often had little to offer the most destitute of the resident poor, and it had even less meaning for those who had been vagabonds in civilian life. Thousands of vagrants had trodden the highways and byways of England before the civil wars, and popular literature had long portrayed them as a catalyst for criminality. In contrast to the lively historiographical debate as to whether the caricatures created by Elizabethan 'rogue' literature induced a moral panic in early modern society, there has been little written on vagrancy between 1639 and 1660.[52] This silence is remarkable, because far from reducing the numbers of vagrants the civil wars exacerbated the problem. Anthony Fletcher has noted that vagrancy 'reached alarming dimensions' during the mid-1640s, and it was not simply a question of numbers: many vagrants were now armed, trained and dangerous.[53] John Awdelay's literary image of the 'ruffler' – the ex-soldier whose 'chiefest trade is to rob poor wayfaring men and market women' – had already linked veterans with vagrancy in the public mind, and the civil wars served to reinforce the perception.[54] A report on the London hospitals in 1644 noted that whereas soldiers wounded in Parliament's service were being cared for in the great institutions of St Thomas's and St Bartholomew's, hundreds of wounded royalists, 'wandering soldiers, and other vagrant people' had been sent to the infirmary at

Bridewell – already notorious as a house of correction.[55] Honourably discharged soldiers were anxious to avoid being mistaken for vagrants: demobilised veterans presented a petition to Parliament in June 1647 pleading for their arrears to be paid before they obeyed a proclamation to leave London, in order that they should not 'perish like vagabonds'.[56]

Looking back on the civil wars, James Howell declared that war was a seminary for thieves.[57] This resonated with the sentiments in Thomas More's *Utopia*, which had been reprinted in 1639: 'Theeves be not the most false and faint-hearted Souldiers, nor souldiers bee not the cowardliest theeves, so well these two Crafts agree together.'[58] Wandering soldiers were increasingly implicated in localised crime waves from 1645 onwards. Buckinghamshire was plagued by a gang of 'wood robbers' who had no loyalty to either side, and plundered indiscriminately. Some gang members who were caught claimed to be royalists, 'but the King will not own them'.[59] The parliamentary committee for Dorset reported widespread criminal activity in their area by January 1646, noting that the gangs were mounted and armed, and causing fear and terror throughout the shire.[60] Wiltshire experienced equally serious lawlessness, which justices there blamed squarely on wandering soldiers. In July 1646 they attempted to restore law and order by ordering towns and villages under their jurisdiction to arrange regular patrols of local roads, bridges and crossroads. Watchmen and tithingmen were to 'apprehend all wandering soldiers and mariners, rogues, vagabonds and suspicious persons that they shall meet with who cannot give good account of their travel'.[61] Heavy penalties were prescribed for communities or officials who neglected to do their duty. Despite an attempted crackdown in the areas under Parliament's control, at least one criminal gang was still causing trouble in Sussex in 1648.[62]

Criminal behaviour continued even when wandering soldiers began to set down roots. In November 1651 the Corporation of Rye described the economic dislocation which had arisen following an influx of disbanded soldiers, and pleaded for outside help to subdue and expel those who had no ties to the locality. Rye's burghers declared themselves powerless to deal with men who daily committed misdemeanours and indulged in 'evil behaviour', and who were 'imboldened to despise and contemne all Government and ministers'.[63] They were not the only authority figures who found themselves unable to cope: order frequently broke down in military camps as well. In June 1645, parliamentarian commanders in Lancashire had found, like so many captains before them, that they had reason to fear their men more than the enemy. They too pleaded for help to placate unpaid and mutinous soldiers, who had 'beaten, struck, wounded, and imprisoned some of us', and were threatening to desert.[64]

Given their superiors' impotence in the face of such malevolence, it was understandable that constables and churchwardens rarely attempted to detain unsupervised soldiers passing through their parishes, despite instructions and threats from above. Soldiers usually deserted their armies in small groups, but sometimes as many as forty or fifty men could be led away by renegade sergeants.[65] Of course, even the seven men who followed Corporal Atkins out of Browne's encampment at Abingdon in January 1645 could intimidate a civilian community.[66] An incident involving West Ham church-wardens, who in February 1648 opted to pay a group of unruly soldiers 'to keep the quiet' rather than attempt any arrests, shows that civilians would do almost anything to avoid trouble.[67] It was not always the wandering soldier who initiated the violence, however: one deserter apprehended following a tense armed standoff between ex-soldiers and locals in a Sussex alehouse in 1648 alleged that he had joined the gang primarily for reasons of personal safety.[68] By the mid-1640s, soldiers on both sides had become adept at extorting food, horses and money from local communities, and many went well beyond their official remit.[69] Such activities fuelled widespread antipathy towards the military, and motivated some civilians to assault wandering soldiers travelling alone.

In view of the numbers of military fugitives who passed through civilian localities in the 1640s and 1650s, it is remarkable how few can be positively identified as wandering soldiers in parish accounts. While it is important not to stray beyond the evidence, it is useful to consider how the fugitives presented themselves, and how churchwardens and constables in turn sought to reduce the risk of a potentially lethal encounter at the same time as they attempted to avoid being punished for dereliction of duty.

The first question to consider is whether parish officials could recognise a soldier when they saw one. Agostini has noted that eighteenth-century deserters regularly adopted disguises or invented stories to hide their identity.[70] Seventeenth-century veterans were held to have discernible features which made such subterfuge difficult. In the New Model, as with many regiments in the armies that preceded it, soldiers tended to be issued with red coats, so much so that the wandering soldier in his ragged red coat became a stock image in ballads and plays.[71] Observers also sometimes referred to soldiers' weather-beaten faces, as these tended to be more scarred, battered and tanned than civilians. Civilians engaged in outdoor occupations had a hard life, but they could sleep beside their hearths in extreme weather whereas soldiers were often bereft of any shelter. It was not until Cromwell's expedition into Scotland in 1650 that common soldiers were issued with tents. As a character in Edward Howard's play *The Man of Newmarket* says: 'I know you have been a Souldier, and deserve a handsome recompense, though men of your Complexion are not always fortunate to finde it.'[72]

Strangers in an unfamiliar locality invariably gave themselves away when they opened their mouths. Barbara Donagan's suggestion that 'deserters, even those far from home, could hope to fade into the general population' perhaps underestimates just how diverse English accents and dialects were during the early modern period.[73] As the war became less regional in character armies campaigned further afield, and deserters were forced to travel ever greater distances to reach familiar territory. The detailed documentation associated with maimed soldiers provides some idea of the distances travelled by their less reputable comrades. Jeremiah Maye's journey from Basing House to his home in Essex, for example, involved a trip of almost one hundred miles.[74] Entries in parish records during Charles I's campaigns in the 1620s show that unsupervised soldiers travelled anywhere up to 400 miles.[75] Former vagrants had a distinct advantage in such circumstances, for, as Paul Slack has shown, the long distances and regular circuits they had travelled before the wars meant that many 'knew the roads of England like the backs of their hands.'[76]

The *patois* developed within the military community was considered exceptionally rough and vulgar. Soldiers 'ought by their Profession to be as good at begging', opined a detractor after the Restoration, but 'they commonly act like themselves, bluntly, without consideration, and are usually denied without much ceremony'.[77] Episodes such as the Sussex alehouse brawl lent weight to this prejudice, but those who had been vagrants before their military service were probably more street-wise. Vagrants routinely exchanged information with others they met on the road, and were thus well aware which categories of traveller received the warmest welcome from parishes. It is therefore entirely possible that some individuals recorded in parish accounts as Irish refugees or victims of piracy may in actuality have been wandering soldiers. Traditional 'rogue' literature asserted that vagrants were practised impersonators, which made it all the more difficult for parish officials to ascertain which stories were genuine and which false. If it was indeed difficult for soldiers to conceal their occupation, it is particularly interesting that parish records of the 1640s should so often feature hybrid descriptions such as 'three distressed Souldiers which came out of Ireland', and 'two poore soldiers taken by the Turkes'.[78] Other variations on the theme include three English soldiers who passed through a Suffolk parish in 1643 claiming to have come from Germany, and the 'poore plundered souldier and his wife' who persuaded Swaffham officials to part with 6d.[79]

Experienced vagrants knew how to fake sickness or injury in order to achieve their aims. To this end, it is instructive to look closely at the specific nomenclature used by parish officials. *Bona fide* maimed soldiers were almost always recorded as such in parish records, not least because the description had a long-established legal status. The condition of others variously described as 'lame soldiers', 'sick soldiers', 'distressed soldiers', 'poor soldiers', and combinations thereof is more ambiguous. Such terms appear to have been used judiciously – and quite possibly with the intention of introducing ambiguity.[80] Soldiers' health was often poor – more than one died on the road through exhaustion and exposure – but it was easy to feign illness.[81] Parish officials had to bear in mind the very real possibility that wandering soldiers might be sick with plague or an equally lethal disease. Such considerations gave officials added incentive to take soldiers' stories at face value, and to usher them through to the next parish as quickly as possible.

The wording of parish records suggests that increasing numbers of individuals travelled without documentation. Even the accounts kept by the ultra-efficient constables of Upton, Nottinghamshire (who diligently recorded passes, commanding officers and other circumstances) suggest that unsupervised soldiers continued to slip through.[82] During the course of the civil wars the gentry were divided by their conflicting loyalties to King, Parliament, religion and county, and by their reactions to the political revolution which followed. This influenced the administration of law and order even in counties not directly affected by fighting. Meanwhile, far more people were taking to the roads than had been the case in peacetime. Parish officials, facing an increasing workload, and confused by conflicts within the normal chain of command, do not seem to have demanded passes with the same alacrity as in previous decades. Maimed soldiers and war widows travelling to their home parishes could usually produce certificates, as the law required them to submit documentary evidence when applying for relief from the county Quarter Sessions. Firth claims that soldiers discharged by Parliament from 1647 onwards were routinely issued with passes, although few have survived.[83] Wandering soldiers, on the other hand, lacked passes but apparently had no need of an organised counterfeiting service, such as that discovered by Chester justices in 1601.[84] Parliamentary ordinances demanding ever greater rigour in apprehending deserters therefore seem to have been somewhat divorced from the realities of parish administration. But then, wandering soldiers posed a different set of problems for those in high places.

John Pym, John Hampden, William Strode, Denzil Holles and several other leading parliamentarians had played a prominent role in the protests against Charles I's imposition of martial law in the 1620s – a measure which had been taken in order to protect civilians from marauding soldiers. They could hardly maintain the moral high ground, nor expect to retain popular support, if they now indulged in the kind of arbitrary action they had so publicly opposed in the past.[85] Parliament's initial response to mass desertion was therefore tentative. MPs' first inclination was to resort to bribery: in November 1642 every soldier who repaired to his colours and attended the earl of Essex's rendezvous set for later that month was promised an additional bounty over and above his normal pay.[86] By the spring of 1643, however, the Commons found it necessary to instruct the authorities in London, Westminster and the provinces to undertake a general search for deserters.[87] Desertion from regional armies was left to local commanders to sort out. Clive Holmes has noted the series of warrants issued by the earl of Manchester, 'backed up by a variety of threats', which were sent to the constables of Croft, Lincolnshire between June 1644 and March 1645, 'ordering them to turn in any deserters who made their way back to the village'.[88]

By the summer of 1644, with Pym and Hampden dead, and Strode dying,

MPs grew sufficiently desperate to draw up the first of a series of ordinances instituting martial law in London, Westminster and other strategically sensitive areas.[89] Presbyterian peers proved squeamish about such measures, even though they were intended to be of limited duration. In July 1644 the Commons felt it necessary to bully the Lords into extending the period of martial law, impressing upon their Lordships the ominous numbers of deserters gathering in and around London.[90] Throughout the winter of 1644–45, the Lords repeatedly attempted to separate the issue of desertion from that of martial law. Meanwhile, those in the Commons urging a more energetic prosecution of the war against the King saw martial law as the only effective solution to desertion.[91] The tide of desertion would only be stemmed if local civilian authorities could be coerced into stemming it.

The creation of the New Model Army intensified this wrangling. Its high desertion rate embarrassed the 'war party' (whose political credit depended largely upon the Army's success), and alarmed the conservative Presbyterian 'peace' faction. It was therefore in their mutual interest to approve a new ordinance in April 1645, detailing draconian punishments for deserters.[92] The mass exodus from the Army after Naseby resulted in more extreme measures: an ordinance passed on 27 June 1645 authorised all county committees to impose martial law within their jurisdiction, and gave them the power to execute deserters.[93] In January 1646 it was found necessary to extend the ordinance for a further nine months. County committees were now instructed to appoint provost-marshals. These were expected to deal with wandering soldiers, as Charles' provosts had done in the 1620s, and also to supervise the confinement of any disaffected individual.[94] Despite these enhanced powers county committees did not execute swathes of deserters, not least because parish officials became ever more circumspect in their record-keeping. There are far fewer mentions of soldiers in the Cratfield churchwardens' accounts from the spring of 1645, for example, but more references to poor lame 'people', groups of 'travellers', and even '7 pore people that came from the hospital in Southerucke'.[95] These seven were surely soldiers claiming to have been patients at St Thomas's hospital.

The issue of wandering soldiers took a further twist following the politicisation of the New Model and its estrangement from a Presbyterian-dominated Parliament. Deserters and demobilised soldiers were still camped in and around London in huge numbers, and there were rumours that Presbyterian MPs intended to form them into an army to counter the New Model. Sir Samuel Luke, Presbyterian governor of Newport Pagnell, was strongly suspected of attracting New Model deserters to his garrison for the same purpose. The New Model was alert to the danger, however, and warned MPs against proceeding further.[96]

Following Pride's Purge in December 1648 and the subsequent execution of the King in January 1649, the new military-backed Commonwealth was unpopular but secure, and able to expedite a gradual restoration of law and order in the provinces. Even so, the regime remained mindful of the political threat represented by wandering soldiers, and took precautions against an expected mass desertion of troops being sent to Ireland in July 1649.[97] Large numbers of ex-soldiers hanging around London continued to excite concern, as did the seepage of troops from the New Model. In 1651 the Council of State warned county commissioners that 'many Souldiers in pay desert their colours, and retire into the country'.[98] However, when two deserters were caught in Sussex, the Council was sufficiently relaxed to order them simply to be delivered to the nearest army conductor, requesting that local officials impress upon the men 'that if they desert their colours again, they will be proceeded against according to law'.[99] In the event, the republic was to be undone not by deserters, but by Oliver Cromwell and the increasingly well-disciplined New Model. There is little mention of wandering soldiers in the legal records of the Cromwellian Protectorate – it would have been particularly embarrassing for a military dictatorship to admit there was a problem – but there are several references to localised concerns regarding vagrancy, felony and highway robbery.[100] After the Restoration of 1660, many more military veterans took to the roads: the returning royalists ejected hundreds of maimed soldiers from London's military hospitals, thousands were discharged from Cromwell's 'Old Army', and many royalist prisoners-of-war are said to have returned from servitude in Barbados. These bodies of men, however, would pose a different set of problems for a very different regime.[101]

This study has sought to approach the complex problem of wandering soldiers from the varying perspectives of the men themselves, local civilian communities, and the parliamentary authorities in Westminster. With respect to the soldiers, it is wrong to assume that deserters, or even discharged veterans simply went home. Even those who did return to their parishes interacted with a series of civilian communities along the way, both positively and negatively. Many others had no permanent place of residence, and their military experience meant that they were substantially different, both in character and capability, from the more harmless vagrants of pre-war years. Nevertheless, David Underdown has argued that 'deserters and other masterless men who took to a life of crime were not engaging in a form of social protest, but simply trying to survive'.[102] Joining a criminal gang was often an act of self-defence. Wandering soldiers feared civilians as much as civilians feared them.

Even in times of peace, petty constables and churchwardens had frequently found themselves squeezed between the prerequisites of their local community and the political imperatives of higher authority. The particular circumstances of the civil wars necessitated a renegotiation of authority, between parish officials and county rulers, and between county rulers and Westminster. The issues surrounding wandering soldiers laid bare many of the fundamental tensions between the lawmakers in Parliament and those expected to enforce their will in the localities. Far from being able to harness the power of localism to solve the problem of the wandering soldier, parliamentarian leaders found local communities unable or unwilling to cooperate. As a result, what began as an embarrassment became a serious threat to the war effort, to parliamentarian unity, and to Parliament's moral authority. The unsettling presence of wandering soldiers in the localities fed into royalist rhetoric regarding incipient societal chaos at the same time as it threatened to undermine Parliament's self-image as the guardian of the people and the Common Law. Inaction would give the impression of incompetence, and unfitness to rule, whereas positive measures courted accusations of tyranny. Charles I's opponents therefore found themselves facing many of the same problems which had bedevilled the King in the 1620s. As they were forced to adopt ever more arbitrary policies, MPs knew that they risked similar opprobrium to that which they had heaped upon Charles. Wandering soldiers did not represent a mere political problem for the parliamentarian leadership as much as an existential crisis.

NOTES

1 Quoted in T. Barnes, 'Deputies not principals, lieutenants not captains: the institutional failure of lieutenancy in the 1620s', in M. Fissel (ed.), *War and Government in Britain 1598–1650* (Manchester: Manchester University Press, 1991), p. 59.

2 I. Gentles, *The English Revolution and the Wars in the Three Kingdoms, 1638–1652* (Harlow: Pearson Longman, 2007), p. 436.

3 C. H. Firth, *Cromwell's Army: A History of the English Soldier during the Civil Wars, the Commonwealth and the Protectorate* (London: Greenhill, 1992, facsimile of 1902 edn), pp. 268–75; C. Holmes, *The Eastern Association in the English Civil War* (Cambridge: Cambridge University Press, 1974), pp. 39, 168, 169; A. Fletcher, *A County Community in Peace and War: Sussex, 1600–1660* (London: Longman, 1975), pp. 341–2; M. Kishlansky, *The Rise of the New Model Army* (Cambridge: Cambridge University Press, 1979), pp. 241, 244–5, 247, 249; C. Carlton, *Going to the Wars: The Experience of the British Civil Wars* (London: Routledge, 1992), pp. 196, 225, 235.

4 R. Bennett, 'War and disorder: policing the soldiery in Civil War Yorkshire', in Fissel (ed.), *War and Government in Britain*, pp. 248–73.

5 I. Gentles, *The New Model Army in England, Ireland and Scotland, 1645–1653* (Oxford: Blackwell, 1992), pp. 33, 37–8, 389, 392, 402; B. Donagan, *War in England, 1642–1649* (Oxford: Oxford University Press, 2008), pp. 263–75.

6 P. Thomas, 'Vagabond soldiers and deserters at Elizabethan Northampton', *Northamptonshire Past & Present*, 9:2 (1995), 101–10; P. Thomas, 'The Elizabethan Privy Council and soldiers at York in a time of war: deserters, vagrants and crippled ex-servicemen', *York Historian*, 13 (1996), 15–24; G. Phillips, 'To cry "Home! Home!": mutiny, morale and indiscipline in Tudor armies', *Journal of Military History*, 65:2 (2001), 313–32; L. Salamon, 'Vagabond veterans: the roguish company of Martin Guerre and Henry V', in C. Dionne and S. Mentz (eds),

Rogues and Early Modern English Culture (Ann Arbor, MI: University of Michigan Press, 2004), pp. 261–93; J. Childs, 'War, crime waves and the English army in the late seventeenth century', *War & Society*, 15:2 (1997), 1–17; N. Garnham, 'Desertion and deserters in eighteenth-century Ireland', *Eighteenth-Century Ireland*, 20 (2005), 91–103; T. Agostini, '"Deserted his Majesty's service": military runaways, the British-American press, and the problem of desertion during the Seven Years' War', *Journal of Social History*, 40:4 (2007), 957–98.

7 J. Sharpe, 'History from below', in P. Burke (ed.), *New Perspectives on Historical Writing* (2nd edn, London: Polity Press, 2001), p. 31; G. Rudé, *The Crowd in History* (London: John Wiley, 1964, revised edn 1981); J. Walter, *Crowds and Popular Politics in Early Modern England* (Manchester: Manchester University Press, 2006); A. Beier, 'Vagrants and the social order in Elizabethan England', *Past & Present*, 64 (1974), 3–29, esp. 3, 26; A. Beier, *Masterless Men: The Vagrancy Problem in England, 1560–1640* (London: Methuen, 1985); S. Hindle, 'Power, poor relief, and social relations in Holland Fen, 1500–1800', *Historical Journal*, 41:1 (1998), 67–96; S. Hindle, *On the Parish? The Micro Politics of Poor Relief in Rural England, c. 1550–1750* (Oxford: Oxford University Press, 2004).

8 P. Burke, 'History of events and the revival of narrative', in Burke (ed.), *New Perspectives on Historical Writing*, p. 291, cited in J. Walter, *Understanding Popular Violence in the English Revolution: The Colchester Plunderers* (Cambridge: Cambridge University Press, 1999), p. 8.

9 I. Gentles, 'Why men fought in the British Civil Wars, 1639–1652', *The History Teacher*, 26:4 (1993), 408.

10 ERO, Q/SBa2/78; BL, Egerton MS 2,647, fo. 166.

11 *Notes & Queries*, fourth series, 11 (1873), p. 430.

12 BL, Thomason E128(30), *A Most Worthy Speech Spoken by the Right Honourable Robert Earl of Warwick* (London, 1642), pp. 1–2; BL, Thomason E127(9), H. Farre, *A Speech Spoken unto his Excellencie the Earle of Warwicke by Captain Farres in the Behalf of the Whole County of Essex* (London, 1642), p. 3; C. Holmes, 'The Eastern Association' (PhD thesis, University of Cambridge, 1969), p. 110; A. Kingston, *East Anglia and the Great Civil War* (Godmanchester: Trotman, 2005), p. 133; BL, Egerton MS 2,647, fo. 241.

13 TNA, SP 28/129, fo. 23.

14 TNA, SP 21/16, fo. 243.

15 *LJ*, VIII, pp. 267–8.

16 Gentles, *New Model Army*, p. 34.

17 TNA, SP 16/501, fo. 152.

18 *LJ*, VIII, pp. 267–8.

19 M. Fissel, *English Warfare 1511–1642* (London: Routledge, 2001), p. 108.

20 Agostini, 'Deserted his Majesty's service', 963; Garnham, 'Desertion and deserters', 101–2.

21 Fissel, *English Warfare*, p. 108.

22 BL, Egerton MS 2,647, fo. 199.

23 Wing A3258, *Another Extract of More Letters Sent Out of Ireland, Informing the Condition of the Kingdome as it Now Stands* (London, 1643), p. 5.

24 TNA, SP 21/17, fo. 173.

25 STC (2nd edn) / 17393, G. Markham, *The Second Part of the Souldiers Grammar* (London, 1643), p. 156.

26 Quoted in Kingston, *East Anglia*, p. 147.

27 BL, Thomason E75(34), *Lawes and Ordinances of Warre, by his Excellency the Earl of Essex* (London, 1643), sig. C; Wing L696A, *Laws and Ordinances of Warre, by Colonell Michael Iones* (Dublin, 1647), sig. B.

28 BL, Thomason E126(13), E. Kightley, *A Full and True Relation of the Great Battle Fought between the King's Army, and his Excellency, the Earl of Essex* (London, 1642), pp. 4–5.

29 ESRO, Danny MS 85, quoted in Donagan, *War in England*, p. 302.

30 BL, Thomason E126(13), Kightley, *Full and True Relation*, pp. 6–7.

31 T. Venn, *Military & Maritine [sic] Discipline in Three Books* (London, 1672), I, pp. 5, 188–9, Markham, *Second Part of the Souldiers Grammar*, p. 123; J. Turner, *Pallas Armata* (London, 1683), p. 223.

32 Denbighshire Record Office, GB 0209 BD/B, cited in D. Evans, *Montgomery 1644: The Story of the Castle and Civil War Battle* (Llanidloes: March Publications, n.d.), p. 31; Holmes, *Eastern Association*, p. 168, n. 46.

33 BL, Thomason E345(2), *Articles for the Delivering Up of Lichfield-Close* (London, 1646), p. 7.

34 Gentles, *The New Model Army*, p. 37; Gentles, *The English Revolution*, p. 103.

35 BL, Thomason E288(46), *The True Informer*, 21 June (London, 1645), pp. 68, [70].

36 BL, Thomason E292(5), *The Scotish Dove*, no. 89, 27 June–4 July (London, 1645), p. 700. According to one old royalist, the prisoners were held in London for four months: HMC, *Manuscripts of Rye and Hereford Corporations, Etc.*, Thirteenth Report, Appendix, Part IV (London: HMSO, 1892), p. 346.

37 G. Foard, *Naseby: The Decisive Campaign* (Whitstable: Prior Publications, 1995), pp. 306–7.

38 Holmes, *Eastern Association*, pp. 38–9.

39 BL, Stowe MS 842, fo. 6; I. Slocombe (ed.), *Wiltshire Quarter Sessions Order Book, 1642–1654* (Wiltshire Record Society, 67, 2014), p. 302; Suffolk Record Office (Ipswich), FC62/A6/211.

40 Fletcher, *Sussex*, p. 341.

41 Lancashire Archives, QSB/1/295/36.

42 L. A. Botelho (ed.), *Churchwardens' Accounts of Cratfield* (Suffolk Records Society, 42, 1999), p. 20.

43 BL, Thomason E1243(2), R. Cotton, *Cottoni Posthuma*, ed. J. Howell (London, 1651), p. 312.

44 Clarke MS 41, fo. 122, quoted in Kishlansky, *Rise of the New Model Army*, p. 214.

45 T. Otway, *Titus and Berenice* (London, 1677), epilogue.

46 STC (2nd edn) / 24760.7, P. Vincent, *The Lamentations of Germany* (London, 1638); BL, Thomason 669 f. 6(12) *The English-Irish Soldier* (London, 1642); BL, Thomason E1448(1) and Wing C6370, J. Cotgrave, *Wits Interpreter* (London, 1655), p. 143.

47 BL, Thomason E69(15), H. Foster, *A True and Exact Relation of the Marchings of the Two Regiments of the Trained Bands of the City of London* (London, 1643), sig. B3.

48 R. Holmes, *Acts of War* (London: Cassell, 2003), pp. 376–80.

49 KHLC, Q/SO E1, fo. 64; SRO, Q/SR E1652, fo. 20; C. Mayo (ed.), *The Minute Books of the Dorset Standing Committee 23rd Sept., 1646 to 8th May, 1650* (Exeter: William Pollard, 1902), p. 80.

50 TNA, SP 12/261, fo. 70, quoted in J. Cockburn, 'Patterns of violence in English society: homicide in Kent 1560–1985', *Past & Present*, 130 (1991), 85; ERO, Morant MS D/Y 2/5, fo. 95, 2/8, fo. 259.

51 Bennett, 'War and disorder', pp. 250, 261, 262. See also SRO, Q/SR M. 1647, fo. 11. For those sceptical of the extent of the violence, see Cockburn, 'Patterns of violence', 85; Barnes, 'Deputies not principals, lieutenants not captains', p. 75.

52 STC (2nd edn) / 12787.5, T. Harman, *Caveat for Common Cursitors* (London, 1567). See the survey of vagrant historiography in P. Clark, 'Migration in England during the late seventeenth and early eighteen centuries', in P. Clark and D. Souden (eds), *Migration and Society in Early Modern England* (London: Hutchinson, 1987), pp. 213–15. One scholar who has considered aspects of the civil-war period is L. Woodbridge, 'The neglected soldier as vagrant, revenger, tyrant slayer in early modern England', in A. Beier and P. Ocobock (eds), *Cast Out: Vagrancy and Homelessness in Global and Historical Perspective* (Athens OH: Ohio University Press, 2008), esp. pp. 71–82.

53 Fletcher, *Sussex*, p. 341.

54 STC (2nd edn) / 994.5, J. Awdelay *The Fraternity of Vagabonds* (London, 1603 edn), sig. A2.

55 BL, Thomason 669 f. 10(2), *A True Report of the Great Costs and Charges of the Foure Hospitals* (London, 1644). London's military hospitals were funded separately, and do not feature in the report.

56 Parliamentary Archives, HL/PO/JO/10/1/235; *LJ*, IX, p. 265.

57 Wing H3119, J. Howell, *Therologia, The Parly of Beasts* (London, 1660), pp. 114, 117.

58 STC (2nd edn) / 18098, T. More, *The Common-wealth of Utopia* (London, 1639 edn), pp. 29–30.

59 BL, Thomason E266(37), *Perfect Occurrences of Parliament*, 2 January (London, 1647), sig. [A4].

60 Mayo (ed.), *Minute Books of the Dorset Standing Committee*, p. 169.

61 Slocombe (ed.), *Wiltshire Quarter Sessions Order Book*, pp. 55–6.

62 Fletcher, *Sussex*, p. 341.

63 HMC, *Manuscripts of Rye and Hereford Corporations*, p. 216.

64 TNA, SP 16/507, fo. 16.

65 TNA, SP 21/17, fo. 165.

66 *Ibid.*

67 ERO, D/P 256/5, fo. 51.

68 ESRO, Sessions Rolls 70/76, fo. 77, 80/64, fo. 65, cited in Fletcher, *Sussex*, p. 341.

69 ERO, Q/SO1, fo. 203v; SRO, Q/SR M. 1647, fo. 11.

70 Agostini, 'Deserted his Majesty's service', 959, 971.

71 BL, Thomason 669 f. 25(58), *The Lamentation of a Bad Market, or the Disbanded Soldier* (London, 1660); Wing S2698, E. Settle, *Love and Revenge* (London, 1672), pp. 1–2; Wing D2789, T. D'Urfey, *Trick for Trick* (London, 1678), prologue.

Red coats are noted in parish records as early as 1625: J. Stocks (ed.), *Market Harborough Parish Records* (London: Oxford University Press, 1926), p. 92.

72 Wing H2969, E. Howard, *The Man of Newmarket* (London, 1678), p. 28.

73 Donagan, *War in England*, p. 271.

74 ERO, Q/SBa 2/78.

75 Stocks (ed.), *Market Harborough Parish Records*, pp. 90, 96, 97.

76 P. Slack, 'Vagrants and vagrancy in England, 1598–1664', in Clark and Souden (eds), *Migration and Society in Early Modern England*, p. 58.

77 Wing B3742, F. Boothby, *Marcelia, or, The Treacherous Friend* (London, 1670), sig. D2.

78 A. Craven (ed.), *The Churchwardens' Account of St Mary's Devizes 1633–1689* (Wiltshire Record Society, 2016), pp. 57, 62; Botelho (ed.), *Churchwardens' Accounts of Cratfield*, pp. 34, 47, 55.

79 *Ibid.*, p. 55; NRO, Swaffham churchwardens' accounts 1627–52, PD52/72, fo. 13 – a reference I owe to the kindness of Patricia Appleby.

80 Numerous instances of each category appear in Craven (ed.), *Churchwardens' Account of St Mary's Devizes*; NRO, PD52/72; ERO, D/P 75/5/1; ERO, D/P 265/5; Botelho (ed.), *Churchwardens' Accounts of Cratfield*; Stocks (ed.), *Market Harborough Parish Records*; M. Bennett (ed.), *A Nottinghamshire Village in War and Peace: The Accounts of the Constables of Upton, 1640–1666* (Thoroton Society Record Series, 39, 1995), pp. 20–1, 23.

81 ESRO, PAR498/1/1/3.

82 Bennett (ed.), *Nottinghamshire Village*, pp. 8, 9, 10, 16, 18.

83 Firth, *Cromwell's Army*, pp. 269–70.

84 Cheshire Archives, QSF/49, fos. 27, 86, 91.

85 Donagan, *War in England*, pp. 171–3. See also J. M. Collins, *Martial Law and English Laws, c. 1500–c.1700* (Cambridge: Cambridge University Press, 2016), chapter 5.

86 *CJ*, II, pp. 841–2.

87 *CJ*, III, pp. 49, 107.

88 Holmes, *Eastern Association*, p. 168, note 46.

89 *LJ*, VI, pp. 673–4, 681; VII, pp. 88, 333–4, 402, 418–19; VIII, pp. 23, 29, 30, 106, 200.

90 *CJ*, III, p. 568.

91 *CJ*, III, p. 693.

92 *LJ*, VII, pp. 334–5.

93 *LJ*, VII, p. 461; BL, Thomason E290(3), *An Ordinance of the Lords and Commons* (London, 1645).

94 *LJ*, VIII, pp. 102–3; BL, Thomason E316(12), *An Ordinance of the Lords and Commons* (London, 1646); Mayo (ed.), *Minute Books of the Dorset Standing Committee*, p. 169; Parliamentary Archives: HL/PO/JO/10/1/199.

95 Bothelho (ed.), *Churchwardens' Accounts of Cratfield*, pp. 63, 64, 70, 71, 72, 77, 79, 92, 95; Carven (ed.), *Churchwardens' Account of St Mary's Devizes*, p. 44.

96 Kishlansky, *Rise of the New Model Army*, pp. 241, 244–5, 249; H. Tibbutt (ed.), *The Letter Books of Sir Samuel Luke, 1644–45* (London: HMSO, 1963), pp. 561, 564.

97 TNA, SP 25/62, fo. 494.

98 TNA, SP 25/96, fo. 35; C. H. Firth and R. S. Rait (eds), *Acts and Ordinances of the Interregnum, 1642–1660*, 3 vols (London: HMSO, 1911), II, p. 349.
99 TNA, SP 25/65, fo. 265.
100 Firth and Rait (eds), *Acts and Ordinances*, II, pp. 1098, 1262; *CJ*, VII, pp. 530, 552, 570–1, 577.
101 D. J. Appleby, 'Veteran politics in Restoration England 1660–1670', *The Seventeenth Century*, 28:3 (2013), 326–8, 333; B. Garside, *Parish Affairs in Hampton Town during the Seventeenth Century* (Richmond: Dimbleby, 1954), p. 48.
102 D. Underdown, *Revel, Riot and Rebellion: Popular Politics and Culture in England, 1603–1660* (Oxford: Oxford University Press, 1985), p. 159.

Chapter 8

'The deep staines these Wars will leave behind': psychological wounds and curative methods in the English Civil Wars

Erin Peters[1]

The lingering effects of physical disability as a direct result of combat in the English Civil Wars has been the topic of several important recent studies.[2] The surviving petitions of ex-soldiers and the official papers of state hospitals provide ready evidence of seventeenth-century conceptualisations of the nature of physical disability. In addition, the establishment, in 1593, of an official state system of benefits for disabled soldiers marks the early modern period in England as the starting point for the consideration of physical injury and resultant disability as a social and political construct.[3] In his study of soldiers' petitions for pensions during the civil-war years, Geoffrey Hudson explains the manner in which the pensioners narrated their injuries as well as the ways in which those injuries were considered to be disabling. He reveals that most pensioners explicitly mentioned that they had been physically disabled as a result of battle, listing injuries such as the loss of a limb, a head wound, visual or hearing impairments.[4] In other words, the various forms of injury incurred through combat were restricted to the realm of the physical. As Hudson points out, this is hardly surprising given that eligibility for hospital and county disability pensions during the civil wars rested on the inability to work and required military certificates and physical examinations.[5] Indeed, what is readily apparent here is the close relationship between contemporary ideals of the healthy body and what constituted injury and disability.

Yet, although under the pension scheme disability was restricted to physical impairment, this period of violence also saw a growth of interest in the conceptualisation and public narration of psychological damage. This chapter will discuss aspects of this development and will suggest that the mid-seventeenth century saw an increase in the awareness of non-physical, non-visible war-wounds and early attempts to address what modern psychology has labelled post-traumatic stress disorder or combat stress disorder. The intention is not to engage in retrospective diagnoses, but rather to explore the early history of psychiatry in mid-seventeenth-century England and in the context of civil war. This chapter will suggest that alongside the official and authorised interpretation of disability as a physical impairment, a popular understanding of the disabling nature of psychological injury developed. This growing awareness can be traced in the unauthorised, non-official, print sources circulating in the mid-seventeenth century.

However, before evidence of a popular cognizance of psychological wounds can be considered, it is necessary to examine some contemporary efforts made towards understanding the damaged mind, the effect such damage was understood to have upon the life and abilities of the individual, and contemporary suggestions of curative methods. Following this, and in relation to it, the discussion will then turn to considerations of some published material which establishes the forms that descriptions of psychologically disabling experiences took. Throughout, the chapter shall demonstrate that the authors of these narratives addressed 'a traumatic collective experience with which it was necessary to come to terms' at a national level.[6] Ultimately, this suggests that there was a high level of fluidity between the manner in which individual and collective trauma was conceptualised as a disabling, injurious force. What will become evident in the course of this chapter is that mid-seventeenth-century print sources indicate that the effects of psychological trauma on the individual were transferred, more or less directly, onto the canvas that represented the national psyche: for example, just as a mentally traumatised soldier suffered the paralysing effects of intense psychological battlefield stress, so the nation as a whole appeared to observers to be in the vice-like grip of unfathomable intestine destruction and its immediate consequences. The connection between contemporary images of the injured individual and the injured body politic becomes apparent here.[7] Moreover, contemporary responses to the disabling nature of psychological trauma demonstrate a developing cognizance of the therapeutic value of attempting to construct a publically available collective trauma narrative.

THE DAMAGED MIND

Theories about the damaged mind and early ideas of psychiatry were already circulating in print in the 1630s. John Sym's *Lifes Preservative Against Self-killing. Or, An Useful Treatise Concerning Life and Self-murder* (1637) is one example of contemporary attempts to categorise and conceptualise psychological impairment. Sym (*c.* 1581–1638) was born in Scotland and became a minister at Leigh-on-Sea in Essex, where he remained until his death. A zealous Calvinist with strong predestinarian beliefs, Sym also believed that he was witnessing an epidemic of suicides in England at the time of his writing, and his aim in the treatise was both to demonstrate that deliberate self-destruction was a dreadful sin and to provide methods to prevent it. *Life's Preservative* is the first full-length work on suicide published in English.[8] In explaining various motives for suicide, Sym writes:

> The third kind of evill, whereupon men take occasion to kill themselves, is that which is upon their minds, as in the immediate subject thereof, which the neerer it is, the more intollerably it doth affect: all other sufferings being as whippings upon the coats, but this as upon the naked skin; and more intollerable than death, which some men choose, and voluntarily inflict, with their own hands, upon themselves, that thereby they may be freed from the trouble of their minds.[9]

Sym's description of psychological suffering as potentially more tormenting, and thus more intolerable, than physical pain and injury is important in that it signals a clear willingness to take seriously ailments that are invisible to the eye, and from which conventional means ('coats') offer no protection. Moreover, this ready recognition of the seriousness of the trouble of the mind is extended by Sym's effort to understand mental disorders and his distinction between different types and their common causes:

> This trouble of the minde is of foure sorts. First, extreame griefe of minde and trouble of conscience ... *The* second sort of the troubles of mind, which occasions self-murder, is mens excessive discontentment ... The third kinde of troubles of minde that sometimes occasions self-murder, is shame and confusion ... The fourth kinde of the mindes trouble, that may occasion self-murder, is servile and excessive feare; wherewith a man may be surprised and possessed, either from the present evills that he suffers, which he conceives are beyond his strength to beare, and out of which hee sees no meanes of delivery, to be freed so soone as he would, but by killing himselfe.[10]

A key aspect of Sym's categorisation, for our present purpose, is his recognition that some mental disorders are caused by matters usually external to the sufferer's corporeality: the first two categories of extreme grief describe an intense experience of loss, while the third cause, 'shame and confusion', is predicated largely on a perceived or actual failure to meet established norms and expectations, social, communal or otherwise.[11] Indeed, these categories in particular suggest a recognition of what, in modern terms, would unhesitatingly be labelled as examples of psychological trauma. Sym's 1637 publication is thus significant for two reasons: it acknowledges mental disorder as a serious, potentially fatal illness and recognises that external factors, such as traumatic events, have the power to cause significant disorders of the mind, that is, psychological damage.

Sym was not, of course, the first man in England to engage explicitly and extensively with matters concerning the afflicted mind: a decade and a half earlier Robert Burton had published what was one of the most widely read seventeenth-century accounts of mental illness, the bestselling *The Anatomy of Melancholy* (1621).[12] In this rather digressive and eclectic survey, it is not so much Burton's recognition of various manifestations and degrees of psychological problems as a disease that is important for the present discussion as the proposed remedies. Discussing the internal workings of the mind, Burton foregrounds the external invisibility and cyclical nature of psychological disorders:

> As children are affrighted in the darke, so are melancholy men at all times, as having the inward cause in them, & still carrying it about ... they keep the mind in a perpetuall dungeon, and oppresse it with continuall feares, anxieties, sorrows, &c. ... Fear makes our imagination conceive what it list, invites the Devil to come to us ... and tyranniseth over our phantasy more than all other affections.[13]

Trapped within and tormented by imaginary fears, anxieties and sorrows, the afflicted individual suffers from a seemingly inescapable cycle of psychological re-traumatisation. What Burton proposes to alleviate the psychological suffering and ultimately to release the sufferer from the trauma cycle has a distinctly 'modern' hue: the verbalisation of the damaging psychological experience. The relevant lengthy passage is worth quoting in full:

> If then our Judgement be so depraved, our reason over-ruled, Will precipitated, that we cannot seeke our own good, or moderate our selves, as in this Disease commonly it is, our best way for ease is to impart our misery to some friend, not to smother it up in our brest ... grief concealed strangles the soul; when as wee shall but impart it to some discreet, trusty, loving friend, is instantly removed by counsell happily, wisdome, perswasion, advice, his good means, which we could not otherwise apply unto our selves ... the simple narration many times easeth our distressed minde, and in the midst and greatest extremities so many have bin relieved by exonerating themselves to a faithfull friend, he sees that which we cannot see for passion and discontent, he pacifies our mindes.[14]

Burton's remedy for the 'disease' of the 'distressed mind' is thus essentially what became known as the Freudian 'talking cure' almost three centuries later: seeking to reinstate the rule of reason and break through repressive habits, it is the repeated narration of the sufferer's grief and mental turmoil that will ultimately bring relief from the affliction. This relief comes from attempting to give meaning to experiences that seem to defy comprehension. Deliberately forming the narration of trauma allows the sufferer to attempt to actively control it. This reduces the risk of unwanted intrusions and so allows for a reflection on past experiences that can be endured, to a certain extent, by the sufferer. Burton, moreover, was not alone in proposing this cure, as Sym similarly recommended the seeking of counsel to alleviate the trouble of the mind. A decade and a half after Burton he suggests that the:

> Antidotes and meanes to be used for prevention of self-murder, is the course that they, that labour under such temptations, are to take jointly with others ... The care of private friends, so farre interessed by confession in this case, should be, not only to advise ... they should often deale with them, and question them about their successe against their temptations: for, what cannot be effected at once, repetition may worke; and the victory be got, and the cure be accomplished; suddaine cures

are commonly unsound: and to leave them over-soone argues too much neglect of them; and also the disease is not fully discovered when they suppose the same is healed. Self-murder is prevented, not so much by arguments against the fact; which disswades from the conclusion; as by the discovery and removall of the motives and causes.[15]

It is thus the repeated verbal expression of the causes and effects of mental disorders, to sympathetic listeners, that early seventeenth-century commentators identified as the key method of treatment for psychological disorders. The treatment proposed by Burton and Sym contrasts significantly with conventional histories of early psychiatry that assume the dominance of demonological ideas in medieval and early modern views of mental illness and that describe the treatment of the afflicted as cruel and inhumane.[16] Indeed, Burton's and Sym's approaches to mental illness and psychological trauma essentially demonstrate a firm grasp of the efficacy of what modern psychotraumatology has conceptualised as Narrative Exposure Therapy (NET) or Testimony Therapy, belying the supposed modernity of psychotherapy. Moreover, while Sym labels his different types of mental disorders as 'evils', there is a noticeable conceptual shift away from understanding psychological damage exclusively in the context of religious ideas of 'good' and 'evil'. Burton and Sym both explicitly recognise that external factors, such as traumatic events, have the power to cause significant, but nevertheless treatable, mental disorders.

The notion that external factors are responsible for affecting the condition of the psyche can also readily be found in treatises dedicated to studying the human condition. For example, Edward Reynoldes' *A Treatise of the Passions and Faculties of the Soul of Man* (1640) suggests that:

Wee may sundry times reade the abilities of the Minde, and the inclinations of the Will: so then it is manifest, that this weaknesse of apprehension in the Soules [minds] of men, doth not come from any immediate and proper darknesse belonging unto them.[17]

Reynoldes (1599–1676), a minister in Northamptonshire during the wars, was interested in the interconnection between emotions and experience and their effects on the human soul and psyche. The popularity of his treatise is demonstrated by the fact that it was republished twice more, in 1647 and 1650. Thomas Povey (c. 1613–1705), colonial entrepreneur, civil servant and non-partisan anti-war writer, was similarly interested in the lingering effects of psychological wounds derived from external experiences, specifically combat. Using the language of sickness and injury, and so demonstrating an awareness that the mind, like the body, can be damaged through experience, Povey explains:

For War, like a strong disease, leaves many dregs and reliques behind it, which (though the maine Forces be disbanded, and it be no more an Army, a Fever) will punish the uncleansed body with several fits and distempers.[18]

Here, the echoes of psychological wounds ('reliques') linger long after the cause ('fever') has been put down. Remarkably, Povey describes the effect of this disease with terms often reserved for mental disorders ('fits and distempters') demonstrating, perhaps, a deliberate association between visible and invisible wounds. The royalist soldier, early neurologist and psychologist Thomas Willis (1621–75) was similarly interested in how the mind might be affected during periods of disorder. His focus on external stimulae that induced feelings of fear, worry and sadness (which he defines as melancholy and delirium, without fever) helped to shift the image of the body from a system of humoral balances to a site of reciprocating dynamics affecting both the body and mind.[19] For Willis, the individual was not permanently fixed and governed by the four humours, but rather was 'a site of nervous dynamism, capable of change both by chance and intention'.[20]

Although Willis did not offer suggestions for treatments or therapies to cope with disorders of the mind, the conceptualisation of psychological distress and the most effective treatment for it did gain a popular foothold during the course of the seventeenth century; as we shall see, the curative methods proposed by Sym and Burton were adopted by some individuals who experienced or witnessed the distressing events of the civil wars. Perhaps the first thing to note concerning available primary sources in print is that discussions of soldiers' psychological responses to their experience of combat and the sights of the battlefield are rare in published descriptions of early modern European warfare. As Sharon Alker has explained, this was due to the predominance of two dominant discourses: the language of historical fact and the language of heroic stoicism.[21] Contextualising her discussion of fictional English Civil War memoires produced within living memory of the conflict, Alker usefully identifies several characteristics shared by both fictional and non-fictional war literature. War accounts were, in the first instance, usually constructed on the basis of a strict adherence to what was considered historical fact, that is, the depersonalised narration of a description of a military encounter. Moreover, by employing the rhetoric of national and personal glory, seventeenth-century accounts of combat typically represented soldierly responses to battlefield atrocities in terms of a Christian acceptance of the will of God, or neo-stoic heroism, which was grounded in contemporary beliefs concerning society and order, and justice and authority. However, in an internecine conflict such as the English Civil Wars, these narrative forms become destabilised by the difficulty of representing the killing of a fellow countryman as a glorious act. The limits of traditional narrative forms that allow for distressing experiences to be rationalised are thus exhausted in a civil-war context, and traditional explanations centred on heroic endurance for a just cause collapse in their moral uncertainty. As Alker explains in respect of the civil wars, 'In the inflamed imagination of the soldier, killing the enemy becomes conflated with killing the self, which, in turn, inflames passions of grief and fear ... the implications of killing without a just cause and without disciplined integrity are horrendous'.[22] While leaders on both sides of the conflict attempted to present their enemies on the field as traitors and rebels to the State, thereby justifying the lawfulness of the war, there was a recognition among the troops that this 'uncivil' war was self-destructive.[23] The enemies were often visibly and linguistically indistinguishable from each other, and were made up, as Thomas Povey explains, of 'brothers, kindred, and friends'.[24] Thus, he acknowledges that although 'the killing of our Country-men must be called valour and a service to the State ... wee must execute the designs of our enemies upon our selves'.[25] Bearing this in mind, the experience of the English Civil Wars was so intense that, in spite of the dominant discourses of soldierly stoicism, descriptions of the horrors of the battlefield, and the subsequent difficulties of coming to terms with the psychological trauma caused by them, occasionally found a place in contemporary pamphlet literature.

Mid-seventeenth-century narrations of distressing events were, of course, reliant upon the culturally produced frames of reference available to them: common reference points included the natural order, a sense of national and communal [in]justice, and divine providence. However, some patterns emerge in civil-war print material that reflect a parallel, if not entirely disconnected, frame of reference which spoke more directly to the experience of psychological trauma. This 'trauma frame' manifested itself in descriptions of confusion and rupture, extreme grief and a fundamental sense of loss, and excessive fear. Even though they are not mutually exclusive, these seventeenth-century categories of traumatic war experiences offer a useful analytical lens through which to read contemporary narratives of psychologically distressing experiences and the curative desires that, sometimes obviously, underscored these writings. One might also note that, while the effects of psychological trauma, by their very nature, resist clear categorisation, these categories nevertheless allow a clearer tracing of an emerging seventeenth-century awareness of the psychological wounds that could be caused by combat experiences as well as contemporary attempts to address and cure these afflictions. Indeed, while it is difficult to measure the occurrences of mental health problems among soldiers and veterans of the wars, there is evidence that county authorities did sometimes provide for traumatised soldiers, further demonstrating contemporary awareness of this affliction.[26] However, before analysing the various expressions of psychological injury evident in print, it is useful to discuss the notion of therapeutic writing as it was conceived in the period.

THERAPEUTIC WRITING

While the authors of documents which describe the distressing nature of events of the mid-seventeenth-century had their own unique experiences of and perspectives on the wars, their published descriptions of the 'troubles of the minde' had one thing in common: they were intended to be printed and circulated widely.[27] What is more, within many of the documents discussed in this chapter, the traumatic elements are repeatedly rehearsed, demonstrating the application of narrative therapies as recommended by contemporary psychoanalysts like Sym and Burton. In 1647, the royalist James Howell offered an explanation for publishing a short pamphlet entitled *Down-right Dealing* in which he styles himself as 'an impartiall observer of the present'. Addressing the reader, Howell explains that his writings 'are not the fruits of discontent ... neither are they intended to kindle that fire, which already (though seemingly smother'd) blazes too fast, but rather to quench it'.[28] His intention is self-evidently therapeutic, he writes in an attempt to extinguish his present distress. In an earlier pamphlet entitled *Englands Teares, for the Present Wars* (1644), Howell again explicitly describes the purpose of his writing. Discussing the destruction caused by the wars and the nation's resultant distress, he invites his reader to 'weep and wayle with me ... in my melancholy', and begs, 'if there be any sparkles of humane compassion glowing in thy bosome, stay awhile and hear my plaints'.[29] In the midst of his narrative, Howell agonises, 'Oh, I feele a cold quame come over my heart, that I faint, I can speak no longer; yet I will straine my selfe to breath out this one invocation'.[30] Readers are thus offered a frank description of the debilitating effects of psychological impairment on the individual (his melancholy). However, Howell also offers an important extension: in describing his own civil-war induced psychological trauma, he invites readers to recognise it and embrace it as their own. Howell's readers are thus engaged in curative reading while the author attempts to relieve his psychological suffering by narrating and sharing it. In other words, Burton's advice that 'the simple narration many times easeth our distressed mind' is put into practice by Howell, who solicits an audience to whom he may repeat his 'plaints'. The intensity of the narrative activity is remarkable: addressing his traumatisation psychologically strains the author even to the point of inducing a psycho-somatic response ('I faint, I can speak no longer'). However, in what may be regarded as an appropriation of the neo-stoic heroism of traditional war literature, Howell carries on with his narration. In two separate publications, then, Howell attempted to deal with his own mental distress in a manner that reflected the curative methods advanced by some early seventeenth-century psychological theorists. Furthermore, in addressing a general readership Howell extended his personal trauma and encouraged it to be incorporated on a collective level.

Another prominent example of the link between psychological damage and narrative expression can be found in a 1643 publication by the parliamentarian soldier Major George Wither. Wither explains his reasons for writing a description about his experiences in the war:

Nor carefull am I, whether Hee or Shee,
Be pleased or displeased with my Muse:

> For, none to sooth or vexe, my musings be:
> But, now I write, because I cannot chuse.
> ...
> The sword hath had his turne, and now the Pen
> Advanced is to play her part again.[31]

While Wither declares that he is not writing with the intention of comforting anyone, including himself, he simultaneously acknowledges that he feels a compulsion to write; he 'cannot chuse' but allow the pen to pick up where the sword left off. He explains:

> And, since it will not onely be an ease
> To mine own heart my numerous thoughts to vent,
> But also may some honest Readers please,
> Ev'n in these times of gen'rall discontent.[32]

Regardless of his earlier protestations, it appears that Wither is attempting a narration of his troubled mind with the hope that he will achieve the calming effects of 'venting' his distress. Like Howell, Wither extends his writings to his readers, inviting them to share in his description and, by that means, experience the same curative benefits. The therapeutic value of narrating one's distressing thoughts is also explicitly touched upon by Thomas Povey. His twenty-eight page pamphlet on the disastrous nature of war in England ends with a sense of relief, as he explains to the reader, 'I was big of these Thoughts, and could not be quiet untill I was delivered of them ... Thus many times doth a minde fill'd with grief find ease by emptying it self in Complaints'.[33]

In a similar address to the reader in 1649, the Quaker Isaac Penington (1616–79) invites: 'Reader behold (if thou be'st able to bear the sight) a few specks of thine own black dark Self, some broken fragments of that filthiness which every man thinks he is free from, and yet the heart of every man is ful of.'[34] Penington offers a description of his own invisible wounds (his 'black' and 'broken' heart) as a mirror to reflect those of the reader, apparently at the limits of the psychologically sufferable. If repeatedly rehearsing the troubles of the mind was considered therapeutic, it appears that writers also considered that reading, and thereby sharing, the trauma of others could help to heal a nation in the grip of collective trauma by reintroducing reason to counteract emotion. Concluding his pamphlet, Wither expresses the hope that his readers 'Take, therefore, counsell from a soldiers Penn/And (while you may) be warn'd, be wise, be men'.[35] In a similar manner, Howell offers his story to his reader because, he explains, 'misery is the schoolmaster to wisdom, and that wit is the best when it is dearly payd for, and truly I beleeve you have payd enough for it'.[36] Howell expresses his hope that readers will acquire the healing potential of understanding ('wisdom') that his trauma narrative can offer. To shed light on how these writings were considered therapeutic, it is necessary to recognise the forms with which expressions of psychological trauma were commonly framed.

CONFUSION AND RUPTURE

Seventeenth-century writers who attempted to construct a therapeutic narrative of their wartime experiences found themselves facing an immediate problem. How can writing adequately and accurately depict an event so distressing that it defies depiction? This is a problem commonly recognised in modern trauma theory. Psychological trauma manifests itself in disjointed and fragmentary ways, and modern traumatology recognises the essential unrepresentability of traumatic recall. In the efforts made by mid-seventeenth-century soldiers and witnesses of the wars to narrate their experiences, this problem is typically attributed to a mental block frequently described as confusion. In attempting to describe his wartime experiences, James Howell labels it as 'Enigmaticall' and writes that 'there was never such a confus'd mysterious civill warre as this'. He goes on to voice his expectation that 'whosoever will be curious to read the future story of this intricate Warre (if it be possible to compile a story of it) he will find himself much stagger'd, and put to a kind of riddle'.[37] Thomas Povey also describes the 'cause' to be 'much like a riddle'.[38] George Wither, too, is confounded by his efforts to describe his experience. He expresses regret that he cannot adequately narrate the wars and an awareness that the times are to blame for that inadequacy: 'Destructive times, distractive musings yield / expect not therefore method now of me'.[39] Similarly, a frantic letter from an anonymous writer in Bristol, published in 1643, explains that his attempts to give an account of his experiences have been obstructed by 'how little time I have had to eate, drinke, or sleepe, or to write, speake, or thinke of anything'.[40] Sharing this experience, Wither finds his time is so taken up that he must do his thinking on the road:

And, whilst we marcht, my heart, with thoughts confus'd,
Was over-fill'd; and thus I sadly mus'd.
Those dreadfull Tragedies, must I, O Lord!
Must I, not onely now survive to see;
Which were so long time fear'd, and so abhorr'd?
But live, in them, as Actor too, to be?[41]

Wither's confusion spreads to an existential crisis as he mourns the loss of peace and the times in which he lived.

In *Intelligence from the Armie* (1643), the anonymous author makes it clear that he does not want to write at all, but nevertheless has 'forced my Pen to this Letter, and myself to deal more freely with you, than the world with me, and to tell you some of my thoughts'.[42] Frustratingly, in his efforts to impart his thoughts on the 'present state of the Common-wealth', he finds that he 'can reduce things to nothing but confusion'.[43] The confusion of the affairs of the nation are reflected in the confusion of the author's narrative. The letter contains several digressions as the writer's scattered attention turns upon various topics. He continuously reins himself back, acknowledging: 'but you require my most serious thoughts concerning the issue of the present business', and 'but something of News you expect from me', and finally, 'Pardon this digression ... I hope some more able pen shall be intrusted with the whole story'.[44] At the end of the document, the author ponders the nature of this confusion in inclusive language: 'It is a sad thing to think how slight a thing we make of this solemn appeal to Heaven, for so War is, and manage it betwixt jests and earnest, as if our thoughts were really comfortable'.[45] The recognition that strategies used to cope with psychological injury (for example, jests) can mask 'uncomfortable' thoughts demonstrates a, perhaps unconscious, recognition that living through horrendous experiences can result in invisible injuries that require mediation and processing.

EXTREME GRIEF AND LOSS

Expressions of grief are common in testimonies about and descriptions of the experience of the wars. This is hardly surprising, as the period was one of destruction and atrocity. What is particularly interesting, however, is that very few chroniclers describe or discuss personal grief. Instead, accounts of the emotional devastation and the utter sadness of the times reflect the seventeenth-century notions of self-control, stoicism, submission to the providence of God and, above all, notions of the collective. Wither describes the sense of communal grief:

> But now, the Breach is made; the Floods break in,
> And we with miseries, are overflowne.
> We shall be losers, though the day we win.
> When spoiles we take, the losse will be our owne.
> Because, from forreign foes, we fear'd no harm,
> God, for our sins, has rais'd us foes at home.
> Our selves, against ourselves, we strongly arme;
> And slaught'rers, of each other, are become
> ...
> Give me, Oh God! Give me those moving teares,
> Those deep-set sighes, and those prevailing groanes.[46]

The sense of loss is a national one, and individual grief and loss are narrated within a framework that focuses on the collective. In terms of the therapeutic potential of these narratives, framing grief and loss as collective emotions allows for individual experiences to be embraced as part of the national narrative of the wars. To put this differently, echoing Burton and Sym, these narratives demonstrate a contemporary awareness of the healing power for the individual of narrating the injuries of the mind, and of reading and recognising the trauma of others for the collective.

An anonymous pamphlet from 1642, entitled *Englands Complaint*, is a further remarkable example of seventeenth-century narrations of suffering that solicits an audience with whom to rehearse the trauma as a curative method. This pamphlet, which was printed by order of Parliament, addresses first the King, and then Parliament, nobles, gentry, commons, judges and clergy and begs for 'mutuall agreement and reconciliation'.[47] It begins with the author's invitation to the reader to recognise his or her own trauma in the narrative ('Behold therefore if there be any sorrow like unto my sorrow') and then compulsively pleads for the reader's attention ('O give eare and listen to my counsel'; 'Give eare and help me'; 'Give eare and pitie me ... commiserate my wofull and distressed condition'). Throughout this eight-page pamphlet the frenzied author begs for the reader's ear nine times.[48] What is more, the writer positions the act of listening (repeatedly using the phrase 'give me eare') with the act of assisting ('listen', 'commiserate', 'help'). Beyond the more specialist tracts by Burton and Sym, and the conceivably polemical intentions of this piece, pamphlets of this kind signal a wider seventeenth-century awareness of the curative effects of narrating one's traumatic experience and considering the trauma of others.

Taking another approach to narrating invisible, psychological injuries, James Howell adopts the voice of the nation in his account of extreme grief. In the role of England, Howell describes the sad consequences of the wars:

> These deep wounds, which Prince, Peere and people have receiv'd, by this; such wounds, that it seems no gentle Cataplasms can cure them, they must be lanc'd and cauteriz'd, and the huge scars they will leave behind them, will, I feare, make me appeare deformed and ugly to all posterity, so that I am half in despair to recover my former beauty ever again. The deep staines these Wars will leave behind, I fear, all the water of the Severne, Trent or Thames cannot wash away.[49]

Howell relates the lingering wounds of war on the national psyche with the language of physical injury. He not only writes of desires to attempt to cure these wounds, but also demonstrates an awareness of the haunting nature of psychological damage with his discussion of scars and stains that cannot be washed away. Finally, in mentioning the three great rivers, Howell extends the scars, deformity and despair across the face of the country. In a similar fashion, Wither questions, 'But what are private Losses, while we view / Three famous Kingdoms, woefully expos'd'.[50]

The notion of excessive despair and grief is also touched upon in print that discusses the rise in suicides. In 1644, Howell noted that self-murder had become a common occurrence, explaining, 'They [the people of England] would not cut their own throats, hang, drown, and do themselves away in such a desperate sort, which is now grown so common, that self-murther is scarce accounted any news'.[51] Despite Howell's contention, death caused by excessive grief occasionally did make the news: for example, a 1647 broadsheet entitled *A Generall Bill or Mortality, of the Clergie of London* lists 'The total of the Ministers of London within the Bills of Mortality (besides Paul's and Westminster) turn'd out of their Livings by Sequestration and otherwise' at one-hundred-and-fifteen. Of that number, twenty-two are listed "dead with grief".[52] While this is likely a polemical point, its circulation in print further testifies to the heightened sense of pervasive and deadly grief brought about by the wars, which could lead, as Howell describes, to desperate acts. This is particularly the case given that suicide was viewed with an increasingly severe attitude in England from the 1530s onward, and law, religion and popular belief were all adamantly opposed to it.[53]

EXCESSIVE FEAR

According to seventeenth-century theory, fear was not considered to be an internal feeling; rather, it was something that affected the body. Examining narratives of fear from the Thirty Years' War, Andreas Bähr suggests that those who experienced fear were considered to have sensed it like a physical disease. The correct approach to overcoming this form of fear and anxiety was through religion.[54] This manner of thinking about the origins and causes of fear is evident in the descriptions from the English Civil Wars, as well. As a physical affliction, fear was often described as a poison (Howell writes, 'Oh, I am deadly sick ... an unknown disease ... a strange kind of infection').[55] Fear and anxiety were sent by God, and the endurance and eventual overcoming of the fear of violence was providential. For example, a 1643 pamphlet entitled *Great Britains Misery; with Causes and Cure* discusses fear and anxiety using the typical seventeenth-century expressions of illness, 'He that knows not his Disease, seeks not for Cure; And diseases are best known by their Causes'.[56] However, in this long pamphlet, the disease, and so the thing to be feared, is divine wrath and the cure is repentance and atonement, 'the efficient and first cause of all misery is God: and the want of serious and due consideration of this: that Gods hand is in every affliction, augments the misery, and hinders the cure'.[57] While this form of religious reasoning is common in the pamphlet literature during this distressed decade, there is also evidence of a baser, increasingly more mortal form of fear in the chronicles that recount traumatising experiences of the civil wars. Here we see descriptions of the fear of death, of violence, of rape, of atrocity and of loss. This was not a philosophical concern for the soul, but an innate, reactionary and distinctly human terror. In 1642, a pamphlet entitled *The Anatomy of Warre* acknowledged this pervasiveness of combat-induced fear:

> None delights in the sound of warlike Drums, or in the Alarmes of Warr; but onely they who never tasted the bitternesse thereof for he who hath once felt the smart of it, will tremble as oft as he thinks of its approach ... If an Army consists of raw, yong, and fresh-water souldiers, who seldome or never saw men wounded or slaine; when they come to see such sights, they will tremble and be confounded with feare.[58]

Here the fear of battle is all-consuming, and extends to both those who have previous fighting experience and to fresh soldiers about to engage in combat for the first time. While perhaps the pamphlet's declaration that battle is a fearsome prospect for soldiers is not unexpected, the real trauma of war and violence is also explained:

> War continued, or long wars make men inhumane ... that is, at first sinne seems to us loathing, but often sinning makes sinne seeme nothing ... where before [a soldier] ever entered into the wars, he thought he could never be so cruell, as to dash the childrens braines against the stones ... but afterwards when he was injured with warre, he did it.[59]

The language of injury is used to discuss the desensitising properties of combat, where the psychological effect of experiencing the violence and atrocities of battle 'made them like savage beasts'.[60] Thomas Povey explains that 'Humanity is almost turned to cruelty', while George Wither also reflected on this consequence, writing that 'ere long, so hardened men in sin will grow / that on his neighbour none will have compassion ... and shall corrupt each other and devoure'.[61] Similarly, James Howell observed that 'people are grown half wild in many places' and that they have become 'wolvish' in a war that 'passeth all understanding'.[62] The invisible injury produced through excessive fear is the loss of humanity, and that, in itself, is portrayed as a cause for fear. In other words, frequent exposure to and engagement in atrocities wound the individual mind to the extent that engaging in acts of extreme violence may 'seeme nothing', yet the injury has the acknowledged capacity to 'devoure[s]' the sufferer. Edward Reynoldes' 1647 treatise on the human condition also offers a reflection on the desensitising nature of fear:

> For as cloth once died from its naturall white, will take no other but a darker colour: so minds once steeped in the bitter humours of this melancholique passion, will seldom admit of any, but more black and fearful conceits. And from this suspicion of fear it is, that timorous men are usually cruel, when they gain any advantage: their jealousie teaching them to do that unto others which they fear from them.[63]

The experience of fear derived from living through a period of extreme violence is also occasionally articulated as paranoia. James Howell writes, 'me thinks I hear my neighbours about me bargaining very hotly for my skin, while like an unruly horse I run headlong to dash out my own braines'.[64] That both Howell and the anonymous author of *The Anatomy of Warre* include a description of a smashed-out brain to discuss the psychological injuries sustained through experiencing trauma is important. The trauma narratives present an image of a fractured head to give a perceptible injury to an invisible wound. Taking this image further, that the victims of the psychologically damaged soldiers are children and animals reflects the notion that an injured mind is a corruption inflicted on the innocent. Nevertheless, in writing about these horrifying imaginings, the authors are actively attempting a curative treatment. As Wither explains, 'Tis time, thought I, that in the gap we stand /

to stop the breach, that else will drown the land ... To make a passage, thorow blood and wounds / for Justice, Truth, and Peace, we forward'.[65]

CONCLUSION

This chapter has demonstrated a mid-seventeenth-century awareness of non-physical, non-visible wounds and early attempts to develop curative methods that emphasised various verbalisation, or narration, techniques. If repeatedly rehearsing the troubles of the mind was considered therapeutic for the individual, it appears that writers and publishers also considered that reading, and thereby sharing, the trauma of others could help to heal a nation in the grip of collective trauma. Thus out of the combat-induced psychological disability of the individual comes that of the nation. Moreover, the existence of individual trauma narratives help further to demonstrate that contemporaries were aware of the disabling nature of psychological impairment and that they were cognizant of the therapeutic value of attempting to construct a descriptive narrative. Indeed, this was the case even before the civil wars, as evidenced by the popular theories and treatises on the damaged mind by men like Sym and Burton.

As narrative therapies, by definition, aim to make sense of the insensible and give meaning to seemingly incomprehensible experiences, the narration of war trauma in the mid-seventeenth century necessarily made use of the culturally produced frames of reference available to them. In order for writers to construct a logically structured rehearsal of the 'troubles of the mind' that adhered to familiar narrative forms – and, perhaps, allowed for a therapeutic experience – the expressions of psychological injury typically manifested in descriptions of confusion and rupture, extreme grief and sense of loss, and excessive fear. Although they are not mutually exclusive, these seventeenth-century categories of describing traumatic war experiences offer a useful analytical lens through which to read contemporary narratives of psychologically distressing experiences as well as the curative desires that often accompany them. What becomes apparent in the print material that discusses the damaging effects of the wars is that this period of violence saw a growth of interest in a holistic approach to the conceptualisation and treatment of combat-related injuries.

NOTES

1 I am very grateful to Andreas Mueller for helpful comments on an earlier version of this chapter.
2 See, for example: G. L. Hudson, 'Arguing disability: ex-servicemen's own stories in early modern England, 1590–1790', in R. Bivins and J. V. Pickstone (eds), *Medicine, Madness and Social History: Essays in Honour of Roy Porter* (London: Palgrave Macmillan, 2007), pp. 105–17; M. Stoyle, 'Remembering the English

Civil War', in P. Gray and O. Kendrick (eds), *The Memory of Catastrophe* (Manchester: Manchester University Press, 2004), pp. 19–30; M. Stoyle, 'Memories of the maimed: the testimony of Charles I's former soldiers, 1660–1730', *History*, 88:290 (2003), 204–26; E. Gruber von Arni, *Justice to the Maimed Soldier: Nursing, Medical Care and Welfare for Sick and Wounded Soldiers and their Families during the English Civil Wars and Interregnum, 1642–1660* (Aldershot: Ashgate, 2001).

3 Hudson, 'Arguing disability', p. 110.

4 *Ibid.*, p. 108.

5 *Ibid.*, p. 111.

6 J. Scott, *England's Troubles: Seventeenth-Century English Political Instability in European Context* (Cambridge: Cambridge University Press, 2000), p. 162.

7 See E. Reynoldes, *A Treatise of the Passions and Faculties of the Soul of Man* (London, 1640), p. 4.

8 M. P. Battin, *The Ethics of Suicide: Historical Sources* (Oxford: Oxford University Press, 2015), p. 296.

9 J. Sym, *Lifes Preservative Against Self-killing. Or, An Useful Treatise Concerning Life and Self-murder* (London, 1637), p. 217.

10 *Ibid.*, pp. 218–24.

11 A mid-seventeenth-century definition for 'shame' has been provided by Henry Cockeram, who lists it along with terms such as 'disparagement', 'dishonour' and 'disgrace'. Confusion is defined as a 'disorderly mingling'. H. Cockeram, *The English Dictionarie* (London, 1639), pp. 22, 30.

12 The popularity of Burton's book is evidenced by the fact that it was republished seven times between 1621 and 1660.

13 R. Burton, *The Anatomy of Melancholy* (Oxford, 1621), pp. 261–3.

14 *Ibid.*, pp. 364–5.

15 Sym, *Lifes Preservative Against Self-killing*, p. 323.

16 For example, G. Zilboorg, *The History of Medical Psychology* (New York: W. W. Norton, 1941). Also see: S. Kemp and K. Williams, 'Demonic possession and mental disorder in medieval and early modern Europe', *Psychological Medicine*, 17:1 (1987), 21–9; R. Neugebauer, 'Treatment of the mentally ill in medieval and early modern England', *Journal of the History of Behavioural Sciences*, 14 (1978), 158–69; R. Neugebauer, 'Medieval and early modern theories of mental illness', *Archives of General Psychiatry*, 36 (1979), 477–83.

17 Reynoldes, *A Treatise of the Passions*, p. 7.

18 BL, Thomason E89(21), T. Povey, *The Moderator Expecting Sudden Peace, or Certain Ruine* (London, 1642), p. 13.

19 J. T. Hughes, *Thomas Willis, 1621–1675* (Oxford: Rimes House, 2009), p. 79; M. Faubert and A. Ingram (eds), *Depression and Melancholy, 1660–1800*, 4 vols (London: Pickering and Chatto, 2012), II, p. x.

20 Faubert and Ingram (eds), *Depression and Melancholy*, II, p. x.

21 S. Alker, 'The soldierly imagination: narrating fear in Defoe's *Memoires of a Cavalier*', *Eighteenth-Century Fiction*, 19:1&2 (2006), 47.

22 *Ibid.*, 62.

23 B. Donagan, *War in England, 1642–1649* (Oxford: Oxford University Press, 2008), p. 132.

24 BL, Thomason E89(21), Povey, *The Moderator*, p. 11.

25 *Ibid.*, pp. 5, 11.

26 See D. J. Appleby, 'Veteran politics in Restoration England 1660–1670', *The Seventeenth Century*, 28:3 (2013), 334.

27 Sym, *Lifes Preservative Against Self-killing*, p. 218.

28 BL, Thomason E408(17), J. Howell, *Down-right Dealing, or The Despised Protestant Speaking Plain English* (London, 1647), pp. 1–3.

29 BL, Thomason E253(10), J. Howell, *Englands Teares, for the Present Wars* (London, 1644), pp. 1–2.

30 *Ibid.*, p. 14.

31 BL, Thomason E1144(4), G. Wither, *Campo-Musae: Or The Field-Musings of Captain George Wither* (London, 1643), pp. 1–2.

32 *Ibid.*, p. 2.

33 BL, Thomason E89(21), Povey, *The Moderator*, p. 28.

34 Wing / P1170, I. Penington, *The Great and Sole Troubler of the Times Represented in a Mapp of Miserie, or A Glimps of the Heart of Man* (London, 1649), p. 2.

35 BL, Thomason E1144(4), Wither, *Campo-Musae*, p. 66. The connection between masculinity and military stoicism, characterised by self-discipline and self-restraint, is common in contemporary writings on the nature of war. Kevin Sharpe explains that the appeal lay in the belief that reason 'might free men from the passions that enslaved them'. Although Sharpe states that 'there has been almost no work on the impact of Stoicism in England', he also explains that 'there is some evidence that, as well as general currency in early Stuart England, Stoic ideas influenced the ethical and political ideas of statesmen'. See K. Sharpe, *Reading Authority and Representing Rule in Early Modern England* (London: Bloomsbury, 2013), p. 124.

36 BL, Thomason E408(17), Howell, *Down-right Dealings*, p. 14.

37 BL, Thomason E253(10), Howell, *Englands Teares*, pp. 1, 6.

38 BL, Thomason E89(21), Povey, *The Moderator*, p. 7.

39 BL, Thomason E1144(4), Wither, *Campo-Musae*, p. 3.

40 BL, Thomason E97(6), Anon., *A Full Declaration of all Particulars Concerning the March of the Forces under Collonel Fiennes to Bristol ... Together with Sundry Letters Annexed* (London, 1643), p. 11

41 BL, Thomason E1144(4), Wither, *Campo-Musae*, p. 13.

42 BL, Thomason E105(16), Anon., *Intelligence from the Armie* (London, 1643), p. 2.

43 *Ibid.*, p. 6.

44 *Ibid.*, pp. 8–13.

45 *Ibid.*, p. 13.

46 BL, Thomason E1144(4), Wither, *Campo-Musae*, pp. 15–17.

47 BL, Thomason E118(47), Anon., *Englands Complaint or the Church Her Lamentation* (London, 1642), p. 1.

48 *Ibid.*, pp. 1–8.

49 BL, Thomason E253(10), Howell, *Englands Teares*, p. 8.

50 BL, Thomason E1144(4), Wither, *Campo-Musae*, p. 16.

51 BL, Thomason E253(10), Howell, *Englands Teares*, pp. 11–12.

52 BL, Anon., *A Generall Bill of Mortality, of the Clergie of London* (London, 1647).

53 Battin, *The Ethics of Suicide*, p. 296.

54 A. Bähr, 'Remembering fear: the fear of violence and the violence of fear in seventeenth-century war memories', in E. Kuijpers, J. Pollmann, J. Müller and J. van der Steen (eds), *Memory Before Modernity: Practices of Memory in Early Modern Europe* (Leiden: Brill, 2013), pp. 270–1.
55 BL, Thomason E253(10), Howell, *Englands Teares*, p. 2.
56 BL, Thomason E250(4), G. S., *Great Britains Misery with the Causes and Cure* (London, 1643), p. 1.
57 *Ibid.*
58 BL, Thomason E128(15), R. Ward, *The Anatomy of Warre, or, Warre with the Wofull, Fruits, and Effects thereof, Laid Out to the Life* (London, 1642), pp. 5–6, 19.
59 *Ibid.*, p. 8.
60 *Ibid.*
61 BL, Thomason E89(21), Povey, *The Moderator*, p. 5; BL, Thomason E1144(4), Wither, *Campo-Musae*, p. 15.
62 BL, Thomason E253(10), Howell, *Englands Teares*, p. 11.
63 Reynoldes, *A Treatise of the Passions*, pp. 291–2.
64 BL, Thomason E253(10), Howell, *Englands Teares*, p. 4.
65 BL, Thomason E1144(4), Wither, *Campo-Musae*, p. 13.

Chapter 9

The administration of military welfare in Kent, 1642–79

Hannah Worthen

The people of Kent experienced the British Civil Wars through local conflicts as well as national military action. Men departed the county to fight
for Parliament and King and so left behind their families. Many of those who
returned were disabled and unfit to work, and fighting inside and outside
the county left women as widows and children as orphans. This chapter
will highlight the response of the governments of the period to the need
that this created, by establishing a county pension scheme to support the
maimed and the widowed in society. The records of this scheme highlight
the ways in which local government interacted with central authorities. These
records also, crucially, give an insight into the ways in which ordinary people
who had suffered great losses because of the wars sought to gain financial
relief for themselves and their families. Thus, this chapter will examine the
administration of military welfare in Kent in order to analyse how the men,
women and children of soldiering families in Kent experienced the civil wars,
Interregnum and Restoration periods.

While Kent was not a major centre of military activity in the form of
large-scale battles and sieges, it is well known for the part it played in the
Second Civil War. The Christmas riots in Canterbury in December 1647
and the battle of Maidstone in May 1648 were significant for the county and
the country, and yet these were not the only outbreaks of fighting in Kent.
During the First Civil War Kent witnessed several small-scale rebellions that
were anti-parliamentarian or royalist in nature. In July 1643 discontented
men rose up in rebellion in Ightham, Sevenoaks, Aylesford, Yalding and
Maidstone against an attempt to administer the Vow and Covenant: a loyalty
oath imposed by Parliament in response to the supposed Waller plot against
London in June of that year.[1] In the early summer of 1644 there was a mutiny
among newly raised parliamentary troops at Sevenoaks and again in April

1645 there was an uprising of parliamentarian soldiers at Wrotham Heath.[2] During this time there was also an abortive attempt to seize Dover Castle and a royalist rising in the Darent valley.[3]

As well as these local events, soldiers fought outside the county. In March 1644 Kent was joined by Parliament with Southampton, Sussex and Surrey to form the South-Eastern Association and soldiers were raised to join Sir William Waller's forces.[4] Kentish men also joined the royalist cause, either at the start of the war or by becoming caught up in one of the local rebellions. For example, some chose to fight on and travel to Colchester in the aftermath of the battle of Maidstone in June 1648.[5] As a result, many families in Kent were left forever changed by the loss of fathers and husbands or by long-term and life-changing injuries.

As a result of a parliamentary initiative at the start of the wars, Kent's JPs handed out military welfare to war widows and maimed soldiers in the form of pensions and one-off gratuities. This financial relief was to be administered via the meetings of the Quarter Sessions court. Those who had been maimed in service, as well as the widows and orphans of those who had died, were required to petition in order to receive this entitlement. After the Restoration, changes in national and local government were reflected in the administration of the county pension scheme in Kent. Very soon after 1660 former royalists and their dependants became the beneficiaries of pensions (instead of the parliamentarians) and pensions continued to be granted to those who had been loyal to the King for the next two decades.

This research is indebted to other pieces of local history research and specific work on the county pension scheme in other areas of the country. The methodology of Alan Everitt's seminal study of civil-war Kent, *The Community of Kent*, has made examining local records, people and processes fundamental to civil-war research. Yet, those responding to his work have raised some important issues. Everitt argued that at the start of the civil war, England 'resembled a union of partially independent county-states or communities'.[6] He went on to argue for a county that was intensely locally focused, even isolated, with strong ties of intermarriage within a cohesive gentry community. More recently, this picture has been challenged. For example, Jacqueline Eales found that 'Everitt's emphasis on the gentry led him to discount the relevance of religious non-conformity amongst other social groups', and Michael Zell argued that 'before 1640 (or 1660) the county of Kent was unified only in certain limited, political and social contexts'.[7] Ann Hughes stated that she found herself 'sceptical about notions of a sharp contradiction between local and general concerns' in this period.[8] It is this final aspect of Everitt's work, which stressed 'the pre-eminence of local allegiance and the gentry's ignorance of and lack of concern for national issues', which will be challenged by this study.[9] Everitt's arguments were in reality more sophisticated than this picture, but this research will add to the assessment that it was local *and* national concerns which influenced the decisions of the gentry in Kent through the lens of a study of military welfare.

Geoffrey Hudson has initiated a focus on the war widows 'negotiating for blood money' during the civil wars, Interregnum and Restoration.[10] This work, which focused especially on the counties of Cheshire, Worcestershire, Nottinghamshire and Wiltshire, found that 'war widows successfully adopted tactics used by the men and in their actions and words demonstrated a keen awareness of entitlement to pensions'.[11] David Appleby has also completed work on the war widows and maimed soldiers who petitioned the Essex Quarter Sessions. He analysed the tactics used by both sets of petitioners and compared those with their relative success.[12] There have also been studies on the experiences of maimed soldiers after the Restoration in Kent and in Devon.[13] This chapter will look at particular aspects of these pieces of research when they can be compared to Kent and, in particular, the ways in which these records have been used by other historians to demonstrate patterns of loyalty. The records for Kent do seem to show a strong link between royalist petitioners and general patterns of allegiance across the county. Nevertheless, the objections of other historians, such as John Morrill, have urged that this approach should be used with caution.[14]

This chapter will examine the administration of military welfare in Kent in the period from 1642, when Parliament first issued a pension ordinance, to 1679, when Parliament allowed the scheme to lapse.[15] Firstly, it will examine the process by which pensions were administered before and after the Restoration, and consider how national orders interacted with local processes in Kent specifically. Secondly, it will look at the ways that people gained a pension. That process began with preparing to construct a petition and ended, the petitioner hoped, with an appearance in the Quarter Sessions and the award of a pension. Using the petitions that exist among the Kent Quarter Sessions' rolls, as well as the incidental detail within the order books, this section will review how maimed soldiers and war widows in Kent accessed the relief promised to them by Parliament. The final section will provide evidence for how many pensions were awarded in Kent, how much they were worth and consider comparisons between the periods before and after 1660. It will also examine the different ways that maimed soldiers and war widows were treated. By scrutinising how pensions were administered, petitioned for and received, this chapter will provide an overview of military welfare in Kent between 1642 and 1679. It will question how far political and military events, local sympathies and parliamentary directives played a part in the changes within the scheme and how maimed soldiers and war widows were able to benefit from it.

ADMINISTERING PENSIONS

The administration of military welfare had roots in Elizabethan legislation and the key principles which underlined the county pension scheme were not much altered throughout the mid-seventeenth century. The Elizabethan government had offered maimed soldiers and mariners financial relief in the form of a pension if they were disabled from working.[16] The money to support this relief was drawn directly from the county and each parish was rated at a certain amount. JPs at Quarter Sessions ordered pensions to be paid to those who had petitioned and whom they deemed eligible for relief. The success-ful petitioners would collect their money quarterly from the Treasurer for Maimed Soldiers: an office held by local men of at least middling-sort status who were 'Subsidy-men, *viz.* of 10 l. in lands, or 15 l. in goods' and therefore considered trustworthy to administer the funds.[17]

In October 1642 Parliament passed an ordinance which reinvigorated this scheme and stated that pensions were to be provided to those who had 'undertaken for the Preservation of the King's Majesty's Person, the Defence of the Religion and Laws of the Realm' and 'who have little or nothing to maintain themselves, their Wives, and Children'.[18] The idea that maimed soldiers formed part of the 'deserving poor' of society was outlined in this section from a 1658 printed pamphlet:

> there are impotent poore, and there are impudent poore: The former are so through Necessity, either by birth; as those borne Creeples, or Blind, or Fatherlesse, &c. or by casualty of losses, sicknesse, as the decaied Housholder, the maimed Souldier and the like: The latter are so through Choice, they are poore, because they are idle and lazy, and so will be poore.[19]

One key difference between the Elizabethan legislation and this civil-war ordinance was that the latter scheme was also intended to provide for the widows and orphans of deceased servicemen. This departure may have been in response to Parliament's need to recruit soldiers to their cause. In the words of the ordinance, it was 'for their [the soldiers'] better Encouragement in their Service'. War widows and orphans were, nevertheless, intended to be provided for only 'over and besides such relief as they shall gain by their work and labour' and after maimed soldiers had first been accommodated.[20]

The county pension scheme was intended to provide only for parliamen-tarian maimed soldiers, widows and orphans. So, potential claimants had to include a certificate of service with their petition to ensure that there were no fraudulent recipients. The royalists did attempt to administer a system of relief to their maimed soldiers, but the treatment and welfare of the King's sick and wounded troops 'compared badly with Parliament's achievements' and they did not attempt a central system of relief for war widows.[21] Consequently, before 1660 many of the widows of royalist soldiers and injured servicemen in Kent probably fell upon parish relief. After the

Restoration, things changed. The Cavalier Parliament passed a new pension Act in 1662 which provided relief to 'every Officer Souldier or Mariner maimed indigent aged or disabled in body for worke in the Service of his said late Majesty or his Majesty that now is during the late Warrs'.[22] The Act also stipulated that only those who 'have continued faithful to his Trust and not deserted the same by taking up Armes against his said late Majesty' were eligible for pensions. Thus the tables turned, and only royalist maimed soldiers and war widows, who could prove that they had always been loyal to the King, were eligible for relief.

Throughout the period the responsibility for administering the county pension scheme fell to JPs at the Quarter Sessions. These men adhered to Parliament's national rule that stipulated who was eligible for relief and how it was to be allocated. In Kent, as in other counties, there are numerous references in the Quarter Sessions' order books to the JPs trying to better order the process. For example, in April 1648 it was recorded that 'it is found by experience that the stocke for the said maymed souldiers falleth short and is not sufficient for their present reliefe'.[23] Similarly, in West Sussex in 1657 it was found that 'the moneys due & payable for maymed souldiers and charitable uses are very much in arrears', and 'it is not certeynly knowne what euery p[ar]ish ought to pay'.[24] As a result of these issues the JPs would reissue orders for parish rates, and audit the recent accounts of the Treasurer for Maimed Soldiers.[25]

Since the JPs had such an important role in administering pensions, the nature and character of the county bench influenced the ways in which the scheme was implemented. This was most apparent at the time of the Restoration when new Commissions of the Peace replaced sitting JPs to bring county administration in line with the new regime.[26] The records for the Commission of the Peace in Kent in 1665 show that of the 123 JPs, only twelve had appeared in the last commission in 1658.[27] That meant a considerable change to the local ruling elite. There was also an abrupt change in the personnel who administered the pension scheme shortly after Charles II's arrival. In June 1660 a memorandum stated that John Fry was required to attend the JPs at the White Hart in Canterbury.[28] He had been appointed the Treasurer for Maimed Soldiers for the eastern part of the county in 1653 following the death of the previous incumbent, and was, unusually, re-appointed annually to the position in the coming years.[29] Fry had also briefly been Treasurer for the County Committee of Kent in the early 1640s and was described as 'a p[er]son faithfull to the Com[m]onwealth interest' by members of the Kentish gentry and County Committee in the letter that recommended his appointment.[30] After the Restoration the man who had been displaced as Treasurer for Maimed Soldiers during the civil wars because of his loyalty to the King, William Russell, demanded his job back. An order from July 1660 confirmed that Russell was to be reinstated as Treasurer for Maimed Soldiers. John Fry lost his position.[31]

Rapid changes to the makeup of the county bench and its treasurers were mirrored by the speed with which parliamentarian pensions were revoked in Kent. In April 1661, there was an order in the West Kent books that all pensions awarded prior to the previous October (1660) were to be suspended.[32] Notably, this preceded the Parliamentary Act and similar orders for other counties. This order did contain one exception: a certain William Ashdown, who was first granted an annuity of £3 in 1648 after serving Parliament in Devon, was allowed to continue to receive his pension. This was not just found in Kent: in East Sussex the order to discharge old pensions contained the exceptions of two men and Appleby has found similar confirmations of parliamentarian pensions in Essex.[33] Perhaps knowledge of the personal circumstances of these men, or the severity of their wartime injuries, may have moved the JPs to retain them on the pension roll. Generally speaking, however, parliamentarian pensioners were quickly replaced by royalist recipients and JPs in Kent dramatically increased their expenditure by rewarding those who came forward to claim that they had fought for the King. In Kent, and West Kent in particular, the fervour of the new administration's loyalty to the present and former Kings' cause was reflected in their generosity towards maimed soldiers and war widows.

PETITIONING FOR PENSIONS

In order to receive a pension or a one-off gratuity from the JPs, maimed soldiers and war widows had to construct a petition. These documents can be found in the Quarter Sessions' rolls among recognizances, indictments and examinations. All of the petitions for Kent were constructed in the familiar secretary hand of government and conformed to the classical style of petitions: an address, followed by the details of the case and finishing with final exhortations.[34] It is very rare to find a petition signed by the petitioner themselves and the petitions would have been constructed by a third party such as a lawyer, clergyman or the Clerk of the Peace. Only four of the maimed soldiers from Kent were styled 'gentleman' in the records (three of these were royalists).[35] Status descriptors were rare among the maimed soldiers' petitions, and there is no indication in those of any war widow. Consequently, it seems likely that most of the men and women who sought relief from the county bench were of low social status and did not have other means to fall back on, besides parish relief, for their financial subsistence. For example, the Kentish war widow Susan North described how she and her family had 'sold & paund such things w[h]ich she had for maintenance' and were now in desperate need of a pension.[36]

These petitions were clearly written to persuade and this presents some challenges when it comes to analysing their content. It is difficult to know what elements of the petition came directly from the petitioner and what from the scribe. Did Susan North, in the above example, specifically request that those words were entered into her petition in that way? Or was the scribe relying on familiar narrative devices used across petitions of that type? Many of these petitions do contain a wide variety of unique and persuasive elements, which could suggest the influence of a distinctive authorial voice. Natalie Zemon Davies's work on French pardon tales in the sixteenth century suggested that historians should do more than just seek historical truth from the archives.[37] Hudson concurred with this analysis but further argued that we must avoid 'total cynicism' with regards to the truth of these petitions. They were indeed constructed to persuade in a collaborative process that involved both the petitioner and scribe, but they had to 'stand up to some scrutiny' because the petitioner themselves had to confirm the story in their own words when they appeared before the Quarter Sessions.[38]

It is clear from the records that there was an expectation that petitioners should appear at a Quarter Sessions' court when they first presented their plea for relief and again to receive their pension quarterly. In Sussex in 1652 the JPs ordered that Jeremy Clark's pension should be suspended 'for his misbehaviour and insolent carryage and speeches toward[es] the Justices of peace at the present sessions', which indicates that he was present at the session.[39] However, his pension was ordered to be paid with arrears at the next session and so his misdemeanours were clearly forgiven, or forgotten.[40] Occasionally there is also evidence that the petitioners themselves did not appear in court but that they sent a representative on their behalf. Thomas Berkhead's petition, for example, contains the pertinent phrase, 'my wife hath Come purposely About this busines'.[41] An order for relief for a war widow also described the process of gaining relief in unusual detail: 'Upon the reading of the petition of Jane Rusbridger with a Certificate of Captayne Clerke and oath made in court by Robert Hopkins'.[42] This could suggest that Jane herself was not present in court but that her petition was put to the court orally and that somebody else stood up under oath on her behalf. Consequently, practices seemed to differ about whether or not a petitioner accompanied their petition to court and stood to defend it or read it. Nevertheless, the JPs clearly wanted to have petitioners, or their representatives, appear before them when they decided whether to grant relief.

Such protocols may have been a mechanism to prevent fraud. Hudson found that several war widows who presented themselves in court to ask for pensions, but were denied them and only given one-off sums, repeatedly re-attended.[43] These people were known as 'importuners'. This was certainly the case in Kent where a considerable number of war widows who were told 'not to expect more' came to court again.[44] The county benches were also suspicious of people trying to gain pensions from more than one place. Kent JPs paid John Blunder a one-off sum of 5s, 'In regard hee cannot make it appeare that hee tooke vpp armes in this County'.[45] Attending the Sessions in person was one way to ensure that petitioners did indeed come from that area, as both the 1643 and 1662 legislation insisted. Pensions could also be suspended by the JPs if they thought the recipient was no longer deserving. For example, the pension of Mr Armstronge was discharged 'for certaine misdemeanors'.[46] One way to bolster the claims of a petition and to protect it from such charges was to include an endorsement with it, perhaps from prominent local people. For example, the petition of the royalist soldier, John Fletcher, was accompanied by the signatures of twenty-nine men who supported his request and who were also probably eager to remove him from their parish's poor rate.[47]

The process of petitioning for a pension was not confined to the petitioner themselves. When their petition was constructed at least one other person was involved, scribing the petition and probably giving advice as to its contents. Then the petitioner, or somebody they trusted, appeared in court to give testimony to their claims. The petition could also be accompanied by an endorsement from local people, military officers, or even some of the JPs who might be adjudicating their case.[48] In Kent, as in other counties, the JPs were concerned about fraud and ensuring that they only gave pensions to those who deserved it. Therefore, the petitioners responded to this requirement to persuade, and constructed petitions in ways that would help them to be the most successful. This does not mean that these documents were inherently fictive. They were an integral part of the administration of military welfare and demonstrate to historians the ways in which maimed soldiers and war widows navigated the process in order to support themselves and their families.

RECEIVING PENSIONS

Early modern Kent had one bench of justices but the four Quarter Sessions for each year rotated between East and West Kent. Epiphany and Midsummer sessions were held at locations in East Kent, and the court moved to West Kent for Easter and Michaelmas. Figure 9.1 illustrates the number of pensions granted in East and West Kent by year, from 1642 to 1679.[49] The dates reflect when a pension was listed as awarded in either the order book or at the bottom of a petition in the sessions rolls. Therefore, it does not show the cumulative number of individuals on the pension roll per year but instead only fresh orders for relief.

Figure 9.1 shows very few pensions being granted to maimed soldiers or war widows in the first few years of the civil wars. This may be partly as a result of the extant records: the order book for East Kent only starts in 1650 so the graph shows no pensions being granted in this part of Kent from 1642 to 1650 but this almost certainly does not reflect the true figure. Despite this gap, there are still some interesting features of the data. The first pension recorded, granted in 1644, was given to the maimed soldier Henry Clerke of Cowden. He was awarded a pension of £4 and the entry described how he 'went forth against the Rebells there [Yalding] for the suppressing of

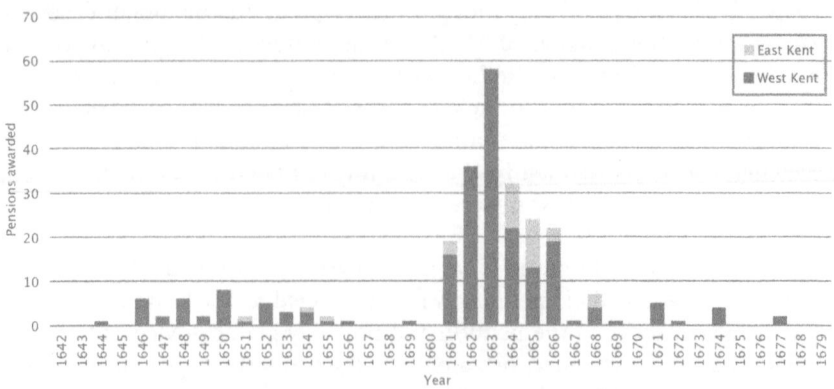

Figure 9.1 Number of pensions awarded in East and West Kent, 1642–79

that Rebellion as also for the safeguard of this Countie'.[50] This pension was, therefore, closely related to the events that took place within the county rather than outside of it. Twenty years later, in March 1664, the widow of Jeremy Tauntington was granted a one-off sum of 40s.[51] Her husband had fought in that same uprising in Yalding in 1643 but presumably on the side of the 'rebels' who had declared allegiance to the King.

While pensions were awarded at a fairly low but consistent rate in Kent before the Restoration, the graph show a marked increase in pensions during the years from 1660 to 1663. 1663 saw the most pensions awarded: fifty-eight men and women were granted money in this year. This was more than seven times the largest amount of pensions given during any one year before the Restoration. This amounted to a high expenditure on behalf of the county stock. The pensions awarded during this year alone amounted to the value of £177. If these were paid out consistently throughout the next few years, something that cannot be certain, then the cost to the county would have been high. By comparison, throughout the whole of the period before the Restoration the total value of pensions listed in the existing order books only came to £120 6s. The graph also demonstrates that the majority of these awards came from West Kent and that without the awards from West Kent there would be no such peak. This illustrates Appleby's point that royalist affiliation was particularly strong among JPs from north and west Kent.[52] This also coincides with the areas where there had been resistance to Fairfax and support for royalism in 1648.

It is clear that Kent's JPs, and in particular those from West Kent, were generous to royalists in the first few years following the Restoration. Yet, the provision of pensions fell largely to maimed soldiers. Of the 212 pensions that were awarded after 1660, only four went to war widows. This is probably because the 1662 Act (like the 1642 Ordinance) gave provision to war widows

Table 9.1 Pensions awarded to maimed soldiers and war widows in Kent, 1642–79

	Parliamentarian (1642–59)			Royalist (1660–79)		
	Total	Percentage	Average	Total	Percentage	Average
Maimed Soldiers	36	81	2li 15s 17d	208	98	2li 8s 2d
War Widows	8	19	2li 14s 0d	4	2	2li 5s 0d

Source: KHLC, Q/SO/E1–E2, East Kent QS Order Books, 1654–79; KHLC, Q/SO/W1–W3, West Kent QS Order Books, 1642–79; KHLC, Q/SB/1–11, Kent QS Sessions Rolls, 1642–79

Table 9.2 One-off grants awarded to maimed soldiers and war widows in Kent, 1642–79

	Parliamentarian (1642–59)			Royalist (1660–79)		
	Total	Percentage	Average	Total	Percentage	Average
Maimed Soldiers	53	71	1li 10s 7d	297	78	1li 5s 5d
War Widows	22	29	2li 4s 2d	83	22	4li 3s 12d

Source: KHLC, Q/SO/E1–E2, East Kent QS Order Books, 1654–79; KHLC, Q/SO/W1–W3, West Kent QS Order Books, 1642–79; KHLC, Q/SB/1–11, Kent QS Sessions Rolls, 1642–79

and orphans but only 'out of the Surplusage of such Stock of Maintenance as shall remain in the hands of the said Treasurers after such Pensions and payment of them made'.[53] This was an area where the Restoration justices in Kent were less generous than their predecessors. Table 9.1 illustrates the percentage of pensions awarded to war widows in both periods.[54]

Kent JPs may not have awarded many pensions to royalist war widows but they did hand out considerable amounts to them in one-off sums. The order books for West Kent contain extensive lists of names for those who were awarded financial relief (many more than petitions survive for) and this included some lists that were reserved just for women and children. They were described as 'widdowes & Orphans of men who in their life tyme did suffer many extremeties by reason of theire loyaltye to his Ma[je]stie in the sa[i]d late tymes' and were rewarded well for their husbands' and fathers' actions.[55] In Kent, eighty-three war widows received one-off sums between 1660 and 1679. Table 9.2 shows that it was not just the number of war widows who received one-off sums that reveals the justices' generosity, but also the amounts that individuals were awarded.

This table shows that the average amount royalist war widows received in one-off grants was considerably higher than maimed soldiers before and after the Restoration (and war widows during the civil wars and Interregnum).

These numbers account for the amount that each maimed soldier or war widow received in total. Consequently, the striking divergence in the final column of Table 9.2 reflects the fact that many widows received multiple one-off awards. For some widows, the JPs awarded one-off sums with such frequency that they could have been pensions. The names of Rebecca St Leger and Elizabeth Ennis appear every year in the order books for West Kent between 1663 and 1671 and they were awarded sums of between £2 and £8 each time (although most frequently they were granted £5).[56] Between them, the county stock of West Kent expended £77. This suggests that the JPs were treating them like pensioners: it was always at the Easter Session that they were granted money and they received it consistently. Hudson's research also found that war widows 'were rarely granted stipends and had to settle for gratuities' and argued that this reflected 'the attitudes of the royalists to women and the armed forces'.[57] Nevertheless, the scarcity of war widows who were granted pensions in Kent after the Restoration does not necessarily show that the justices were ungenerous towards them. The JPs seemed to have made a special case for certain widows: their names were frequently set apart in order books and some received one-off sums regularly. Therefore, after the Restoration war widows may have also benefitted from the political persuasion of the local administration even though they were not awarded pensions to the same extent as maimed soldiers.

Finally, the records which state how many people received pensions can be used to outline patterns of allegiance. Most of the order book entries and petitions also refer to the parish of origin of the petitioner and so, as has been argued by Mark Stoyle, 'the maimed soldiers' petitions can shed crucial light upon patterns of popular allegiance'.[58] David Underdown also used order books and petitions to measure the distribution of wartime loyalty.[59] This approach has attracted criticism largely because the parish of origin stated in a petition or in an order book entry may not have been the parish that the maimed soldier originally left to take up arms. This is a particular problem with the royalist petitioners who received relief long after the wars were over and thus the chances of them having moved in the intervening years were higher. John Morrill has also suggested that it may be the case that these records instead reveal something about the history of poor relief.[60] Perhaps the patterns in the parishes of maimed soldiers and war widows indicate where there were areas of financial dearth rather than popular loyalty. This certainly seems to have been the case in Essex where the bulk of petitioners came from the impoverished hundreds of the county.[61] The Quarter Sessions records are also not complete records of who served either Parliament or King within the county. Consequently, this discussion of Kent will not argue that these records alone can reveal where in Kent loyalty to King or Parliament was strongest. Despite this, it will be made clear that there are strong links between where royalist recipients of relief resided after the Restoration and areas of the county that were

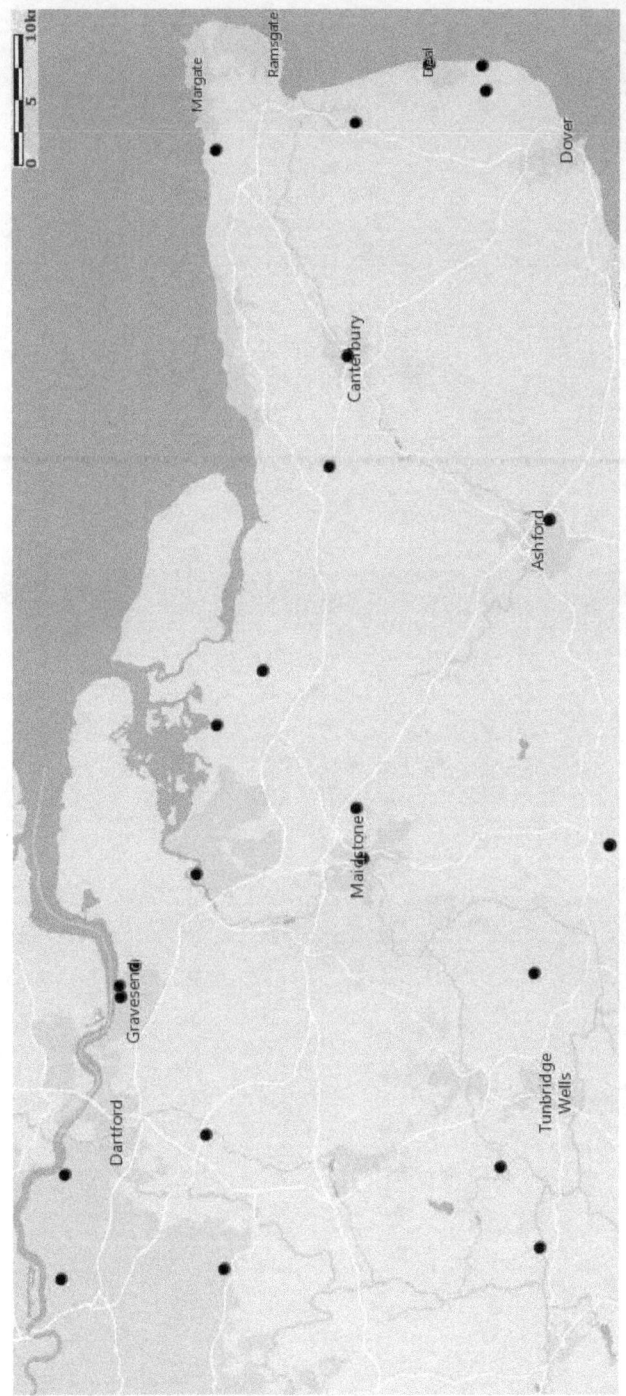

Figure 9.2 Parish of origin of parliamentarian maimed soldiers and war widows in East and West Kent, 1642–59

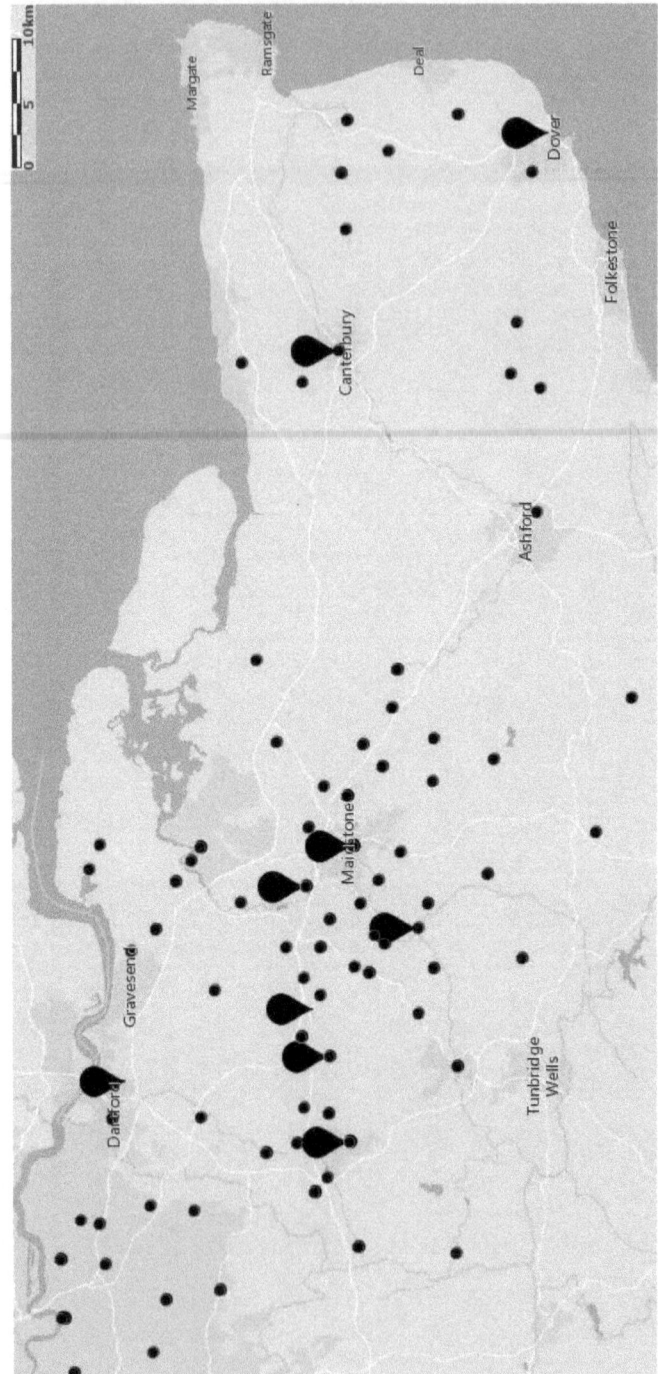

Figure 9.3 Parish of origin of royalist maimed soldiers and war widows in East and West Kent, 1660–79

involved in uprisings during the civil wars. This therefore indicates, like Stoyle's findings for Devon, that there were more factors influencing the geographical spread of petitioners than simply 'the incidence of post-war poverty'.[62]

Figure 9.2 shows the parish of origin (when it was stated) of maimed soldiers and war widows who were granted pensions and one-off sums between 1642 and 1659. The map shows some clusters around coastal areas but there is not enough evidence from the petitions alone to assume that these petitioners were seamen. There are gaps in central west Kent, Sevenoaks and the areas surrounding Maidstone, where few maimed parliamentarian soldiers and war widows resided, so it is possible that people from these areas were less likely to submit petitions for relief before the Restoration. Nevertheless, there are several limitations to these conclusions. The overall numbers of parliamentarian entries from Kent are too low to produce significant correlation and the missing East Kent Order Book may have contained additional entries to change the results.

By contrast, the numbers of royalists who received pensions and one-off sums after 1660 was considerable. Thus, it is possible to see clearer patterns emerging from their geographical spread.

Comparing Figures 9.2 and 9.3 clearly shows the space in West Kent being filled with a substantial number of claimants. This is not just significant because many of these parishes did not have previous parliamentarian recipients of relief residing in them. They were also clustered around some of the sites of Kent's royalist uprisings (marked with black points on the map), in Yalding, Sevenoaks and Maidstone, and areas of strong royalist support such as Dartford and Greenwich. Some areas had particularly high numbers of royalist recipients of relief. For example, taken as pairs the neighbouring parishes of Greenwich and Deptford, and Sevenoaks and Chevening each had thirty-seven royalist maimed soldiers or war widows residing there. It is possible that these soldiers were former parliamentarians from the First Civil War who switched sides when rebellion broke out in Kent in 1648. This situation, as well as more widespread evidence of side changing during the wars, presents further problems with using these records as accurate evidence of military service.[63]

The evidence for pensions awarded after the Restoration in Kent shows that there was clearly a link between local patterns of allegiance and military welfare. This does not mean that these records provide complete evidence for how the county divided during the civil wars. Certain parishes had higher numbers of royalist recipients of relief residing in them but that may reflect the financial needs of the area rather than its loyalty. Presumably these men and women had been compelled to rely on parish relief for their subsistence in previous decades, so it is unsurprising that there was a rush from former royalist soldiers and war widows for financial aid at the Restoration. Additionally, these records do not just reveal information about the loyalties of those who petitioned for relief. It is important to remember that the political allegiances of the JPs who administered the system, and were willing to grant relief in such proportions, must also have been a significant factor. Despite these limitations, it is still possible to argue that the records of military welfare are a valuable resource for understanding the patterns of wartime loyalty in the localities. The county of Kent, with its high numbers of royalist pensioners and interesting geographical correlation, adds to that case.

CONCLUSION

The county pension scheme provided an important means of financial subsistence for those maimed or bereaved as a result of the civil wars. In Kent, pensions were granted to a substantial number of claimants (although not nearly as many as that recorded in Devon), and JPs seemed eager to grant relief.[64] The records of this process tell historians about poverty and need within the county as well as about wartime loyalty and allegiance. They are an invaluable source for local historians of Kent as well as important evidence for the ways in which early modern governments treated their military dependants. Analysing this process demonstrates that an integrated research approach is required, which takes into account both local and national concerns. There are clearly some aspects that were peculiar to Kent. This is made clear by the large amount of pensions that were awarded in the first few years after the Restoration, and the number of claimants who resided in parishes associated with unrest in the previous decades. Nevertheless, the system did not exist in a vacuum. It was directed by acts and ordinances of Parliament, and the counties which bordered Kent operated their own county pension schemes. When it came to accessing relief, both parliamentarian and royalist claimants, men and women, had to construct petitions to represent their experiences. They also had to actively participate in this particular arena of local, public politics. Therefore, these documents demonstrate the tenacity with which many maimed and bereaved Kentish people fought to survive once the wars had ended.

NOTES

1 A. Everitt, *The Community of Kent and the Great Rebellion, 1640–60* (Leicester: Leicester University Press, 1966) pp. 190–1.
2 *Ibid.*, pp. 204, 215.
3 *Ibid.*, pp. 213, 215.
4 C. H. Firth and R. S. Rait (eds), *Acts and Ordinances of the Interregnum, 1642–1660*, 3 vols (London: HMSO, 1911), I, pp. 413–18.
5 B. Donagan, *War in England, 1642–1649* (Oxford: Oxford University Press, 2008), pp. 316–17.
6 Everitt, *The Community of Kent*, p. 13.

7 J. Eales, *Community and Disunity: Kent and the English Civil Wars, 1640–1649* (Faversham: Keith Dickson Books, 2001), p. 5; M. Zell, 'Introduction', in M. Zell (ed.), *Early Modern Kent: 1540–1640* (Woodbridge: Boydell, 2000), p. 5.

8 A. Hughes, *Politics, Society and Civil War in Warwickshire, 1620–1660* (Cambridge: Cambridge University Press, 1987), p. xi.

9 C. Holmes, 'The county community in Stuart historiography', *Journal of British Studies*, 19:2 (1980), 55.

10 G. L. Hudson, 'Negotiating for blood money: war widows and the courts in seventeenth-century England', in J. Kermode and G. Walker (eds), *Women, Crime and the Courts in Early Modern England* (London: University College, 1994), pp. 146–69.

11 *Ibid.*, p. 162.

12 D. J. Appleby, 'Unnecessary persons? Maimed soldiers and war widows in Essex, 1642–62', *Essex Archaeology and History*, 32 (2001), 209–21.

13 D. J. Appleby, 'Veteran politics in Restoration England, 1660–1670', *The Seventeenth Century*, 28:3 (2013), 323–42; M. Stoyle, '"Memories of the maimed": the testimony of Charles I's former soldiers, 1660–1730', *History*, 88:290 (2003), 204–26.

14 J. S. Morrill, 'The ecology of allegiance in the English Revolution', *Journal of British Studies*, 26:4 (1987), 466.

15 G. L. Hudson, 'Disabled veterans and the state in early modern England', in D. Gerber (ed.), *Disabled Veterans in History* (Ann Arbor, MI: University of Michigan Press, 2000), p. 122.

16 *Ibid.*, pp. 118–22.

17 E. Wingate, *An Exact Abridgment of all Statutes in Force and Use from the Beginning of Magna Carta until 1641* (London, 1666).

18 Firth and Rait (eds), *Acts and Ordinances of the Interregnum*, I, pp. 36–7.

19 N. Rogers, *The Good Samaritan: Or An Exposition on that Parable* (London, 1658), p. 91.

20 Firth and Rait (eds), *Acts and Ordinances of the Interregnum*, II, pp. 938–40.

21 E. Gruber von Arni, *Justice to the Maimed Soldier: Nursing, Medical Care and Welfare for Sick and Wounded Soldiers and their Families during the English Civil Wars and Interregnum, 1642–1660* (Aldershot: Ashgate, 2001), p. 37.

22 'Charles II, 1662: An Act for the releife of poore and maimed Officers and Souldiers who have faithfully served His Majesty and His Royal Father in the late Wars', in J. Raithby (ed.), *Statutes of the Realm: Volume 5, 1628–80* (London, 1819), pp. 389–90.

23 KHLC, QO/SO/W1, West Kent Order Book, April 1648, fo. 182r.

24 ESRO, QO/1/5/3, West Sussex Order Book, April 1657, fo. 31v.

25 For example: KHLC, Q/SO/W1, West Kent Order Book, April 1656, fo. 152v; KHLC, Q/SO/E2, East Kent Order Book, January 1676, fo. 26r.

26 R. Hutton, *The Restoration: A Political and Religious History of England and Wales, 1658–1667* (Oxford: Clarendon Press, 1985), p. 129.

27 KHLC, Q/J/C/10, Commission of the Peace, 1665.

28 KHLC, Q/SO/E1, East Kent Order Book, June 1660, fo. 46.

29 In Sussex the Treasurer for Maimed Soldiers changed every year: B. C. Redwood (ed.), *Quarter Sessions Order Book, 1642–1649* (Sussex Record Society, 54, 1954), p. xvii.

30 Everitt, *The Community of Kent*, p. 175; KHLC, Q/SB/4/72, Correspondence, 18 April 1653.

31 KHLC, Q/SB/7/68–9, Order, 24 July 1660.

32 KHLC, Q/SO/W2, West Kent Order Book, April 1661, fo. 71r.

33 Appleby, 'Veteran politics in Restoration England', 334; ESRO, QO/1/5/4, East Sussex Order Book, January 1662, fo. 30v.

34 J. Daybell, *The Material Letter in Early Modern England Manuscript Letters and the Culture and Practices of Letter-Writing, 1512–1635* (Basingstoke: Palgrave Macmillan, 2012), p. 70.

35 KHLC, Q/SO/W1, West Kent Order Book, August 1647, fo. 168v; KHLC, Q/SO/W2, West Kent Order Book, April 1663, fo. 99r; KHLC, Q/SO/W2, West Kent Order Book, April 1665, fo. 113r; KHLC, Q/SO/E1, East Kent Order Book, January 1666, fo. 103r.

36 KHLC, Q/SB/3/26, Petition of Susan North, 1652.

37 N. Zemon Davis, *Fiction in the Archives: Pardon Tales and their Tellers in Sixteenth-Century France* (Stanford, CA: Stanford University Press, 1987), pp. 2–3.

38 Hudson, 'Negotiating for blood money', p. 156.

39 ESRO, QO/1/5/2, East Sussex Order Book, July 1653, fo. 34r.

40 ESRO, QO/1/5/2, East Sussex Order Book, April 1654, July 1655, April 1658, fos. 24r, 34r, 60r, QO/1/5/3, fos. 4v, 51r.

41 West Sussex Record Office (WSRO), Q/R/W80, Petition of Thomas Berkhead, October 1654, fo. 4.

42 ESRO, QO/1/5/2, West Sussex Order Book, October 1651, fo. 21r.

43 Hudson, 'Negotiating for blood money', p. 158.

44 For example: KHLC, Q/SO/W2, West Kent Order Book, April 1656 and April 1657, fos. 31r, 38r.

45 KHLC, Q/SO/W2, West Kent Order Book, April 1653, fo. 14r.

46 KHLC, Q/SO/W1, West Kent Order Book, October 1649, fo. 193r.

47 KHLC, Q/SB/8/54, Petition of John Fletcher [1662].

48 For example: KHLC, Q/SO/W2, West Kent Order Book, October 1661, fos. 75v–76r.

49 Note that while data was collected up to 1679, the last pension awarded in this period was in 1677.

50 KHLC, Q/SO/W1, West Kent Order Book, April 1644, fo. 147r.

51 KHLC, Q/SO/W2, West Kent Order Book, March 1664, fo. 103r.

52 Appleby, 'Veteran politics in Restoration England', 334.

53 'Charles II, 1662: An Act for the releife of poore and maimed Officers and Souldiers', in Raithby (ed.), *Statues of the Realm*, pp. 389–90.

54 The average amount has been calculated using the mean and the total reflects the number of individuals who received awards (rather than the total number of awards).

55 KHLC, Q/SO/W2, West Kent Order Book, April 1663, fo. 91r.

56 KHLC, QO/SO/W2, West Kent Order Books, 1663–72, fos. 91r, 103r, 113r, 120r, 125r, 131r, 135r, 141v; QO/SO/W3, fos. 6r, 13v.

57 Hudson, 'Negotiating for blood money', p. 151.

58 M. Stoyle, *Loyalty and Locality: Popular Allegiance in Devon during the English Civil War* (Exeter: Exeter University Press, 1994), p. 79.

59 D. Underdown, *Revel, Riot and Rebellion: Popular Politics and Culture in England 1603–1660* (Oxford: Clarendon Press, 1985), pp. 191–8.
60 Morrill, 'The ecology of allegiance', 466.
61 Appleby, 'Unnecessary persons?', 212.
62 Stoyle, *Loyalty and Locality*, p. 89.
63 A. Hopper, *Turncoats and Renegadoes: Changing Sides during the English Civil Wars* (Oxford: Oxford University Press, 2012), pp. 78–99.
64 Stoyle, *Loyalty and Locality*, p. 80.

Chapter 10

———

'To condole with me on the
Commonwealth's loss': the widows
and orphans of Parliament's military
commanders

Andrew Hopper

The pioneering work of Geoffrey Hudson and Eric Gruber von Arni into military welfare has inspired a recent new wave of civil-war scholarship that highlights the experiences of war widows.[1] So far, these studies have been either regionally based or focused on the administration of the county pension scheme to the widows of junior officers and common soldiers.[2] Another study has examined how royalist widows sought to protect their estates from a hostile regime.[3] These scholars have been broadly sympathetic to the notion that women became more actively engaged with politics as a consequence of the wars, deploying languages of loyalty and suffering to win over those in authority. Their works have tended to agree that Parliament's granting of pensions to its war widows was a landmark moment in welfare history. Parliament's motives in granting such relief were to mobilise further support, as well as to demonstrate their legitimacy and authority. These concerns were intensified when dealing with the widows and orphans of their fallen commanders. These men were well-known national figures, celebrated in print for specific political purposes, so Parliament had to be seen to reward their exemplary sacrifice. In 1647 Josiah Ricraft set out slain parliamentarian commanders in order of rank. This chapter will investigate how the circumstances of their deaths drew their widows into more public political roles.[4] Such widows looked directly to Westminster for aid. They sought payment of their late husbands' arrears of pay, frequently amounting to thousands of pounds. Their overriding concern was to mitigate the wider loss of status incurred by widowhood. Four principal means of redress were open to them: obtaining the wardship of their eldest son, presenting themselves as particularly deserving in their addresses to authority, mobilising influential contacts and networks in their favour, and finally, seeking recompense from enemy estates. This chapter will compare how these widows employed some or all of these means to safeguard the future of their families, livelihoods and estates.

Only two parliamentarian peers were killed during the conflict, leaving two widowed baronesses: Arabella, Lady St John, daughter of John Egerton, first earl of Bridgewater, and Katherine, Lady Brooke, daughter of Francis Russell, fourth earl of Bedford. Their husbands Oliver St John, fifth baron St John of Bletso and Robert Greville, second baron Brooke, were both slain on active service early in the war, and because of their status as peers were listed as first and second respectively on Josiah Ricraft's list of slain parliamentarian worthies.[5] Lord St John was mortally wounded at Edgehill, supposedly having 'declared at his death a full satisfaction and cheerfulness to lay down his life in so good a cause'.[6] This may have reflected Edmund Ludlow's concern, or that of his 1690s editor, John Toland, to keep the circumstances of St John's death from staining the posterity of the parliamentarian cause. The royalists reported his death very differently. Bernard de Gomme wrote that during the battle St John 'had the Kings horse by the Bridle'.[7] Such an act against the King's sacred person would have attracted widespread horror. The earl of Clarendon expanded upon St John's rotten character, pointing out he had been deeply in debt, and that 'his course of life [was] licentious and very much depraved'. Rather than dying a noble death for his cause, St John's 'canting' last words were that 'he did not intend to be against the King, but wished him all happiness'. This contest over St John's memory reflects the importance contemporaries attached to last words, but Clarendon also asserted cowardice: that St John 'had received some wounds in running away' before dying in royalist custody the following morning.[8] So, an awkward discomfort may explain Parliament's inaction in celebrating St John's memory or supporting his widow. St John died in debt with no male heir. His widow, Arabella, was buried at Melton Mowbray in 1669.[9] Her will suggests a secluded and modest retirement, hardly in keeping with her status as a peeress of the realm.[10] The contrast with Lady Brooke's experience can hardly have been greater.

The circumstances of Lord Brooke's death elevated him into the pantheon of parliamentarian martyrs. While besieging Lichfield on 2 March 1643, he was shot through the eye by a sharpshooter stationed in the cathedral's tower.[11] He was buried 'a month or six weeks' later in the first Lord Brooke's vault in the chapter house of St Mary's, Warwick.[12] Thomas Spencer, the puritan vicar of nearby Budbrooke who was probably present, recorded that the funeral was 'performed in honourable and warlike fashion', with 'his Bodie being interred in the same vault or Sepulchre, with his Noble Predecessour'.[13] Although several of the funeral bills were addressed to Katherine, Lady Brooke, and included her own mourning attire, convention dictated that all mourners had to be male at the heraldic funeral of a nobleman.[14] Therefore it remains doubtful that Katherine participated, although it appears her four young sons did so as the bill for their mourning gloves survives.[15] With the funeral over, Katherine resided at Brooke House in Holborn, a large London mansion of forty-four rooms attended by thirty servants.[16]

The circumstances of Brooke's death invited Parliament to intervene more strongly than they had done for Lady St John. The royalists celebrated that Brooke, who had been so vehement against bishops, had been shot on St Chad's Day, the patron saint of Lichfield Cathedral.[17] It was even said that Brooke had prayed the very morning that he was shot 'that if the cause he were in were not right and just, he might be presently cut off'.[18] Rejoicing that Brooke's death was providential could not go unanswered. Thomas Spencer exhorted Parliament not to forget 'in the midst of your most weightie ymployments' Brooke's 'fair and hopeful yssue'.[19] Only four days after his death, the House of Lords ordered that the £1,000 Brooke had lent upon the Propositions be repaid to his executors.[20] In time Parliament pledged further aid for Brooke's widow and their unborn son Fulke, for whom the deceased lord had made no provision, not knowing his wife was then pregnant.[21] Yet this assistance was not immediate. Katherine's brother William, fifth earl of Bedford, brought suspicion upon the family by his temporary defection to the royalists in August 1643. When Bedford returned to London in January 1644 he failed to recover his seat in the Lords, and was confined in Brooke House, where Lady Brooke resided with her sons.[22] The upkeep of Bedford, his servants, coach and horses brought considerable expense.[23]

Worse still than Katherine's anxieties about her brother, was that widowhood endangered noble patrimonies, especially during a time of civil war. Charles I continued to exercise wardship, granting that of her eldest son, the young Francis, to his principal secretary of state, Lord Digby on 13 March 1644.[24] This endangered both Francis's person and his inheritance. In such circumstances, wards' estates were 'frequently exploited rather than managed', and recovering lands from wardship was a lengthy, expensive and difficult process.[25] The grant of wardship to Digby was drawn up by Richard Chamberlain, clerk of the royalist incarnation of the Court of Wards at Oxford, whose Warwickshire home had been turned into a garrison by Brooke's soldiers.[26] Katherine received a letter from the King dated 15 April 1644, erroneously addressed to 'Dame Anne Brooke widdow' demanding she hand over the custody of Francis to Digby upon pain of a fine of £5,000.[27] To prevent her son falling into enemy hands, Katherine petitioned Parliament to claim wardship for herself. This involved paying fees to nineteen different individuals in Parliament and the Court of Wards, totalling £78 5s 5d. One 'Mr Sprigg'[28] was paid for drafting two petitions and a cousin was sent with payment to John Browne, clerk of the Parliament to draw up the ordinance. Lady Brooke's petition was read in the Commons on 27 August 1644, and the House voted to repudiate Digby's claims and settled on her Francis's guardianship. In retaliation, the Commons granted Digby's fashionable residence on Queen Street, London, to Lady Brooke for her youngest son, Fulke. The case prompted the Commons to order a further ordinance to discharge from wardship the heirs of all those who died in Parliament's service.[29] In 1646, Parliament abolished the Court of Wards altogether.[30] Yet Lady Brooke continued to be troubled by wartime exactions. A royal order to her tenants in June 1644 commanded them to pay Digby all their rents and arrearages since Brooke's death, upon pain of being fined £5,000.[31] This made collecting her rents more difficult. Some of the family estates were in royalist-held territory. Unsurprisingly, rents fell short of their pre-war value of £5,000 per annum.

Lady Brooke's social status allowed her to petition the House of Lords directly. She did this on numerous occasions and her petitions were carefully managed to represent her in the most favourable and deserving light. On 3 August 1647, the Lords intervened to protect her horses from being enlisted into the intended defence of the city against Fairfax's New Model Army.[32] On 22 October 1647 Katherine reminded them of the pledge by the House of Commons in August 1644 to provide for Fulke's future, pointing to her own forbearance in not bothering them hitherto: 'Your Petitioner ever since (in regard of the weighty Affairs of the Kingdom) hath been therein silent.'[33] This was part of her representation as the stoic and patient puritan widow, who put suffering in the cause before her personal interests. Katherine's portrait in mourning apparel does much to project this image, and was in attire that she had certainly paid for, and likely chosen herself.[34] Now held at Warwick Castle, it is attributed to Theodore Russell. The painting depicts her holding a posy of flowers that include pink laurel, which was to represent honour, triumph and eternal life, along with rosemary to signify remembrance.[35] How long she wore this remains unknown; she may have appeared in it at Tower Hill for the execution of her husband's old foe, Archbishop Laud.[36]

Lady Brooke was thrust into playing the role of Parliament's premier war widow because of her husband's dramatic death, and his aggrandisement in their propaganda. Thomas Spencer remarked how Brooke's death had become the subject of 'many nimble Pennes'.[37] One tract lamented, 'Weep thou, his vertuous Lady, cry yee, pretty children (his own pictures)'.[38] Ricraft later explained this outpouring of grief was because parliamentarians tended to 'expect more from him then God would suffer him to perform in the time God afforded him'.[39] This point was later echoed by Clarendon who recalled how Brooke's death 'was exceedingly lamented by that party, which had scarce a more absolute confidence in any man than in him'.[40]

Owing to her extensive familial contacts among the godly, Katherine received much spiritual comfort and many letters of condolence. One minister presented her with verses from her husband, while Katherine stoically refused a portrait of her husband, paying off the painter.[41] Thomas Spencer wrote Katherine a kind letter, hoping she would find solace in her children, and alluding to Psalm 128, 'God Almightie enlarge his graces upon your Selfe, and all your noble olive Branches, and fill you all with His strength.'[42] Among the many elegies to Brooke, one was personally addressed to Katherine by John Wallis, the cryptographer, and chaplain to another famous godly military widow, Lady Mary Vere. His condolences were particularly fulsome, exhorting that her personal grief was owned and shared by the kingdom:

We first your Losse, and then your grief bemone;
(Some Ease, in Sadnesse, not to weep Alone:)
Our Teares (ambitious) make their sad addresse;
(We'd bear a part, that You might weep the lesse.)[43]

Even after the regicide, Lady Brooke continued to enjoy close contacts with the republican regime. In September 1649, she spent four days visiting the prominent councillor Alexander Popham at Littlecote, while she rented Digby's Queen Street house to General Fairfax.[44] Her godly household played host to the Countess of Carlisle, while her sons, equipped with books for sermon notes, frequented the library at Sion College. In March 1649 Katherine took her eldest son Francis to the trials of the duke of Hamilton, the earl of Holland and Lord Capel, later purchasing for him their scaffold speeches.[45] Although her receivers managed the rents, Parliament dealt directly with Katherine over her late husband's estates. In 1649 the Council of State requested she pay the arrears of the pension settled by the first Lord Brooke on Dr Isaac Dorislaus, 'barbarously murdered in the service of the commonwealth', leaving a son and two daughters.[46] Katherine authorised payment of £170 to Dorislaus's son.[47] The Council of State reciprocated by sending surveyors to Warwick Castle and recommending a grant of £1,000 for its renovation.[48] With such widespread recognition of her husband's sacrifice, ultimately, Katherine was handsomely rewarded for her sufferings as an exemplary godly war widow. Her activities strongly suggest that she continued to enjoy close connections with men at the centre of the republican regime, not merely because of her husband's memory, but perhaps also owing to her own godly credentials. For instance, after the Restoration, she was implicated in the failed Northern Risings of 1663, having been accused of allowing the arch-conspirator Dr Edward Richardson, to preach in her house.[49]

During the Wars of the Roses, some war widow peeresses were recompensed with the lands of executed nobles from the other side.[50] This precedent of forcing the enemy to pay for a widow's welfare was embraced by the Long Parliament, and nowhere more conspicuously than for Lady Brooke. On 14 January 1648 both Houses ordered the payment of £5,000 for her son Fulke, out of the revenues from the sequestered estates of the earl of Antrim and his wife, the duchess of Buckingham. These payments required the cooperation of the local sequestrators over a prolonged period.[51] It is a tribute to their diligence that on 23 April 1650 only £1,921 remained due and the Committee for the Sale of Delinquents' lands recommended payment of this final sum.[52] Katherine's household accounts show that the sum was paid in full by February 1651.[53] This reflects how Parliament wanted to continue to be seen to honour Lady Brooke after the regicide. Unlike most widows, Katherine's financial position grew stronger with the passing of time. Every year she signed off the household accounts, which were ordered annually by the anniversary of her husband's death.[54] Lord Brooke's death reduced outgoings, allowing Lady Brooke's receivers to stabilise the estate; substantial sums were even found to pay the late Lord's debts in 1643 and 1644.[55] On top of her jointure of £400 per annum, her husband and sons settled on her several manors in Gloucestershire, Oxfordshire and Warwickshire, as well as a mansion house in Hackney.[56] Through these means, Katherine accumulated a sizeable estate in her own right that removed any need to remarry. Four months after her burial in December 1676, her fifth son, Fulke, succeeded as fifth Lord Brooke, ensuring the family line continued into the next century.[57]

The sense that a widow's grief was owned and shared by the wider parliamentarian cause as an exemplar of sacrifice and fortitude is echoed by the case of Lady Frances Fairfax of Steeton. She was the widow of Commissary-General Sir William Fairfax, the cousin of Sir Thomas Fairfax, the parliamentarian commander-in-chief. In 1642, Frances and her daughters left their Yorkshire home for the safety of London, residing with her brothers Thomas and James Chaloner on Queen Street near Charing Cross. A series of moving wartime letters to Frances from her husband were transcribed by Sir Clements Markham in 1885. In them Sir William addressed his wife as if she were a fellow participant in the cause, informing her of his political hopes and military exploits. He wrote a hurried note on the battlefield at Marston Moor to assure her of his survival, while with Prince Rupert vanquished, his last letter of 7 September 1644 made arrangements for her to return to Steeton remarking: 'there is hopes we shall live quietly this winter'.[58]

Yet Sir William was mortally wounded at Montgomery Castle on 18 September 1644, placing him third on Ricraft's list of slain worthies.[59] One newsbook remarked that because of his refusal to retreat, Sir William was wounded twelve or thirteen times, of which injuries he died sixteen hours later. His last words were reported as a desire for Sir William Brereton to tell Parliament 'He thought his life well bestowed in the service of the Parliament, and in that Cause they did maintain, and to desire them to have a care of his wife and children.' The newsbook was concerned to stress how 'accordingly the Parliament hath ordered immediate care be taken for them'. To underline this, it grandly announced: 'This may be said of a Fairfax and a Sheffield, that there is not one of either of those two names in England, but are engaged for the service of the Parliament.'[60] Another newsbook added: 'Sir William Fairfax, one neer allyed to the Lord Fairfax, who is since dead of his wounds; of whose losse, the Parliament hath expressed a great sence.'[61] Gilbert Mabbott's *The London Post* extolled 'Heroick' Sir William, who died, like Epaminondas of Thebes, happy in the knowledge of victory.[62]

Sir William had indeed proved one of Parliament's most experienced and effective field officers, and his commanding general at Montgomery, Sir John Meldrum, felt it incumbent upon him to press Lady Fairfax's case. Meldrum prevented the surgeons taking Sir William's gold bracelet and diamond ring, and sent them to Frances instead.[63] He urged the Committee of Both Kingdoms to see to her welfare:

> I would recommend to your Lordships the distressed estate of Sir Wm. Fairfax's lady, who being left with many fatherless children and much behind in her husband's personal entertainment, doth challenge me in point of duty, her husband dying honourably under my charge. I hope that you, in point of honour, being sensible of her calamities, will use such means for the relief of herself and her children as you may think a business of this nature requires. As an example, it will conduce much to the encouragement of all gallant gentlemen, and by consequence to the advancement of the public service, so will it reflect much in point of glory on your Lordships as instruments of keeping conscience and virtue undespised.[64]

Meldrum rehearsed the principal argument that due care towards widows would strengthen the war effort, but in this case provision for Lady Fairfax and her orphaned children was especially urgent because Sir William Fairfax had died intestate. On 23 September 1644, when news reached Parliament of his death, the Commons hurriedly ordered the Committee of Yorkshire to bring in an ordinance to settle maintenance on Lady Fairfax and her children, and to grant her the wardship of her son, 'without Charges, yearly Rent, or Composition for Fine'.[65] This was possible because of the wardship ordinance of the previous month triggered by Lady Brooke's case. Only a month later, on 24 October 1644, Parliament passed the ordinance granting Lady Fairfax and her brother Thomas Chaloner, MP, the wardship of her sons William and Thomas.[66]

In a similar way to Lady Brooke, Frances Fairfax presented herself as the stoic, godly widow. Her responses to Sir William's gruesome death were tempered by his family's restraint towards outpourings of grief. Parliament's general in the north, Ferdinando, Lord Fairfax, reflected on 'the mortal wounds of my dear nephew', concluding, 'blessed be God, the victory over our enemies doth abate my sorrow for any particular friends'.[67] Having just lost his second son Charles at Marston Moor, and with his eldest son Sir Thomas lying dangerously wounded at the siege of Helmsley, Lord Fairfax's forbearance was exemplary and instructive. Accordingly, Frances emulated Ferdinando, supposedly remarking that she 'grieved not that he died in the cause, but that he died so soon that he could do no more for it'.[68]

Another glimpse of her self-representation is afforded by her petition to Cromwell and the Protectoral Council of 22 March 1655. It explained that upon her husband's death, Parliament had sent Sir Thomas Widdrington, MP, to her in London, 'to Condole the Comon wealths loss as well as that of her owne in his death', and assure her 'that his faithfull services to ye

Parliam[en]t should bee gratifyed & yo[u]r pet[itione]r & her children p[ro]vided for'. She reminded Cromwell that Sir William had died without making provision for his younger children, leaving her with 'nothing but a small Joynture to live upon and many debts to pay.' She maintained, rather indignantly and not entirely truthfully, that eleven years later she had 'never received one penny' of her husband's arrears, but had remained 'unwilling to trouble yo[u]r Highness & Councell while matters of soe great Concernm[en]t to ye Publique was in Consideracon'.[69] Here, Frances was emulating Lady Brooke's posture of godly forbearance, a facet of honour highly prized by her male relatives, in a direct appeal to Cromwell's religion.[70] Her petition went on that 'her Necessityes doe now constrain her on behalf of herself and younger children unprovided for', to which was added in another hand, 'and is still indebted for Armes her husband bought'. She appealed to Cromwell's piety by signing off: 'And yo[u]r pet[itione]r and her younger Children shalbee bound to bless God for soe seasonable Reliefe & Act of Justice to your pet[itione]r.'[71]

As with the case of Lady Brooke, Frances was allowed recompense from enemy estates. On 19 June 1646, she was given the opportunity of presenting any 'delinq[uen]t of the North' to the Committee for Compounding to receive the £300 remaining of a greater sum formerly ordered her by the Committee at Goldsmiths Hall.[72] On 16 January 1647 the Commons authorised her to receive £1,500 out of Sir Henry Griffiths's composition fine.[73] Yet Sir Henry proved slow to compound, and a year later in January 1648, Parliament ordered Lady Fairfax be allowed the rents from Griffiths's estate until the £1,500 was satisfied.[74] The choice of Griffiths may be linked to Sir William Fairfax's brief detention on his estates while delivering Lord Fairfax's message to Henrietta Maria after she landed at Bridlington in February 1643. When Parliament ordered widows money out of sequestered estates it often remains uncertain whether any such sums were paid, but in this case a certificate survives from the East Riding sequestrators of 18 May 1649 that stipulates £443 had been paid.[75] Frances's petition to Cromwell of 1655 again proposed that she be paid out of the discoveries she would make of several people 'who have many thousand pounds in their hands belonging and due to ye Commonwealth'.[76] The Protector's Council referred it to John Lambert, Nathaniel Fiennes and her late husband's cousin, the earl of Mulgrave. Finally, the Council ordered on 7 September 1655 that Lady Fairfax receive £2,000 in full satisfaction of Sir William's arrears and disbursements from discoveries she was to make of concealed land, monies and goods.[77]

Although Lady Fairfax had family embedded in the regime, this did not prevent the relief she received proving dilatory and piecemeal. Her brother Thomas Chaloner, MP, was a prominent Rumper and a regicide, while her younger brother, James Chaloner, MP, who had married Sir William Fairfax's sister, Ursula, sat on the Northern Committee. This committee recommended on 8 June 1652 that she receive £2,000 in final settlement of her husband's arrears, but the sum remained unpaid for three years.[78] The Long Parliament and Protectorate attempted to honour the grand claims made at her husband's death, but they fell far short of fully settling his arrears of pay which amounted to £4,677.[79] Frances was left with two sons and two daughters to support, and a half century of widowhood at Steeton ahead of her. Her two sons became officers in Cromwell's army during the 1650s, and she long outlived her eldest son and daughter, not dying until 1692.[80]

Missing from Ricraft's list because he died from fever rather than wounds sustained in combat, was Sir William Fairfax's predecessor as Commissary-General of Horse in the North, Sir Henry Foulis of Ingleby in Cleveland, baronet. In December 1642 Foulis lamented the royalist takeover of the North Riding, writing: 'Cleaveland is Turned a Wildernesse, my wife and children sole Governours, not one else left either from fear or malignanty.'[81] That Sir Henry's wife, Mary, and his family chose to remain at Ingleby left them at the mercy of the earl of Newcastle's forces, styled 'the popish army of the north' in parliamentarian propaganda. Sir Henry died of fever on active service in Lincolnshire in September or October 1643, his death passing largely unmarked in the press.[82] Lady Foulis had to wait a year before, prompted by the cases of Ladies Brooke and Fairfax, the Yorkshire Committee finally authorised an ordinance granting her the wardship of her eldest son 'without Charge, Fine or Composition' on 24 September 1644.[83]

Several petitions and letters survive for Lady Foulis, allowing more insight into her representation as a deserving war widow. In them she employed an imagery of womanly victimhood that drew on stereotypes of Cavalier cruelty established in the popular press such as William Warren's *News from Exeter*, which depicted drunken Cavaliers engaging in extortion, plunder and violence. While violence against women was not specifically mentioned, the choice of woodcut of a forlorn woman for the frontispiece was intended to represent a Devonshire ravaged by Cavalier brutality. Warren also accused the Cavaliers of herding naked civilian victims into a pond, reminiscent of accusations against the Irish rebels.[84] The allegations in Lady Foulis's petitions to Parliament describing the sack of Ingleby were highly comparable. These linguistic echoes may have been coincidental, but Foulis described how the enemy plundered and defaced her house, carrying off all the horses, cattle and sheep, slaying and wounding her servants, imprisoning her brother, with 'your petitioner & 8 small children driven from thence'. The house was occupied by the enemy and became a minor garrison.[85] With overtones of the Irish atrocities described by Henry Jones,[86] she maintained the household was stripped 'even to their very necessaryes & wearing apparell'. Perhaps because Sir Henry did not share the heroic deaths of Brooke and Fairfax, Mary's petition stressed her husband's resolute and faithful services, and how he had raised his troop from his own credit. Mary remarked that her husband's death 'deprived your petitioner of a kinde & loving husband, and eight small children not only of a carefull father, but of all meanes & man[ner] of livelihood'. She ended with the customary stress upon her and her children's dependency, 'having no other meanes whereby to subsist do wholly cast themselves upon your Justice & goodness'.[87] Such pleading is comparable to the petitions of widows of common soldiers, especially in stressing the tender age of her orphaned children. This was because unlike Brooke and Fairfax, Lady Foulis had at least for a short time become a refugee. With her late husband's estates hugely in debt, and no provision made for her seven younger children, their continuance within the gentry was a pressing and doubtful matter.[88]

She petitioned the House of Commons on 15 November 1643, pleading for her husband's arrears of pay.[89] She wrote to the royalist Sir Ferdinando Leigh describing the sack of Ingleby, because a curt response from Leigh rebuked her for discharging some of her tenants so as to minimise revenues available for the royalists to collect: 'what lands you shall make appeare by wrytings to be truly your ioyncture, none for me shall euer meddle with, but you must not vnder false pretenses protect lands and receiue rents to mayntayn your brothers in actuall rebellion, and there-by to hinder the king of assesments'.[90] On 25 February 1644, Edmund Clough substantiated Leigh's charges, insinuating that Mary had disguised rents worth £500 per annum as her jointure, adding: 'if it be gone in seruice ag[ains]t his ma[jes]tie it is euill spent'. Clough rebutted Mary's pleas for her children, reprimanding that her husband should have considered their future before hazarding it by his rebellion. Far from throwing her and her diminutive children naked into the wilderness, the royalists claimed to have allowed her a jointure of £200 per annum.[91]

The Foulis estates had been worth £1,400 per annum, but £600 per annum had already been mortgaged to pay a £3,000 Star Chamber fine to the earl of Strafford. Sir Henry's pay arrears stood at over £1,000, and Sir Henry's administrator, Thomas Westrop, reckoned the estate's losses from plunder and confiscation to be £3,100. Mary's rents were paid to the royalists until July 1644, and once they were restored to her she faced paying parliamentary assessments to support the rapacious Scottish occupation well in excess of the rent her tenants could pay.[92] The loss of these rents was set out in detail, and Westrop estimated the estate's total debts were £10,000. Several of Sir Henry's creditors were imprisoned for his debts, and others threatened with the same.[93] In this desperate position, Mary followed up her petition with several letters that admonished Parliament for failing to answer her husband's petitions about the fine in Star Chamber, and for failing her late husband's imprisoned creditors. She drafted a petition in her own hand for these bondsmen, and demanded not only Parliament pay Sir Henry's arrears, but also see to a more general 'settling of the estate'.[94] Sitting uneasily alongside this curtness, Mary endeavoured to maintain the stoicism of the godly widow, in a similar manner to Brooke and Fairfax. She accepted her husband's death with the language of providence, noting, 'it pleased God to visit him with a violent feaver'.[95] Later, she reminded Parliament's Revenue

Committee that 'from the duty of good manners', she 'did forbeare to mul-tiply trouble unnecessarily upon' them, 'either by her petition, certificate, or letter on her behalfe', not doubting that she would be relieved by parliamen-tary ordinance.[96]

Again like Brooke and Fairfax, Lady Foulis sought to use her contacts to extract recompense from royalist estates. In particular, she demanded revenue from the estates of Sir Ferdinando Leigh and Sir Ingram Hopton, because they had been granted her Ingleby rents.[97] On 22 January 1645, she wrote to her brother-in-law John Foulis at Fleet Street, pressing him to push for Sir Henry's arrears, and to pursue her case against Hopton, having decided that Leigh was too poor to pursue.[98] Another brother-in-law, Robert Foulis, delivered her petition against Hopton to Sir Thomas Widdrington, supported by Lord Fairfax's attestation of Foulis's pay arrears. She also sent a copy of the certificate from the Committee at York showing for how long Hopton had taken the estate, with instructions that it be given to Widdrington, keeping the original herself 'for fear of miscarriage'. She requested John Foulis draw up a further petition for her with her cousin Chaloner's aid. This was most likely Thomas Chaloner, soon to be returned as MP for Richmond, who was already involved in efforts to relieve his widowed sister, Frances Fairfax.[99]

Mary also sought recompense from the crown itself. On 28 May 1646 when the Committee for the North Riding demanded seven and a half years of arrears of fee farm rents for Sir Henry's estates at Greenhow, estates that were mortgaged to pay the crown's fine to the earl of Strafford, Mary indignantly replied she conceived 'it to be the full intent of the parliament that those who have been such great sufferers should not be molested in this matter'. Maintaining that she had already paid three years' worth, she petitioned to be respited the rest, as this was the time the estate was under royalist and then Scottish occupation: 'Your petitioner well knowing by expe-rience that after payment made in this kind, it is more easie to obtain an acknowledgement of hard measure then a reimbursement.' Instead of the estate being in debt for this, Mary proposed the opposite: that the 'very great debt due from the Crowne' to the estate, because of the fine for Strafford, was now in the interest of her children.[100] To this end, in 1645 Mary instructed Robert Foulis while he was in London to prepare a further petition for her to receive compensation out of Strafford's estates.

Largely owing to Mary's tireless activism on behalf of her offspring, they did not lose their gentry status, despite her early death in 1657. The eldest, Sir David, succeeded his father as third baronet and was MP for Northallerton in 1685. Mary's will established her three surviving daughters as her execu-trices, bestowing on each of them sizeable portions of bonds worth £700. At least two of them married into northern gentry families. Her second son Henry received from her a purse of gold and became a Fellow of Lincoln College, Oxford. Her fourth son Thomas received bonds to make his portion £500 and became a naval officer killed in the Dutch Wars.[101]

Less is known about the other widows near the top of Ricraft's list of fallen commanders. Sir John Meldrum and Charles Fairfax are fourth and fifth, but both were unlikely to have left widows; Meldrum's only kin mentioned in his will was his nephew Robert Meldrum to whom he left all his arrears. In February 1647 Parliament stipulated that £2,000 towards his arrears was to be paid to Meldrum's executors, not mentioning a widow.[102] Ricraft's sixth worthy was Colonel Charles Essex, who was shot at Edgehill.[103] He was buried in St Mary's, Warwick, on 26 October 1642, after a solemn thanksgiving and Stephen Marshall's sermon on Jeremiah 51:5.[104] In December 1642, the Commons ordered that £500 should be granted to his widow and sister, reminding the Treasurers at War to settle this payment the following June.[105] The most surprising omission from Ricraft's list was John Hampden. His widow was his second wife, Lettice, the daughter of Sir Francis Knollys. She bore him no children and was unmentioned in his will. Instead, Hampden's executors were his mother and Edward Symeon, his first father-in-law. His orphans were between them ordered to receive support similar to that granted solely to Fulke Greville; the House of Commons voted them £5,000 in January 1647.[106]

The most prominent parliamentarian widow of the Second Civil War was Margaret, widow of the Leveller Colonel Thomas Rainborowe who was killed by royalists at Doncaster on 29 October 1648. Margaret had intervened on her husband's behalf previously when he was captured at the siege of Hull, having petitioned Parliament to arrange a prisoner exchange for him in November 1643.[107] The unusual circumstances of Rainborowe's death pressured Parliament to act for his widow and children, with allegations that a rival parliamentarian officer, Colonel Sir Henry Cholmley, was implicated in his assassination, and that Rainborowe's last words were that 'he was betrayed'. The newsbook *The Moderate* moved the soldiery to seek vengeance.[108] One correspondent wrote at news of his death: 'I heare his wife is now in London, I pray God give her strength to take it patiently, which is one general use we are to make of such trialls and afflictions.'[109] Rainborowe died intestate and encumbered by debts, leaving Margaret's patience to be tested by a Parliament fearful of her late husband's legacy.[110]

Honouring Rainborowe's widow and family became a national political issue in the growing division between the Army and its enemies at Westminster. During the height of his Council of Officers' debate over Henry Ireton's Remonstrance, General Fairfax wrote to Speaker Lenthall on 13 November 1648, warning him that Parliament had not fully considered Rainborowe's service and losses. Desperate for a conciliatory gesture from Parliament to soothe the Army's anger, Fairfax pledged that he stood 'ingaged at the instance of Mistris Rainborrow to tender her petition unto you and desire it may receive yo[u]r favourable answere w[i]th all convenient speede'.[111] Fairfax's letter remained unread in the Commons for five weeks.[112] By this time, Rainborowe's extraordinary funeral procession had passed through the City to his burial in Wapping. It included 3,000 mourn-ers, 300 horsemen and several hundred women packed into fifty coaches. Ian Gentles has argued that the funeral was a 'revolutionary pageant' that fuelled radical politics and Leveller defiance.[113] It was not until well after the purge and regicide that Fairfax's letter had the desired effect. On 13 February 1649 the Commons ordered the full payment of Rainborowe's arrears, which stood at over £1,300. On 20 July 1649 the Commons ordered Margaret to receive a further £3,000 due to her out of the royalist Sir Francis Doddington's estate. An act for bestowing lands on Margaret was read twice on 22 June 1650, and she eventually received lands in Somerset and Lancashire with an annual stipend of £200 per annum paid in quarterly instalments in the meantime. It seems that Margaret's need and persistence eventually met with goodwill from the Rump, but not until the Levellers had ceased to present a political threat.[114]

The writings and petitions of these elite war widows display similarities and differences with those of the rank and file. All shared a legal entitlement to petition for relief. Nearly all had their petitions drafted by men; clergy or parish officers served poorer widows, while family or political contacts obliged the widows of the elite. These men combined the roles of 'amanu-ensis, co-writer and spin-doctor', and they employed conventional formulae at the beginning and end.[115] Poor widows were often readier than maimed soldiers to quote legal and moral precedent to the justices, and this tendency was even more pronounced among the widows of commanders. Their peti-tions carried more weight not just because of their social status, but because they were swifter to voice feelings of grievance and entitlement. They were often petitioning the friends or acquaintances of their late husbands, and while they understood the need for humility and submission, their petitions display signs of being more particularly informed, manipulative and calcu-lating. Officers' widows could be more explicit in what they claimed were their personal views too. Ann, widow of Captain Benjamin Bale, petitioned Dorset's County Committee for the value of her goods plundered by the royalists, maintaining they had targeted her not because of her husband's military service, but because they knew of her affections to Parliament.[116]

The most obvious contrast between the relief offered to rich and poor war widows was one of scale. The thousands received by Lady Brooke dwarfed the £2 or £3 per annum that a common soldier's widow could hope to receive. Commanders' widows could be more proactive by acting as informants and discoverers of un-confiscated royalist estates, often with their husbands' arrears promised out of such discoveries. As seen in the cases of Brooke, Fairfax and Foulis, this required money, wherewithal and connections that were beyond the means of poorer widows. Their example was emulated by royalist widows after 1660 who sought recompense from parliamentar-ians' estates and vengeance against their late husbands' enemies.[117] When widows of common soldiers sought more assertive means of redress they merely alarmed MPs into taking a more repressive stance. On 16 July 1647 soldiers' widows lobbied Westminster, provoking the House of Commons into discussing how their 'clamours and disturbances ... and their coming to the Doors of the Houses' with consequent 'insolencies and contempts' might best be punished.[118]

Ultimately, the conduct and deportment expected of commanders' widows, and the ways in which they procured favourable responses from authority reflects their active participation within Parliament's war effort. They appreciated how their condition and that of their orphaned children reflected upon Parliament's honour. In turn, Parliament owned them as participants in its cause in a way that was different from the royalists whose focus on a passive loyalty to one's sovereign was less manifestly reciprocal in nature. The widows of Parliament's commanders proved themselves adept at deploying religious and political language to elicit support. They stressed their families' sufferings, thereby affirming their own loyalty and activism alongside that of their husbands. Brooke, Fairfax and Foulis all employed the supplicant's customary language of humility and dependence, but they combined it with a stoic forbearance that accorded with godly notions of honour, public duty, sacrifice and service. The potency and success of their self-representation is evident in the response it provoked from the enemy. Royalist pamphleteers pointed to a threat to the gender order, depicting the wives of parliamentarian commanders as domineering, adulterous and conspiratorial, a set of hypocritical puritans on the make, who were unnatural and unwomanly in their political assertiveness.[119]

NOTES

1 G. L. Hudson, 'Negotiating for blood money: war widows and the courts in seventeenth-century England', in J. Kermode and G. Walker (eds), *Women, Crime and the Courts in Early Modern England* (London: University College, 1994), pp. 146–69; E. Gruber von Arni, *Justice to the Maimed Soldier: Nursing, Medical Care and Welfare for Sick and Wounded Soldiers and their Families during the English Civil Wars and Interregnum, 1642–1660* (Aldershot: Ashgate, 2001).

2 D. J. Appleby, 'Unnecessary persons? Maimed soldiers and war widows in Essex, 1642–62', *Essex Archaeology and History*, 32 (2001), 209–21; H. Cheatle, 'War widows in civil-war Hertfordshire, 1642–67' (BA dissertation, University of Nottingham, 2010); E. Wilbur Alley, 'A humble petition: Lancashire war widows, 1642–79' (MA dissertation, University of Leicester, 2014); S. Beale, 'War widows and maimed soldiers in Northamptonshire after the English Civil Wars', *East Midlands History and Heritage*, 1 (2015), 18–20; I. Peck, 'The great unknown: the negotiation and narration of death by English war widows, 1647–60', *Northern History*, 53:2 (2016), 220–35.

3 H. Worthen, 'Supplicants and guardians: the petitions of royalist war widows during the Civil Wars and Interregnum, 1642–1660', *Women's History Review*, 26:4 (2016), 528–40.

4   Wing / R1436, J. Ricraft, *A Survey of England's Champions and Truths Faithful Patriots* (London, 1647). BL, Thomason 669 f. 11(30), *A Catalogue of the Earles, Lords, Knights, Generalls, Collonels, Lieutenant Collonels, Majors, Captains, and Gentlemen of Worth and Quality Slain on the Parliament and Kings Side, since the Beginning of our Uncivil Civil Warrs* (London, 1647).

5   Wing / R1436, Ricraft, *A Survey of England's Champions*, p. 116.

6   S. Kelsey, 'Oliver St John, fifth Baron St John of Bletso (*bap.* 1603, *d.* 1642)', *ODNB*; Wing / R1436, Ricraft, *A Survey of Englands Champions*, p. 116; C. H. Firth (ed.), *The Memoirs of Edmund Ludlow, Lieutenant-General of the Horse in the Army of the Commonwealth of England, 1625–1672*, 2 vols (Oxford: Clarendon Press, 1894), I, pp. 41–8.

7   'Note on the Battle of Edgehill by Sir Bernard de Gomme', photographed in M. Ashley, *The English Civil War* (Stroud: Sutton, 1996), p. 71.

8   Edward Hyde, 1st earl of Clarendon, *The History of the Rebellion and Civil Wars in England Begun in the Year 1641*, ed. W. Dunn Macray, 6 vols (Oxford: Clarendon Press, 1888), II, pp. 369–71.

9   Kelsey, 'Oliver St John', *ODNB*.

10 TNA, PCC PROB 11/330/18.

11 A. Hughes, 'Robert Greville, second Baron Brooke of Beauchamps Court (1607–43)', *ODNB*.

12 No precise date for the funeral survives owing to the disappearance of the St Mary's parish register of 1538–1650 and the lack of surviving bishops' transcripts. I am grateful to Maureen Harris for alerting me to James Cooke's approximate dating in his *Mellificium Chirurgiae, or, The Marrow of Chirurgery an Anatomical Treatise* (London, 1685), p. 252.

13 P. Styles (ed.), 'The genealogie, life and death of the right honourable Robert Lorde Brooke', in R. Bearman (ed.), *Miscellany I* (Publications of the Dugdale Society, 31, 1977), p. 191.

14 WRO, Castle Records (CR) 1886, BL4725–BL4742; I. Gentles, 'Political funerals during the English Revolution', in S. Porter (ed.), *London and the Civil War* (Basingstoke: Macmillan, 1996), pp. 211, 212, 215.

15 WRO, CR1886/BL4736; D. Greville, *Warwick Castle and Its Earls from Saxon Times to the Present*, 2 vols (London, 1903), II, pp. 862–3.

16 WRO, CR1886/BL2712, Inventory taken at Brooke House, Holborn, 28 July 1643; WRO, CR1886/TN12 Brooke House Accounts, 1643–44.

17 BL, Thomason E247(20), *Mercurius Aulicus*, 10th week (Oxford, 1643), sig. T4r.

18 Clarendon, *History of the Rebellion*, II, p. 474; BL, Thomason E94(28), L. Womock, *Sober Sadness: Or Historicall Observations Upon the Proceedings, Pretences, & Designs of a Prevailing Party in Both Houses of Parliament* (Oxford, 1643), preface. These claims were later circulated in W. Dugdale, *Antiquities of Warwickshire*, 2 vols (2nd edn, London, 1730), II, p. 767.

19 Styles (ed.), 'The genealogie', p. 192.

20 *LJ*, V, p. 640.

21 Brooke's will was dated 17 June 1640, with a codicil of 5 March 1642 to include his fourth son, Algernon: WRO, CR1886 (BB541) BL2833.

22 LJ, VI, p. 361; BL, Thomason E81(14), The Weekly Account, no. 19, 3–10 January (London, 1644), p. 6.

23 WRO, CR1886/TN12, Brooke House Accounts 1643–44, fo. 8v; WRO, CR1886/TN13, Brooke House Accounts 1644–45, fos. 25–6.

24 WRO, CR1886 (BB757) BL2840A.

25 P. Roebuck, 'Post-Restoration landownership: the impact of the abolition of wardship', Journal of British Studies, 18:1 (1978), 70.

26 A. Hughes, 'Politics, society and civil war in Warwickshire, 1620–50' (PhD thesis, University of Liverpool, 1979), p. 511.

27 WRO, CR1886/BL4663.

28 This may have been Joshua Sprigg who was then preacher at nearby St Mary Aldermary.

29 CJ, III, pp. 608, 611; WRO, CR1886/TN13, Brooke House Accounts 1644–45, fos. 23–5.

30 Roebuck, 'Post-Restoration landownership', 71.

31 WRO, CR1886/BL4662.

32 LJ, IX, p. 369.

33 LJ, IX, p. 488.

34 WRO, CR1886/TN12, Brooke House Accounts 1643–44, fo. 8v.

35 For laurel as a symbol of victory see C. Ripa, Iconologia, or Moral Emblems (London, 1709), p. 51. For rosemary during funerals, see T. Adams, A Commentary or Exposition Upon the Divine Second Epistle General Written by the Blessed Apostle St Peter (London, 1633), p. 1239; Gentles, 'Political funerals during the English Revolution', p. 220.

36 Laud was executed at Tower Hill on 10 January 1645, around which time 10s were paid to John Fisher 'for money he laid out for my Lady at tower hill': WRO, CR1886/TN14, Brooke House Accounts 1645–46, fo. 3.

37 Styles (ed.), 'The genealogie', pp. 164–5.

38 BL, Thomason E92(18), England's Losse and Lamentation Occasioned by the Death of that Right Honourable Robert Lord Brooke (London, 1643), sig. A3r.

39 Wing / R1436, Ricraft, A Survey of England's Champions, p. 33.

40 Clarendon, History of the Rebellion, II, p. 475.

41 WRO, CR1886/TN12, Brooke House Accounts 1643–44, fos. 1r, 4r.

42 Greville, Warwick Castle, II, p. 722.

43 BL, Thomason E93(22), J. Wallis, On the Sad Losse of the Truly Honourable Robert Lord Brook: An Elegie, to his Vertuous and Noble Lady (London, 1643), frontispiece, sig. 2r.

44 WRO, CR1886/TN17, Brooke House Accounts 1649–50, fo. 5; TN18, Brooke House Accounts 1650–51, fo. 13.

45 WRO, CR1886/TN16, Brooke House Accounts 1648–49, fos. 9, 11; TN17 Brooke House Accounts 1649–50, fos. 6, 15.

46 WRO, CR1886 (BB551) BL2713; TNA, SP 25/62, fo. 339; SP 25/64, fo. 447; SP 25/94, fo. 443.

47 WRO, CR1886/TN17, Brooke House Accounts 1649–50, fo. 28.

48 W. B. Stephens (ed.), A Victoria History of the County of Warwick: The City of Coventry and Borough of Warwick, 8 vols (London: Institute of Historical Research, 1969), VIII, p. 460.

49 TNA, SP29/86, fo. 104.
50 J. T. Rosenthal, 'Other victims: peeresses as war widows, 1450–1500', *History*, 72 (1987), 222.
51 *LJ*, IX, pp. 661–2; Historical Manuscripts Commission, 7th Report, Appendix (London, 1879), p. 3; TNA, SP 23/247, fo. 8.
52 *CJ*, VI, p. 401.
53 WRO, CR1886/TN18, Brooke House Accounts 1650–51, fos. 25–7.
54 WRO, CR1886/TN12–14, Brooke House Accounts 1643–46.
55 WRO, CR1886/TN13, Brooke House Accounts 1644–45, fo. 32; WRO, CR1886/TN14 Brooke House Accounts 1645–46, fo. 23.
56 WRO, CR1886/BL6757; CR1886 (BB541) BL2833; CR1886/BL2837; CR1886 (BB328) Box 539.
57 Katherine, Lady Brooke, was buried on 23 December 1676, and Robert fourth Lord Brooke was buried on 20 March 1677: WRO, DR 447/1, Parish Register of St Mary's Warwick, fo. 111v.
58 C. R. Markham, *The Life of Admiral Robert Fairfax of Steeton, 1666–1725* (London: Macmillan, 1885), pp. 14–23.
59 Wing / R1436, Ricraft, *A Survey of England's Champions*, p. 116.
60 Sir William's mother was Frances Sheffield, daughter of the earl of Mulgrave: BL, E10(7), *The Kingdomes Weekly Intelligencer*, no. 73, 17–24 September (London, 1644), pp. 588–9.
61 BL, Thomason E10(6), *The Weekly Account*, no. 56, 18–24 September (London, 1644), p. 448.
62 BL, Thomason E10(5), *The London Post*, no. 5, 24 September (London, 1644), frontispiece and p. 8.
63 Markham, *Life of Admiral Robert Fairfax*, p. 23.
64 TNA, SP 16/503, fos. 257–8.
65 BL, Additional MS 31,116, Journal of Lawrence Whitacre, 1642–47, fo. 161v; *CJ*, III, p. 636.
66 *LJ*, VII, p. 33.
67 TNA, SP 16/503, fos. 260–1.
68 Markham, *Life of Admiral Robert Fairfax*, p. 23.
69 TNA, SP 18/97, fo. 15.
70 A. Hopper, *'Black Tom': Sir Thomas Fairfax and the English Revolution* (Manchester: Manchester University Press, 2007), chapter 8.
71 TNA, SP 18/97, fo. 15.
72 TNA, SP 23/3, fo. 145.
73 TNA, SP 23/1, fo. 160; SP 23/266, fo. 17; B. Whitelocke, *Memorials of the English Affairs* (London, 1682), p. 238.
74 *CJ*, V, p. 439; TNA, SP 23/247, fo. 9.
75 TNA, SP 23/86, fo. 11.
76 TNA, SP 18/97, fo. 15.
77 TNA, SP 18/100, fo. 238; SP 25/76, fo. 277.
78 TNA, SP 18/97, fo. 19.
79 TNA, SP 18/97, fo. 15; SP 18/100, fo. 238.
80 A. Hopper, 'Sir William Fairfax (*bap.* 1610, *d.* 1644)', *ODNB*; Markham, *Life of Admiral Robert Fairfax*, pp. 10–11, 24–5.

81 Wing (2nd edn) / F1639A, H. Foulis, *An Exact and True Relation of a Bloody Fight* (London, 1643), p. 3.

82 *The Complete Baronetage* dates Sir Henry Foulis's death as 13 September 1643 and Foster dated his burial at Boston, Lincolnshire on 11 October 1643: G. E. Cockayne (ed.), *Complete Baronetage 1611–1800*, 6 vols. (Exeter, 1900– 1909), I, p. 135; J. Foster, *Pedigrees of the County Families of Yorkshire*, 3 vols (London, 1874), III. However his Inquisition Post Mortem among the family papers dates his death as 31 October 1643: KHLC, U1886, T1, Bundle B (Bundle 9, No. 34), Inquisition Post Mortem of Sir Henry Foulis, Second Baronet (Stokesley, 6 September 1645).

83 *CJ*, III, p. 637.

84 BL, Thomason E70(13), W. Warren, *Strange, True, and Lamentable Newes from Exceter* (London, 1643), sigs. A2r–v, A4r.

85 KHLC, Foulis MSS, U1886/O6/3,11. By kind permission of Viscount De L'Isle from his private collection.

86 BL, Thomason E110(9), *A Remonstrance of the Beginnings and Proceedings of the Rebellion in the County of Cavan, within the Province of Ulster in Ireland, from the 23 of October, 1641. untill the 15. of June 1642*, 11 August (London, 1642).

87 KHLC, Foulis MSS, U1886/O6/3, 12.

88 *Ibid.*, U1886/O6/4.

89 *CJ*, III, p. 311.

90 KHLC, Foulis MSS, U1886/C7.

91 *Ibid.*, U1886/C9.

92 *Ibid.*, U1886/C11.

93 *Ibid.*, U1886/O6/6–11.

94 *Ibid.*, U1886/O6/9.

95 *Ibid.*, U1886/O6/3.

96 *Ibid.*, U1886/O6/16a.

97 *Ibid.*, U1886/O6/15–16; U1886/C11.

98 Leigh pleaded his estate was so impoverished by annuities that it was scarcely worth confiscating: J. W. Clay (ed.), *Yorkshire Royalist Composition Papers, Vol. 3* (Yorkshire Archaeological Society, Record Series, 20, 1896), p. 100.

99 KHLC, Foulis MSS, U1886/C11.

100 *Ibid.*, U1886/O6/14, 16a.

101 For Mary's will see J. W. Clay (ed.), *Abstracts of Yorkshire Wills* (Yorkshire Archaeological Society, Record Series, 9, 1890), p. 123; KHLC, Foulis MSS, U1886/T63/1. For her sons and daughters see W. Dugdale, *The Visitation of the County of Yorke* (Surtees Society, 36, 1859), p. 193; B. D. Henning (ed.), *The House of Commons, 1660–90*, 3 vols (London: History of Parliament Trust, 1983), II, pp. 349–50; S. Carr, 'Henry Foulis (*bap*. 1635, *d*. 1669)', *ODNB*.

102 TNA, PCC PROB 11/200/494; Whitelocke, *Memorials*, p. 241.

103 P. Young, *Edgehill 1642* (Moreton-in-Marsh: Windrush Press, 1998), pp. 65, 248, 268, 292.

104 Styles (ed.), 'The genealogie', p. 183.

105 *CJ*, II, p. 910; *CJ*, III, pp. 121–3.

106 *CJ*, V, p. 56; Whitelocke, *Memorials*, p. 238; C. Russell, 'John Hampden (1595–1643)', *ODNB*.

107 *CJ*, III, p. 302.
108 BL, Thomason E472(15), *The Moderate*, no. 17 (London, 1648), sig. R4v; BL, Thomason E472(4), *The Moderate*, no. 18 (London, 1648), sig. S4v.
109 BL, Thomason E470(4), *A Full and Exact Relation of the Horrid Murder Committed Upon the Body of Col. Rainsborough* (London, 1648), p. 4.
110 W. R. D. Jones, *Thomas Rainborowe (c. 1610–1648), Civil-War Seaman, Siegemaster and Radical* (Woodbridge: Boydell, 2005), pp. 128–30.
111 Bodl. MS Tanner 57, fo. 411.
112 *CJ*, VI, pp. 99–10, 104.
113 Gentles, 'Political funerals during the English Revolution', pp. 207, 217; BL, Thomason E473(8), *Mercurius Militaris*, 14–21 November (London, 1648), p. 37.
114 *CJ*, VI, 139, 265, 429–30; Jones, *Thomas Rainborowe*, pp. 129–30.
115 M. Stoyle, '"Memories of the maimed": the testimony of Charles I's former soldiers, 1660–1730', *History*, 88:290 (2003), 210.
116 C. H. Mayo (ed.), *The Minute Books of the Dorset Standing Committee, 1646–1650* (Exeter: William Pollard, 1902), p. 112.
117 A. Button, 'Royalist women petitioners in south-west England, 1655–62', *The Seventeenth Century*, 15:1 (2000), 55–7; S. Beale, 'War widows and revenge in Restoration England', *The Seventeenth Century* (2017), www.tandfonline.com/eprint/3MYx4WRejrXqhbNEFXhj/full (accessed 18 January 2017).
118 *CJ*, V, p. 245.
119 For royalist invective against the wives of Sir William Waller, Thomas Lord Fairfax and Oliver Cromwell see: J. Taylor, *Crop-eare Curried, or, Tom Nash his Ghost* (Oxford, 1645), p. 20; BL, Thomason E10(20), *Mercurius Aulicus*, 36th week (Oxford, 1644), p. 1147; BL, Thomason E447(19), *The Cuckoo's Nest at Westminster, or the Parlement between the Two Lady-birds, Quean Fairfax, and Lady Cromwell, by Mercurius Melancholicus*, 15 June (London, 1648); Bodl., Wing T2018B, *A Tragi-Comedy Called New-market Fayre* (London, 1649); BL, Thomason E590(12), *The Man in the Moon*, 23–31 January (London, 1650); BL, Thomason E594(7), *Mercurius Pragmaticus*, 19–26 February (London, 1650).

Chapter 11

'So necessarie and charitable a worke': welfare, identity and Scottish prisoners⸳sof⸳ war in England, 1650–55

Chris R. Langley

On 3 September 1650 the English army, led by Oliver Cromwell, routed the Scottish force of David Leslie just south of Dunbar. In the aftermath of the battle, Commonwealth army leaders secured much of the Scottish baggage train and captured a significant proportion of the Scottish army.[1] Receiving the news in London, the English MP Bulstrode Whitelocke described the total nature of the victory: .

> We killed ... above four thousand, and ten thousand prisoners taken; among them the Laird of Liberton, lieutenant-general James Lumsden, colonel sir William Douglas, the lord Grandison, Sir Jo[hn] Brown, colonel Gordon, twelve lieutenants, seventeen cornets, two quartermasters, one hundred and ten ensigns, fifteen sergeants, two hundred horse and foot colours, thirty-two pieces of ordinance, small and great, and leather guns, all their arms, ammunition, tents, bag and baggage.[2]

Upon hearing the news, Scottish Church leaders met in Perth to discuss a response. In *A Short Declaration and Warning*, the ministers asked 'all the Inhabitants of the Land, to search out their iniquities, and to be deeplie humbled before the Lord; that Hee may turn away His Wrath from us. The Lord hath wounded, and chastised us sore, which sayeth, that our iniquities are many, and that our sinnes are increased'.[3] They ordered parishes across the country to participate in a day of national humiliation. Meanwhile, those taken prisoner at Dunbar headed south on the road to Berwick. Their plight would become central to the Kirk's narrative of divine wrath and chastisement.

The Covenanting revolution of the 1640s created unprecedented space for political debate in Scotland.[4] Scottish political and religious leaders maintained this trend by responding to Cromwell's invasion in a similarly public way. Scottish clerics rethought their understandings of providence by concluding that the English Commonwealth's victory at Dunbar was part of

God's design to chasten the ungrateful, yet nevertheless chosen, people of Scotland.[5] The special relationship forged between England and Scotland in the previous decade quickly ebbed away as both sides accused the other of betraying the Solemn League and Covenant – the mutual oath that aimed at uniting British and Irish Protestants in 1643.[6] Religious leaders in Scotland condemned the English policy of religious toleration and blasted the English army for its treatment of Scottish preachers.

These public arguments belied the more practical implications of the English invasion. Church courts scattered, often for weeks on end, and faced a disciplinary backlog upon their return. The English military quickly came to occupy all the garrisons of Lowland Scotland with consequences for local law and order as well as tax collection, social relationships and trade. Historians have disagreed over the manner in which congregations returned to normal business. It was once a mainstay of studies of this period to suggest that Presbyterianism was a spent force by the 1650s which had little parochial relevance.[7] More recent studies have revised this claim by suggesting that, in the worst-case scenario, Presbyterianism entered a kind of 'survival mode' while more optimistic assessments have revealed a fully functioning Presbyterian system of worship that continued to operate with great vigour until the Restoration.[8]

We now appreciate far more about how communities dealt with the human cost of conflict in this post-bellum period. The Covenanting leadership did not create a centralised system of welfare during the conflicts of the 1640s as one observes in England. Instead, parishes remained in charge of providing for widows and orphans or disabled veterans unable to return to work, relying on local generosity and occasional supplementary payments from authorities in Edinburgh.[9] In facing this task, parishes responded strongly. Weekly collections quickly returned to pre-invasion levels and communities absorbed local men who limped home from the battlefields of Dunbar and Worcester.[10] The Kirk's structure proved remarkably robust when dealing with increasingly large numbers of supplicants. Parish-based kirk sessions and, above them, regional presbyteries and provincial synods proved increasingly adept at providing aid for injured servicemen.

It remains unclear how the highly charged political climate in Scotland responded to these charitable campaigns. Hitherto, the two subjects have remained separate. This chapter explores the political and religious background of the campaign to gather help for those men taken captive at Dunbar and imprisoned in Newcastle, Durham and then Tynemouth Castle. Far from their home parishes, these soldiers remained in the thoughts of political leaders in Scotland. The Kirk's clarion call to support these individuals sheds light on much more than mere charitable benevolence. Indeed, collections for Scottish soldiers imprisoned in England were caught up in the Kirk's own internal disputes over how best to respond to the English invasion and occupation of Scotland.

PRISONERS AND COLLECTIONS

Following the execution of Charles I in January 1649, the leadership of the
Scottish Kirk and State installed his son Charles Stuart as King of all of Britain
and Ireland. Despite siding with the English Parliament against Charles at
various times during the 1640s, Kirk leaders were uncomfortable with the
'prevailing party' of Independents in England. In a bid to secure its borders,
the newly minted English Republic set out to quell remaining royalist opposition in Ireland in 1649 and then crossed the Tweed in July 1650 to subdue
its former northern ally. The invading army found many parishes abandoned
and elsewhere, in those places where communities had remained, discovered a native population overwhelmingly hostile to them. Cromwell's troops
marched along the south-eastern coast until they cut inland in East Lothian
towards Edinburgh. The Covenanter army was arrayed in a line defending
Edinburgh and its environs. For two months, Cromwell's troops attempted
to draw out the Scottish force but the Covenanters were unwilling and the
unusually wet campaigning season took its toll on Cromwell's troops.

The English force engaged with the Covenanter army in earnest on 3
September 1650 on the East Lothian coast near to Dunbar. Cromwell's troops
had returned to the coast to restock their supplies and to ferry sick soldiers
back to England. The Scottish army, commanded by David Leslie, followed
and established itself between the English army and the main road south to
Berwick. Although the Scots force outnumbered the English army, Leslie
gave up his defensive position on Doon Hill, just south of Dunbar, and
attempted to squeeze the English formation. On the morning of 3 September,
the Cromwellian cavalry clashed with the right wing of the Scottish army.
The result was a rout. Leslie fled back to Edinburgh and the road to the capital
was wide open for an English advance.[11]

The English had almost obliterated the entire Scottish army in one encounter. Cromwell reported how his forces conveyed around 5,000 Scottish prisoners south and freed another 5,000 who they deemed too sick to travel.[12]
Modern estimates suggest that the English army captured a total of 6,000
troops and, therefore, sent around 3,000 south.[13] The English commanders published the names of the leading officers and troops taken at the
battle to show authorities south of the Border how the battle had crushed
the Covenanter leadership.[14] Colonel Francis Hacker's regiment of cavalry
conveyed the healthiest of the prisoners south towards Newcastle.[15] Once at
Berwick on 14 September, the English governor provided sustenance for the
travelling prisoners but over a thousand had died by the time they arrived
in Newcastle in November.[16] Cromwell ordered the majority of the officers to Tynemouth Castle and those who remained of the rank and file went
either to Durham by foot or by boat to London to await transportation to New
England.[17]

Authorities in England repeatedly complained about the cost of supporting the prisoners the army had taken at Dunbar. Seeing the value of the prisoners, Cromwell ordered the governor of Newcastle and Tynemouth Castle, Sir Arthur Hesilrige, to 'lett humanitie be exercised' towards the prisoners as he was 'perswaded it wilbe comely' and bode well for future endeavours.[18] It is possible that Cromwell sought to use the prisoners as a bargaining chip in case of a Scottish insurgency.[19] Unfortunately, the prisoners proved a heavy burden. Hesilrige had already paid substantial amounts of his own money to the marshal of Tynemouth Castle to provide prisoners already there with personal allowances for meat and drink days before the Scottish prisoners arrived.[20] Increasing the number of prisoners only exacerbated this problem. The burden was so great that a few prisoners were shifted to Trinity Hospital in Newcastle to spread the cost of their support.[21] Evidently struggling to cope with the costs involved in supporting the Scottish prisoners, Hesilrige requested assistance from Westminster in July 1651.[22] In response, the Council of State provided a proportion of £20,000 sterling allocated to the army in the north of England to support the Scottish prisoners in September of the same year.[23]

News of the prisoners' journey and the conditions in which they found themselves quickly reached Scotland. At some point between 3 September and the end of October 1650, the Committee of Estates – meeting in Stirling far from the English advance – sent William Brown, 'ane honest young man', to check on the conditions in which the prisoners found themselves. On 23 October 1650, Brown's report reached the Commissioners of the General Assembly who noted how Brown 'hath been latelie at Newcastle and Durhame, where most of them lye, and hath taken inspection of their condition, and doth informe us that above fyve hundred of them are already dead, and these who are living in a deplorable estate, pyning away for hunger and cold, for want of victualls and cloathes'.[24] The Commissioners acknowledged that, while parishes were already under heavy burdens, 'our relations and bonds to these prisoners being so strait, and their necessities being so great, and there being no uther probable way of supplie for them, we conceave that people will streatch them selves to the utmost in so charitable a worke'.[25] They appointed a nationwide charitable venture and ordered local presbyteries to deliver contributions from all of their parishes to the Provost of Stirling by 14 November.

Parish sessions and ministers announced the collections throughout the autumn or as soon as they received the order. There is some evidence that parishes near Edinburgh pre-empted the Commissioners' announcement and started collecting immediately after the battle.[26] Elsewhere in Scotland, however, the Commissioners' order was the primary means of communicating news of the soldiers' imprisonment. Cupar Presbytery received instructions from the Commission of the General Assembly at the end of October 1650 describing the 'sad and sorrowfull estate of many of our prisoners in Ingland', noting 'that about 500 of them ar dead' and those who were alive suffered from 'hunger, cold and want of confortable supplies'.[27] Areas further north, like Dyce and Forres, received the orders much later and started collecting funds in November and December respectively.[28]

Kirk leaders framed charitable giving as a way to appease God's wrath. The prisoners played an important role in the Kirk's continuing war of words with the English army and helped galvanise those parts of Scotland unaffected by the English advance.[29] In November 1650, the minister at Dyce, Aberdeen Presbytery, exhorted his parishioners to give liberally 'for the releiff of our distressed souldiers taken at Dunbar and keipit in prison by the enemie starving for hunger and cold'. The minister in 'exciting the people to charitable benevolence, notwithstanding of present pressouris', preached on Ecclesiastes 11:1, 'ship your grain across the sea; after many days you may receive a return'.[30] The Commission of the General Assembly took this idea a step further and urged congregations to remember the plight of those suffering at the hands of the English invaders that:

> all ingenuous, honest, and godlie hearts, to consider these things, 1. How many of our deare brethren, flesh of our flesh, and bone of our bone, are slain with the sword, innocentlie, and without cause, and how manie carried into Captivitie, and therein sterved with hunger and cold, & sent away as slaves.[31]

The Commissioners simultaneously attacked the behaviour of the Commonwealth army while obliging Scottish communities to help those who had fought for God's cause. Moreover, by the time of their declaration, the Commissioners were aware that a small group of the prisoners taken at Dunbar were already on their way to New England to act as indentured servants in the plantations. This language of slavery and bondage, combined with the image of inhumane living conditions, served to attack the moral basis of the English invasion.

Despite this zeal, local sessions struggled to pool parish resources to meet the 14 November deadline. The most efficient parishes or those least affected by the English invasion – like Abbotshall in Kirkcaldy Presbytery – completed their collections by the final week of November, thus missing the deadline by at least a week.[32] St Andrews Presbytery managed to bring together the contributions of four of its local parishes on 4 December 1650 extending to over £400 Scots.[33] As if to underline the consequences of such delays, the Commissioners of the General Assembly received a petition from a Lieutenant Wilson regarding the 'lamentable condition' of the prisoners two weeks after the deadline had passed. The Commission, unable to hasten parishes any further, passed the petition to the Scottish Parliament 'for some effectuall course for a remedy'.[34] Members of Parliament heard the report the following day but could only wait for parishes to complete their collections.[35]

Most parishes had contributed to the initial collection by mid-February 1651. William Brown, the young intermediary who had witnessed the conditions in which the prisoners found themselves, was given a small stipend to support him as he delivered the money to England. The Provost of Stirling wrote to the Commissioners of the General Assembly noting that some presbyteries had not contributed fully. The Commissioners ordered the Provost to continue but warned that he should not use the remaining money for domestic matters, 'for we thinke it a great sin to intervert thar charitie upon any pretence'.[36] The next day, the Commissioners sent a letter to presbyteries across the country to urge the completion of the prisoners' collection.[37] This final call to charity brought in an additional £270 Scots within the next month. Again, William Brown was deputed to take the money across the Border.[38]

The Kirk leadership's attempts to gather a collection for prisoners taken to England were not unusual. The previous decade witnessed large-scale collections for those fleeing from the Irish Rebellion, for ministers injured by royalist rebels and, in the largest central aid effort of the period, for the wives and children of dead servicemen.[39] Indeed, the collections for the prisoners used well-established mechanisms, provided the laity with similar updates on the conflict and gave Kirk leaders the opportunity to convey their side of the argument. Ministers exhorted their flocks to give generously by urging the desperate condition of the soldiers and showing how charity could help appease divine wrath. Despite efforts in raising funds in this charitable drive, though, Parliament received another petition from 'poor prisoners at Newcastle' on 19 March 1651.[40] The prisoners may have been in England but they remained a fixture in domestic discussions in Scotland.

ECCLESIASTICAL UNITY

The prisoners' suffering became embroiled in a larger dispute among those collecting aid for them. Behind the anti-English rhetoric, the Kirk was experiencing its own specific series of problems. A small group of ministers dissented from official Kirk policy and rejected the legality of the leadership's actions. This disagreement, which divided parishes, litters the surviving records of presbytery meetings, but it did not detrimentally affect attempts to collect aid for the prisoners in England. Instead, the prisoners' suffering acted as a common point of concern for both sides in the dispute. The common interest was not mere rhetoric, though. Indeed, in most cases, ministers of all stripes cooperated in the considerable logistical efforts involved in helping the prisoners. Collecting financial aid for the Scottish prisoners in England quickly became the first point of contact in efforts to bring the two sides to the negotiating table.

Between October 1650 and July 1651, ministers in the Kirk debated how best to respond to the English invasion. Key to this debate was the position of Charles Stuart – son of the executed Charles I – and those who had fought *against* the Covenanters in the previous decade. In late October 1650, a group in the south-west signed a pact, 'the Remonstrance', asserting that they would fight for the National Covenant but would not uphold the interests of Charles Stuart whose commitment to Presbyterianism they distrusted. Kirk leaders largely condemned the Remonstrance and continued discussing Charles Stuart's coronation and the reintegration of former royalists to oppose the English invasion – a series of policies termed the Public Resolutions. In July 1651, twenty ministers withdrew from the General Assembly meeting of the Kirk to protest against the Public Resolutions on the grounds that the reintegration of former royalists would invoke further divine retribution against Scotland. Those protesting ministers who withdrew refused to acknowledge the legality of future General Assemblies until fully purged of devoted royalists. These ministers returned to their parishes, disputed with their presbyteries and, in the case of a small body of clerics near Linlithgow, created their own rival church courts in protest.[41]

Collections for prisoners in England coincided with the controversy. On 19 March 1651, the Commissioners appointed a nationwide day of humiliation to take place the following month on Sunday, 13 April. The Commission produced a long list of causes explaining why congregations should humble themselves before God. Point six lamented the 'rysing and great differences of judgement upon the unclearnesse of some [concerning] the Publict Resolutions' while point seven reminded readers of the 'the cruel and barbarous usage of our brethren that are prisoners' in England.[42] As if to remind the Commissioners that the prisoners' sufferings were providentially linked to the divisions within the Kirk, the same day, Parliament received a petition from 'poor prisoners at Newcastle' and recommended that the Commissioners of the General Assembly discuss the issue at their meeting.[43] The following day, the Commissioners made this link explicit in A Shorte Exhortation and Warning. Its opening paragraphs spoke at length about soldiers taken at Dunbar, lamenting:

> the sade conditione of our countreymen in the southe pairts of the kingdome, growing under the grivous oppression of strangers, devoringe ther substance and enslaving ther persons; the sade silence in maney congregations, quhosse teachers are drivin into corners by the violence of the enimies, contemners of Gods ordinances, and mockers of his messingers... the innocent blood of our brethreen, murthered by the sword of a merceyles enimey; the sighing of the prissoners, inhumanlie and cruelly ussed by thosse quho keepe them prissoners.[44]

A Shorte Exhortation's authors combined the language of imprisonment and bondage with a desire for ecclesiastical unity. Indeed, A Shorte Exhortation emphasised how the suffering of the prisoners was directly linked to the health and safety of the Kirk itself by stating 'the caire of preserving our posteritie from being sunke under the darke dungeon of error, and fast bound with the heavey chaines of bassest slaverey, do cray so loud in the eares of all quho have eares to heire, and a heart to understand ... and from the watch tower quherone wee are sett, to give warning to the professors and ministers of the gospell througheout the land, and to waken them upe to ther deutey'.[45] The prisoners were a clarion call for further reform. Subsequent days of fasting and humiliation contained the same language. In December 1651, the session of Dalkeith announced a fast for the first week of January 1652 to mourn for 'the divisiones in the kirk and state and for the distresses of our prisoners'.[46]

Unlike the divisions caused by the Public Resolutions, however, most ministers accepted the plight of the prisoners uncritically. Those charged with organising additional collections for the prisoners' relief came from both sides of the dispute. In February 1652, the Synod of Lothian and Tweeddale appointed Robert Trail, a Protester, to receive the region's charitable contributions.[47] The following month, the Synod went a step further and appointed one minister from each of the province's presbyteries to organise local collections. Far from being a move to isolate Protesters like Trail, the ministers selected by the Synod represented the full gambit of opinion concerning the Public Resolutions.[48] The ministers' seniority – and their ability to effectively manage the collection – mattered far more than political opinion. The Synod underlined the importance of the collection by appointing:

> Letters to be written to the Presbytries of St Andrews and Glasgow in name of the Synod, intreating their concurrance in so necessarie and charitable a worke and that theise presbytries may communicat this matter to the rest of the presbyteries within their provinces. And Mr Norman Leslie correspondent is desired to recommend it to the Presbytrie of the province of Merse and Teviotdaill, Messers Andrew Fairfoull and Robert Lawrie nominat to draw the letters.[49]

This was a powerful gesture. Not only were the Synod's own ministers uniting, but they were deliberately reaching out to neighbouring synods that contained very different views on the Public Resolutions.

Elsewhere, Protesters actively led the process of collecting money. These senior ministers received the collections of individual parishes and then passed them to an individual entrusted to deliver the funds to the prisoners. Cupar Presbytery's efforts to help Scottish prisoners in England were led by John Makgill, minister of Dunbog, who previously registered his uncertainty regarding the Public Resolutions.[50] Similarly, John Davidson, minister of the Borders parish of Southdean (Charteris), led the charitable efforts of Jedburgh Presbytery despite his own scruples over the Resolutions. Efforts to gather money for imprisoned soldiers represent one of the main activities where Protesters and Resolutioners most freely cooperated. Areas that wholeheartedly rejected the power of the Commission of the General Assembly accepted the Commission's instructions regarding charitable collections.

Instead of becoming a political pawn within the Kirk's increasingly fractious dispute, the plight of the Scottish prisoners in England became a point of agreement between churchmen of differing opinion. Indeed, the practical business of organising and collecting financial aid was one of the main methods that dissenting ministers used to maintain links with their Resolutioner neighbours. Thus, divisions within the Church did not serve to undermine efforts to gather funds to support the soldiers south of the Border and, particularly, the officers in Tynemouth Castle. The main complicating factor in gathering adequate support, as we will see, occurred not as a result of internecine feuds but because of increasing pressure on local parishes.

LOCAL RESPONSES

Parishes across Scotland faced unprecedented levels of demand for charity as the 1650s progressed. Several disastrous reversals for the Covenanter leadership in 1651 were particularly influential in shifting the focus away from the prisoners taken at Dunbar. Initially, these events were also associated with the concept of imprisonment but, increasingly, subsequent charitable drives added unwanted burdens for local parishes. Thus, centralised campaigns – like those to support the prisoners in 1650 and 1651 – were increasingly difficult to execute. In this new charitable landscape, the prisoners in England represented a rather distant and ongoing burden. Collections for their help continued but they reduced in size and frequency. Parishes, moreover, were less diligent in their collections.

Other centrally organised charitable ventures emerged from mid-1651 but continued to invoke the concept of imprisonment. When the English army disrupted a Committee of Estates meeting at Alyth, Perthshire, in August 1651, the army leadership took more high-profile prisoners. Initially, the English army shipped these ministers and prominent Scottish nobles to Tynemouth Castle and then conveyed them to the Tower of London.[51] While the English military leadership had removed them from Scotland because of their 'dangerous ... influence upon the people there', Scottish preachers responded by lamenting the English use of imprisonment.[52] Provincial synods hurriedly organised collections to help obtain the release of these men and, in contrast to the officers in Tynemouth Castle, managed to secure the release of a number of high-profile individuals.[53]

Presbyteries across Scotland continued to refer to the concept of imprisonment after the sack of Dundee and the defeat at Worcester in September 1651. In both encounters, the English army took a large number of prisoners.[54] In November 1651, Aberdeen Presbytery ordered a fast to 'furnish the prisoners with patience, corrage and constancie and provyd a way for ther delyverance that [God] wald give stedfastness and perseverance to all Covenanted bretheren'.[55] The following month, the records of Brechin Presbytery noted 'the lamentable conditione of some prisoners in Dundie pyning away for hunger and cold, whose sadd conditioun pleads for charitie'.[56] Ministers across the Synod of Mearns continued to preach for the 180 prisoners in Dundee 'who are in greatt necessitie' until mid-1654.[57]

Parishes responded to these further calls for charity. In October 1651,

Jedburgh Presbytery permitted the minister of the Borders town of Jedburgh to give the money raised for the officers in Tynemouth Castle 'to poore distressed soldiers comeing threwe the town' and the surgeons who helped them.[58] Another local minister took the opportunity to ask the Presbytery for additional help to support the 'multitude' of injured soldiers making their way through his parish. The northern parish of Speymouth was still dealing with returning soldiers in March 1652, paying a local man, William Yeman, 'for curing of fortie or fiftie wounded prisoners come from Dundie'.[59] Even in Dundee, parishioners donated significant amounts of money to help the local men taken prisoner at the storming of the town, despite their own personal hardships.[60]

The language of imprisonment stopped abruptly after fire destroyed large parts of Glasgow in June 1652. Glasgow Town Council ordered the Provost, John Bell, to ride to Ayr and then Edinburgh to inform military and ecclesiastical leaders of the damage incurred to the city 'that all helpe and supplie may be gottin thairby that may be for supplie of such as hes thair landis and guids burnt'.[61] The Council's message reached the General Assembly that met in July 1652, although the minutes of the meeting do not survive.[62] The presbyteries in Kirkcaldy and Jedburgh responded by announcing collections in August 1652.[63] Dalkeith Presbytery did likewise and successfully dispatched its collections to Glasgow at the start of October.[64] The response of these sizeable presbyteries was based on a very different idea of suffering than that surrounding the prisoners taken at Dunbar in 1650.

Authorities exerted significant amounts of pressure on parishes to deliver their charitable contributions for Glasgow. Indeed, the collection for Glasgow quickly became the most significant centralised collection for any cause in Scotland. In November 1652, petitioners from Glasgow implored the Synod of Lothian and Tweeddale 'to tak some speedie course for delivering what money the Lord hes moved their congregations to conferr upon and contribut for the relieff of the said distressit people and bee cairfull to caus collect and delyver what is not delyvered'.[65] Later in the month, the Commissioners of the General Assembly received a similar petition asking presbyteries for:

> their contributions for releef of their distressed brethren in the said brugh, recommended to their charity by the late Generall Assembly, to these who are appointed to receive them. The Commission desires a particular list of the presbyteries deficient in that duetie to be exhibited to them from the receivers, that accordingly they may take course for quickening them to so necessary and charitable a work.[66]

Both the Synod of Lothian and Tweeddale and the Commissioners of the General Assembly alluded to the original act of the General Assembly from July 1652. More importantly, both promoted the importance of swift action to help Glasgow.

This other charitable business delayed any concerted effort on behalf of the officers taken captive at Dunbar. Within this mêlée, parish records show that local authorities only renewed their efforts to gather charity for the prisoners taken at Dunbar in 1652. Provincial synods across the Central Belt ordered fresh charitable contributions for the prisoners in Tynemouth Castle in early 1652 with similar orders finding their way to Fife at the same time. The Synod of Glasgow and Ayr renewed its efforts on behalf of the prisoners in mid-1652.[67] The Synod of Fife ordered another province-wide collection in June 1653 with parishes receiving the orders the following month.[68] Organising help for the prisoners became increasingly difficult with the financial and organisational pressures of the Glasgow collection. Parishes in Jedburgh Presbytery struggled to collect for the prisoners in 1652 – dragging their feet until early 1653 – while one observer noted how the parish of Kilpatrick, at the eastern edge of Dumbarton Presbytery, 'haid no houp' of gathering the collection for the prisoners in March 1653.[69]

Parishes took advantage of leeway that allowed them to gather collections for prisoners in England as they saw fit. Faced with these competing pressures, ministers in Cupar Presbytery concluded that individual parishes could adopt their 'owne way of contributing for the prisoners at Dondie' in October 1651.[70] Upon this recommendation, the session at Dairsie decided to delay helping the prisoners in Dundee until the minister 'seik an acompt forst of that contribution quhich was for the use of the prisoners in Ingland'.[71] Evidently, the session did not wish to further burden the parish if their previous collections had not reached their destination. The session of Kinglassie, Kirkcaldy Presbytery, simply combined the collections for the prisoners in Dundee and Tynemouth Castle in early 1652 to reduce the charitable strain placed on the congregation.[72] In September 1653, Dumbarton Presbytery recorded how the money they delivered to Captain Robert Macaulay 'was conceaved not to exceed his proportion of these contributions gathered through Scotland'. Instead, the Presbytery Clerk noted how the contribution should deliberately 'come short' when compared to the collections of other areas.[73] Parishes, burdened by other needy causes, diluted the prominence of collections for the prisoners.

The prisoners in Tynemouth Castle may have temporarily united a fractious Kirk but the practical implications of collecting such large amounts of money served to cause the biggest problems. Faced with a wider range of charitable burdens, parishes were increasingly selective in how they supported the prisoners taken at Dunbar. Parishes combined collections for multiple causes or deliberately delayed collecting for two different causes in quick succession. The ways that local authorities gauged the appetite of congregations for charitable ventures shows how supposedly national causes required considerable amounts of local cooperation.

PERSONAL PETITIONS

Ensuring charitable support for those soldiers still imprisoned in the north of England was difficult. However, because of the regular contact between the prisoners and their homeland, officers responded to the changing circumstances in Scotland. Instead of relying on centrally organised collections, the prisoners appointed proxies to target specific parts of Scotland. A handful of officers crisscrossed lowland Scotland soliciting for aid. As the 1650s progressed, the frequency of their petitions reduced and conditions in which the prisoners found themselves became less relevant to both parishes and ecclesiastical authorities in Scotland. Moreover, the Kirk leadership's grand statements about imprisonment and bondage became increasingly irrelevant the longer the English occupation lasted.

For their part, the prisoners were aware of the breakdown in centrally organised calls to support them. From early 1652, local judicatories in Scotland received petitions directly from the prisoners in England. In February 1652, St Andrews Presbytery recorded a note 'from diverse prisoners at Tinmouth and Durhame since Dumbar desireing supplie in ther great want and necessitie'.[74] Similarly, parishes in the adjacent Presbytery of Kirkcaldy received petitions from 'some persones at Tinmouth Castel'.[75] Later in the same year, parishes in Glasgow Presbytery recorded similar petitions from 'the prisoners at Tinmouth (quho wer taikin at Dumbar) and representit to the Presbyterie for support becaus they wer in ane sterving conditione'.[76] While we cannot verify precise details of the soldiers' living conditions, parishes in Scotland received such petitions regularly and grew increasingly aware of the prisoners' plight.

These petitions frequently arrived by proxy and targeted individual areas. The most prominent of these figures was Robert Bannatyne who was active throughout the Central Belt between 1652 and 1653. Bannatyne was probably the effective commander of Castle Stuart's regiment of horse that was routed at Dunbar. Bannatyne managed to escape to Stirling and then to Burntisland in Fife.[77] His presence gave Scottish prisoners in England a direct point of contact with the changing context of an occupied Scotland and a method to hasten the collection of financial support. In February 1652, Bannatyne appeared before the Synod of Perth and Stirling, deputed by the prisoners in Tynemouth Castle to deliver the money to them, noting he was a man 'in quhom they trust and have sent hither'.[78] Bannatyne made a similar appearance before Jedburgh Presbytery in October 1652 and confirmed the receipt of payments from Dunbar Presbytery the following month before returning the following year.[79] Figures like Bannatyne ensured that the plight of the officers involved in the Dunbar campaign continued to garner attention in Scotland.

The officers deployed intermediaries to ensure charitable payments reached them south of the Border and to apply pressure to parishes that failed to provide support. In mid-1651, the Synod of Perth and Stirling directed all parishes to pay any outstanding money to the prisoners in England via 'James Blair prisoner & sore wounded by the enemie'.[80] The Synod scribe described Blair as holding the rank of major and directed commissioners from each presbytery to pay Blair up to the agreed value of £10 sterling. In September 1653, a Lieutenant Duguid appeared before St Andrews Presbytery with a commission. Duguid was himself 'one of the Prisoners of Tinmouth Castle' and had come to collect collections for the officers from around St Andrews. The Presbytery handed over £200 Scots to Duguid and ordered 'the rest of that contribution to be broght in with all diligence'. To that effect, the Presbytery reminded ministers of the need for charity and even sent a minister to the vacant parish of Kemback to announce the collection for the first time.[81] The presence of an emissary from Tynemouth Castle served to quicken the pace of tardy collections and act as a direct link to the officers.

Those acting on behalf of the prisoners were not always licensed to do so by the government of the English Commonwealth. The House of Commons received a letter from army leaders in Leith in November 1651 complaining that 'there are many of the Scottish Prisoners that do repair into Scotland, and there endeavour to raise new Troubles'. Westminster ruled that 'such Scotts Prisoners who have been placed or disposed of by the Parliament or Council of State, or by their Authority, or by any of the Officers of the Army, as have, or shall run away from the Places where they are so disposed, or go into Scotland *without Leave or Licence* had from the Parliament, or Authority under the Parliament, shall suffer Death'.[82] It may have been that the marshal of Tynemouth Castle preferred soldiers to petition for maintenance from parishes in Scotland rather than providing it himself.

Intermediaries could confirm, in writing, that charitable payments had reached their destination. In these cases, it is quite clear that the intermediary often acted as the agent delivering the money *directly* to the officers. Presbyteries and synods across Scotland expected to receive acknowledgement that the prisoners had received their payments in full from these men. In September 1652, Kirkcaldy Presbytery received a 'letter of thanks' from the prisoners that announced that all of the money gathered in the region had arrived safely.[83] The following month, the ministers of Dunbar Presbytery asked Lieutenant Robert Bannatyne to 'produce an discharge from the prisoneris at Tinmouth Castle for what monies he hes receaved for ther use'.[84] As far as we can tell, most of the money raised in Scotland for the use of Scottish officers in Tynemouth Castle actually reached them.

Leading officers would frequently endorse the receipts and their names litter local records in Scotland. Such receipts showed that the money was used accordingly. In April 1652, the ministers of St Andrews Presbytery informed the prisoners by letter that 'they desire quhat is collected heir for [them] at Tinmouth be equallie divyded amongst them'.[85] Subsequent receipts confirmed that *all* the officers had benefitted from the Presbytery's help. Perth Presbytery received a receipt from twenty-one officers imprisoned in Tynemouth Castle in the autumn of 1652, confirming that they had received over £500 Scots from Robert Bannatyne on behalf of the Presbytery at the start of July.[86]

Rumours spread across parishes that Scottish prisoners would be transported away and the charitable collections for them would go missing *en route*. Commonwealth responses to the Scottish threat increased in severity during the royalist rising led by William Cunningham, earl of Glencairn, and John Middleton between mid-1653 and 1654.[87] Moreover, space in Tynemouth Castle was restricted as the Commonwealth used the garrison as a prison for Dutch sailors during the First Anglo-Dutch war between 1652 and 1654. Contemporaries in Edinburgh reported that the army intended to transport prisoners taken at the defeat of the royalist rising in Dalnaspidal on 19 July 1654 to Barbados.[88] While George Monck reported that transporting prisoners overseas had broken the spirit of the Highland rebels, the news hampered collections for officers still imprisoned in Tynemouth Castle.[89] The session of Whitekirk, Dunbar Presbytery, reported that 'ther was some word that the prisoners war to be transported away'. In the uncertainty, the session immediately suspended any further collections.[90] Despite asking the Presbytery for advice on the matter, the meeting failed to record any discussion relating to the prisoners' whereabouts. It is unclear if prisoners from Tynemouth Castle were included in the shipments of soldiers transported in 1654. It is clear, however, that the Commonwealth government sent nine of the prisoners who remained alive in Tynemouth Castle to Barbados in 1655.[91] Following this decision, Scottish parishes no longer received communications from the officers at Tynemouth, most of whom had, by that point, died or moved to plantations in North America as indentured servants.

Petitions from the Scottish prisoners in England served to connect them with the place of their birth. In return for financial aid, parishes expected information on the destination of their charitable support. Uncertainty over the whereabouts of the soldiers – or their ultimate destiny – served to undermine the impressive charitable campaign pursued by local ecclesiastical authorities in the aftermath of the defeat at Dunbar. By the mid-1650s, the number of officers imprisoned at Tynemouth Castle was dwindling and the English army had established itself as the settled government of Scotland. In such a context, the example of the prisoners' suffering for the Covenanted cause became less poignant and another burden for parishes in an increasingly crowded charitable landscape.

CONCLUSION

The men discovered by archaeologists beneath the Palace Green Library in Durham and their companions-in-arms in Tynemouth Castle continued to play an important role in Scottish politics long after their original capture on the fields of Dunbar in September 1650. Parishes frequently heard announcements relating to the whereabouts of the soldiers and the physical conditions of their imprisonment. The same announcements also provided a touchstone for unity: the prisoners became a device with which the Kirk could criticise the English military and one that could help heal divisions between ministers.

The split between Protesters and Resolutioners in the 1650s did not discourage ministers from working together on issues of common concern. While the plight of the prisoners was an issue that pre-dated the split within the Kirk, it represented a topic where Protesters and Resolutioners could coexist and interact throughout the first half of the 1650s. Loose coalitions of ministers – whose opinions encompassed the full range of political thought within the Kirk – mobilised themselves around organising financial aid for the prisoners.

The collections for prisoners in England underline the strength of parochial structures of charitable support in mid-seventeenth-century Scotland. Once active following the brief interruption of the initial invasion period, local kirk sessions and presbyteries played a key role in organising and distributing charity. They remained responsive to the orders of senior judicatories like the General Assembly and the Commissioners of the General Assembly. The lines of communication that had developed over the previous half century of Presbyterian governance continued to operate effectively despite the upheavals of invasion and occupation.

Unfortunately, the amount of charitable support one parish could provide was limited. The competing demands of other charitable ventures – both at a local and national level – served to detract parishioners' attention from the suffering of the prisoners taken at Dunbar. Initially, the language Kirk leaders used to describe Covenanter reversals at Alyth and Worcester continued to emphasise the idea of imprisonment and bondage: the same language that had made the first collections for the prisoners taken at Dunbar so poignant. However, local pressures and the need to support those affected by the disastrous fire in Glasgow in mid-1652 added a further drain on charitable resources. While it is impressive that parishes continued giving to all the causes facing them, parish ministers and their sessions frequently altered the nature of collections to make them more manageable.

Local authorities chose, increasingly, to limit the charity that they were willing to pay to support their prisoners in England. Faced with high demand and a litany of other charitable concerns, local authorities narrowed the initial open call for charity to one that discriminated between parishes which had local soldiers in prison and those that did not. Kirk session minutes and the records of regional presbyteries increasingly discussed providing an adequate 'portion' of support rather than raising as much money as possible. Although parishes sought central intervention in other cases, parishes sought no help from central government to help the prisoners as, being so remote in England, they posed no immediate financial problem.

A combination of two things served to end charitable help for Scottish prisoners in Tynemouth Castle. Firstly, the petitions of soldiers became less frequent as they invariably succumbed to the brutal conditions they faced in Tynemouth Castle or were slowly shipped to plantations in New England to reduce the risk of further rebellion. Secondly, local charitable business started to take precedence as the poignancy of the prisoners' plight lessened. As the English occupation progressed, Scottish communities had less reason to hold up the prisoners as examples of Scottish suffering and, instead, began complying and interacting with the English authorities. Briefly, however, the prisoners provided a point of unity in an increasingly divided political context.

NOTES

1 W. Scott (ed.), *Original Memoirs Written during the Great Civil War; Being the Life of Sir Henry Slingsby, and Memoirs of Capt. Hodgson* (Edinburgh: J. Ballatyne, 1806), p. 149.

2 B. Whitelocke, *Memorials of the English Affairs from the Beginning of the Reign of Charles I to the Happy Restoration of King Charles II*, 4 vols (Oxford: Oxford University Press, 1853), III, p. 237.

3 The Commissioners of the General Assembly of the Kirk of Scotland, *The Causes of a Public Fast and Humiliation* (Aberdeen, 1650), pp. 10–11.

4 C. R. Langley, *Worship, Civil War and Community, 1638–1660* (London: Routledge, 2016); D. Stevenson, *The Scottish Revolution 1637–1644* (revised edn, Edinburgh: John Donald, 2003); L. A. M. Stewart, *Rethinking the Scottish Revolution: Covenanted Scotland, 1637–1651* (Oxford: Oxford University Press, 2016).

5 R. S. Spurlock, *Cromwell and Scotland: Conquest and Religion 1650–1660* (Edinburgh: John Donald, 2007), pp. 36–7; K. M. MacKenzie, 'Oliver Cromwell and the Solemn League and Covenant of the Three Kingdoms', in P. Little (ed.), *Oliver Cromwell: New Perspectives* (Basingstoke: Palgrave Macmillan, 2009), pp. 156–63.

6 C. Gribben, 'The Church of Scotland and the English apocalyptic imagination, 1630 to 1650', *Scottish Historical Review*, 88:1 (2009), 53–6.

7 A. I. Macinnes, 'Covenanting ideology in seventeenth-century Scotland', in J. Ohlmeyer (ed.), *Political Thought in Seventeenth-Century Ireland* (Cambridge: Cambridge University Press, 2000), pp. 191–2.

8 K. M. MacKenzie, 'Presbyterian Church government and the "Covenanted interest" in the Three Kingdoms 1649–1660' (PhD dissertation, University of Aberdeen, 2008), p. 30.

9 C. R. Langley, 'Caring for soldiers, veterans and families in Scotland, 1638–1651', *History*, 102:349 (2017), 5–23.

10 J. McCallum, 'Charity and conflict: poor relief in mid-seventeenth-century Dundee', *Scottish Historical Review*, 95:1 (2016), 43–5.

11 F. Dow, *Cromwellian Scotland, 1651–1660* (Edinburgh: J. Donald, 1979), pp. 8–11; S. Reid, *Dunbar 1650: Cromwell's Most Famous Victory* (Oxford: Osprey, 2004), pp. 69–77; D. Stevenson, *Revolution and Counter-Revolution in Scotland, 1644–1651* (revised edn, Edinburgh: John Donald, 2003), pp. 147–9.

12 C. H. Firth, 'The Battle of Dunbar', *Transactions of the Royal Historical Society*, new series, 14 (1900), 46.

13 Reid, *Dunbar 1650*, p. 81.

14 J. Rushworth, *A True Relation of the Routing of the Scottish Army near Dunbar* (London, 1650).

15 T. Carlyle (ed.), *The Letters and Speeches of Oliver Cromwell*, 3 vols (London: Methuen & Co., 1904), II, p. 113; M. Wanklyn, *Reconstructing the New Model Army* (Solihull: Helion and Company, 2016), p. 72.

16 Whitelock, *Memorials*, III, pp. 239–57.

17 R. Annis, 'Human remains found at Palace Green, November 2013' (unpublished report, Durham University, 2015); D. Dobson, *Directory of Scots Banished to the American Plantations, 1650–1775* (Baltimore: Clearfield, 1983); M. L. Hamilton, *Social and Economic Networks in Early Massachusetts: Atlantic Connections* (Pennsylvania: Pennsylvania State University Press, 2009), pp. 41–4.

18 Record Office for Leicestershire, Leicester and Rutland, DG21/275/q, Oliver Cromwell to Sir Arthur Hesilrige, 9 September 1650.

19 B. Donagan, 'Prisoners in the English Civil War', *History Today*, 41:3 (1991), 30; E. Murphy, 'Atrocities at sea and the treatment of prisoners of war by the Parliamentary navy in Ireland, 1641–1649', *Historical Journal*, 53:1 (2010), 26–32.

20 TNA, SP 46/95, fo. 88, Warrants from Sir Arthur Hesilrige, September 1650.

21 J. Brand, *The History and Antiquities of the Town and County of the Town of Newcastle upon Tyne*, 2 vols (Whitehall: B. White & Son, 1789), II, p. 480.

22 *CJ*, VI, pp. 615–17.

23 *CJ*, VII, pp. 20–2.

24 J. Christie (ed.), *The Records of the Commissions of the General Assemblies of the Church of Scotland* (Edinburgh: Edinburgh University Press, 1909), III, pp. 86–7.

25 *Ibid.*, III, p. 87.

26 Langley, *Worship, Civil War and Community*, pp. 145–6.

27 NRS, Edinburgh, CH2/82/1, Cupar Presbytery minutes, fo. 181.

28 NRS, CH2/117/1, Dyce kirk session minutes, fo. 75; NRS, CH2/1448/1, Forres kirk session minutes, fo. 19.

29 Spurlock, *Cromwell and Scotland*, p. 35.

30 NRS, CH2/117/1, Dyce kirk session minutes, fo. 75.

31 Commissioners of the General Assembly, *A Solemn Warning to all Members of this Kirk from the Commission of the Generall Assembly* (Aberdeen, 1651), p. 8.

32 NRS, CH2/225/1, Abbotshall kirk session minutes, fo. 2.

33 NRS, CH2/1132/18, St Andrews Presbytery minutes, fo. 229.

34 Christie (ed.), *The Records of the Commissions*, III, p. 137.

35 *RPS*, ed. K. M. Brown *et al.* (St Andrews, 2007–14), M1650/11/11, www.rps.ac.uk (accessed 24 August 2016).

36 Christie (ed.), *The Records of the Commissions*, III, p. 280.

37 *Ibid.*, p. 286.
38 *Ibid.*, pp. 304–5.
39 C. R. Langley, 'Sheltering under the Covenant: the National Covenant, ortho-doxy and the Irish Rebellion, 1638–1643', *Scottish Historical Review* 96 (2017); J. R. Young, '"Escaping massacre": refugees in Scotland in the aftermath of the 1641 Ulster Rebellion', in D. Edwards, P. Lenihan and C. Tait (eds), *Age of Atrocity: Violence and Political Conflict in Early Modern Ireland* (Dublin: Four Courts Press, 2007), pp. 220–2.
40 *RPS*, M1651/3/8.
41 K. D. Holfelder, 'Factionalism in the Kirk during the Cromwellian invasion and occupation of Scotland, 1650 to 1660: The Protester-Resolutioner controversy' (PhD dissertation, University of Edinburgh, 1998), pp. 182–3.
42 Christie (ed.), *The Records of the Commissions*, III, pp. 340–1.
43 *RPS*, M1651/3/8.
44 A. Peterkin (ed.), *Records of the Kirk of Scotland, Containing the Acts and Proceedings of the General Assemblies, from the Year 1638 Downwards* (Edinburgh: Peter Brown, 1842), p. 640.
45 Parishes in southern parts of Scotland did not receive these orders until mid-August 1651. See NRS, CH2/295/4, Peebles Presbytery minutes, fo. 33.
46 NRS, CH2/84/1, Dalkeith kirk session minutes, fo. 73.
47 C. R. Langley (ed.), *The Minutes of the Synod of Lothian and Tweeddale, 1648–1659* (Woodbridge: Boydell, 2016), p. 38.
48 *Ibid.*
49 *Ibid.*
50 NRS, CH2/82/1, Cupar Presbytery minutes, fos. 189–90, 193; H. Scott, *Fasti Ecclesiae Scoticanae* 6 vols (Edinburgh: Oliver and Boyd, 1915), V, p. 150.
51 J. Balfour, *The Historical Works of Sir James Balfour*, ed. J. Haig, 4 vols (Edinburgh: W. Aitchison, 1825), IV, pp. 314–5.
52 *CJ*, VII, pp. 13–15.
53 Langley (ed.), *Minutes of the Synod of Lothian and Tweeddale*, pp. 40–2.
54 H. Cary (ed.), *Memorials of the Great Civil War in England from 1642 to 1652*, 2 vols (London: H. Colburn, 1842), II, pp. 366–7.
55 NRS, CH2/32/2, Belhelvie kirk session minutes, fo. 124.
56 NRS, CH2/40/1, Brechin Presbytery minutes, fo. 347.
57 NRS, CH2/40/1, Brechin Presbytery minutes, fo. 311.
58 NRS, CH2/198/3, Jedburgh Presbytery minutes, fo. 231.
59 NRS, CH2/839/2, Speymouth kirk session minutes, fo. 7v.
60 McCallum, 'Charity and conflict', p. 48.
61 J. D. Marwick (ed.), *Extracts from the Records of the Burgh of Glasgow*, 10 vols (Scottish Burgh Records Society, 12, 1881), II, p. 244.
62 Peterkin (ed.), *Records of the Kirk of Scotland*, pp. 591–3.
63 NRS, CH2/224/1, Kirkcaldy Presbytery minutes, fo. 626.
64 NRS, CH2/424/3, Dalkeith Presbytery minutes, fo. 469.
65 Langley (ed.), *Minutes of the Synod of Lothian and Tweeddale*, p. 51.
66 Christie (ed.), *The Records of the Commissions*, III, pp. 525–6.
67 NRS, CH2/171/5, Glasgow Presbytery minutes, fo. 104; NRS, CH2/1277/1, Govan kirk session minutes, fo. 52.

68 NRS, CH2/154/2/1, Synod of Fife minutes, fo. 254; NRS, CH2/150/1, Ferry-Port-on-Craig kirk session minutes, fo. 84.
69 NRS, CH2/198/3, Jedburgh Presbytery minutes, fos. 248–9; 252; 260–4; NRS, CH2/546/1, Dumbarton Presbytery minutes, fo. 225.
70 NRS, CH2/82/1, Cupar Presbytery minutes, fo. 193.
71 NRS, CH2/427/1, Dairsie kirk session minutes, fo. 48.
72 NRS, CH2/406/1, Kinglassie kirk session minutes, fo. 84.
73 NRS, CH2/546/1, Dumbarton Presbytery minutes, fo. 233.
74 NRS, CH2/1132/18, St Andrews Presbytery minutes, fo. 249.
75 NRS, CH2/406/1, Kinglassie kirk session minutes, fo. 84.
76 NRS, CH2/1277/1, Govan kirk session minutes fo. 35.
77 E. M. Furgol, *A Regimental History of the Covenanting Armies 1639–1651* (Edinburgh: John Donald, 1990), pp. 305–6.
78 NRS, CH2/449/2, Synod of Perth and Stirling minutes, fo. 156.
79 NRS, CH2/198/3, Jedburgh Presbytery minutes, fo. 248; NRS, CH2/99/1, Dunbar Presbytery minutes, fo. 21; Langley (ed.), *Minutes of the Synod of Lothian and Tweeddale*, pp. 72–8.
80 NRS, CH2/449/2, Synod of Perth and Stirling minutes, fo. 150.
81 NRS, CH2/1132/18, St Andrews Presbytery minutes, fo. 278.
82 *CJ*, VII, p. 37. Emphasis added.
83 NRS, CH2/224/1, Kirkcaldy Presbytery minutes, fo. 626.
84 NRS, CH2/99/1, Dunbar Presbytery minutes, fo. 21.
85 NRS, CH2/1132/18, St Andrews Presbytery minutes, fo. 252.
86 NRS, CH2/299/3, Perth Presbytery minutes, fo. 225.
87 K. M. MacKenzie, 'The conundrum of marginality: *Mercurius Politicus*, order and the politics of Glencairn's Rising', *Journal of Irish and Scottish Studies*, 6:2 (2013), 102–6.
88 J. Nicoll, *A Diary of Public Transactions and Other Occurrences, Chiefly in Scotland, from January 1650 to June 1667*, ed. D. Laing (Edinburgh: Bannatyne Club, 1836), p. 134; *A Perfect Account of Daily Intelligence* (26 July–2 August 1654), pp. 1485–6.
89 T. Birch (ed.), *A Collection of State Papers of John Thurloe Esq*, 7 vols (London: Thomas Woodward, 1742), II, pp. 560–2.
90 NRS, CH2/359/1, Whitekirk kirk session minutes, fo. 23.
91 W. N. Sainsbury (ed.), *Calendar of State Papers Colonial, America and West Indies* 39 vols (London: Her Majesty's Stationery Company, 1860), I, pp. 421–3.

Conclusion

David J. Appleby and Andrew Hopper

Aside from the Black Death, the civil wars were the most unsettling experience the British and Irish peoples have ever undergone. The chapters
in this volume help demonstrate why this was the case. They provide a
powerful reminder that the consequences and human costs of war do not
end with treaties and peace settlements, but linger for generations. This was
particularly the case with the civil wars, whose divisive legacy was prolonged
by contested memories of the conflict.[1] This volume's contributors have been
at the forefront of recent endeavours to broaden the scope of the military
history of this conflict, attracting new audiences and extending its meth-
odological reach.[2] Inspired by the pioneering works of Geoffrey Hudson and
Eric Gruber von Arni, it is hoped that *Battle-scarred* will add to this momen-
tum, stimulating further scholarship and opening up new approaches to the
history of mortality, medical care and military welfare.

It has long been recognised that the civil wars extended the threat of
mortality beyond the battlefield to encompass the thousands of civilians who
came into contact with the military.[3] Marching armies have been regularly
portrayed as carriers of epidemic disease, but the experience of towns such
as Newark remind us that populations within besieged and overcrowded garrison towns were especially vulnerable. As civilians are likely to have associated the presence of soldiery in their midst with the increased possibility of
untimely death (as well as anti-social behaviour), it is perhaps unsurprising
that so few soldiers seem to have been afforded decent burials in parish
churches and churchyards. Typhus, plague and 'camp fever' quickly became
weighty considerations for commanders. Such concerns came to influence
not just military–civilian relations, but high-level military strategy, as did
anxieties about mass desertion and the consequences of suffering exces-
sively heavy combat casualties. Lieutenant-General James King warned the

earl of Newcastle in April 1643 that storming Leeds would ruin his army 'by too severe a slaughter'.[4] Further south the royalists learnt this through bitter experience; after incurring terrible losses when storming Bristol in July 1643, the King's Council of War became more cautious about costly assaults, opting thereafter to besiege towns and if possible to subvert enemy garrison commanders.[5]

Despite these attempts to minimise casualties, Ian Gentles has estimated that 120,000 soldiers were wounded in England, Wales and Scotland.[6] This necessitated a dramatic expansion of the numbers of medical professionals and those delivering nursing care. While the period witnessed the establishment of the first professionally staffed, permanent military hospitals in London at the Savoy and at Ely House, not all medical provision measured up to these impressive standards. As Gruber von Arni has shown in this volume, the royalists invariably struggled to match Parliament's administration of care to their soldiery. Nevertheless, more research is needed on the medical practitioners and recovery facilities that served the English and Welsh provincial armies of both sides, as well as the situation in Scotland and Ireland. Ismini Pells has begun this work, constructing a prosopography of regimental surgeons and frontline medical personnel arising from her work with 'The Medical World of Early Modern England, Wales and Ireland 1500–1715' project at the University of Exeter.[7] More research is needed to find out how some of these individuals, such as Elizabeth Alkin, Thomas Clarges and John Troutbeck, rose through their civil-war medical service to become individuals of national political importance.[8]

The essays in this volume also support the contention that the civil wars were a landmark moment in the history of medicine. Medical personnel had many more opportunities to practice their trade and learn from observation as hundreds of them were mobilised to serve in the armies on both sides. Physicians, surgeons and apothecaries gained a wealth of experience. As a result, many medical textbooks were published. The surgical instruments employed appear remarkably similar to those in use today, and performed similar functions. While the standard of medical care might vary according to the status of those wounded, the thousands of petitions that survive from maimed soldiers are a testament to the successes of medical personnel in saving the lives of even the humblest among the rank and file. These petitions often detail the terrible injuries that soldiers carried for years, even decades afterwards. Many of these survivors mentioned their damaged limbs, suggesting that lower survival rates were likely for those injured in the head or torso. The number of petitioners declaring multiple wounds from successive engagements should remind historians that soldiers did not permanently cease to be combatants once they were first wounded.

A comprehensive examination of these petitions on a national level has now become possible. The editors are grateful to the Arts and Humanities Research Council, who in January 2017 announced funding for a four-year project entitled 'Welfare, Conflict and Memory during and after the English Civil Wars' to examine these petitions. The editors will be joined by Lloyd Bowen and Mark Stoyle, with the aim of constructing a national, freely accessible website of photographs and transcriptions of these petitions for relief, along with the medical certificates that often accompanied them. It is currently estimated that 4,000 such petitions survive, presented on behalf of maimed soldiers, war widows and orphans of the civil wars in England and Wales, stretching from 1642 to beyond 1700. These petitions encompass appeals to Parliament, Cromwell, Charles II, the Privy Council, parliamentarian county committees and military governors as well as the county pension scheme administered by JPs from 1642 to 1679. This research will help facilitate a national overview of the geographical distribution of supply and demand for military welfare arising from the civil wars. It will promote a more informed understanding of how ordinary men and women looked back on the conflict. Details of wounds in the petitions and their treatments will enable a deeper understanding of the range of medical care available, particularly for common soldiers. Narrative strategies in the petitions will illuminate how the wounded and bereaved negotiated with various authorities and represented their past service to the Crown or the Commonwealth. Their stories will indicate how they fashioned themselves (or were fashioned by others) as deserving cases worthy of relief. Quarter Sessions order books and the account books of county treasurers for maimed soldiers will help uncover how welfare systems attempted to cope with the enormous strain of supporting so many victims of war. The project will also address how political considerations and contested memories of the conflict influenced the provision of military welfare to the wounded and bereaved of both sides.

In encouraging men to enter military service, Parliament's leaders used the promise of medical care and pensions to strengthen their war effort and shore up support for their cause. In doing so, the Long Parliament established for the first time the important principle that the State should care for those maimed and bereaved in its service. In practice, such care was often less than generous and far from ubiquitous. This was still the case after 1660 when the Restoration regime attempted to honour the Crown's debt to royalist maimed soldiers and widows. In the wake of twentieth-century wars, and more recent conflicts in Iraq and Afghanistan, this principle continues to be enshrined in the UK – not always perfectly – in the Armed Forces Covenant. It may be, as the contributors to *Battle-scarred* have implied, that the seventeenth century still has much to teach us today about the provision of medical care and military welfare.

NOTES

1 M. Stoyle, 'Remembering the English Civil War', in P. Gray and O. Kendrick (eds), *The Memory of Catastrophe* (Manchester: Manchester University Press, 2004),

pp. 19–30; M. J. Braddick, 'The English Revolution and its legacies', in N. Tyacke (ed.), *The English Revolution c. 1590–1720: Politics Religion and Communities* (Manchester: Manchester University Press, 2007), pp. 27–42.

2 A. Hopper, 'The armies', in M. J. Braddick (ed.), *The Oxford Handbook of the English Revolution* (Oxford: Oxford University Press, 2015), pp. 269–71.

3 J. Dils, 'Epidemics, mortality and the Civil War in Berkshire, 1642–1646', *Southern History*, 11 (1989), 40–52; C. Carlton, 'Civilians', in J. Kenyon and J. Ohlmeyer (eds), *The Civil Wars: A Military History of England, Scotland and Ireland, 1638–1660* (Oxford: Oxford University Press, 1998), pp. 272–305.

4 G. Trease, *Portrait of a Cavalier: William Cavendish, First Duke of Newcastle* (London, 1979), p. 115.

5 A. Hopper, *Turncoats and Renegadoes: Changing Sides during the English Civil Wars* (Oxford: Oxford University Press, 2012), p. 130.

6 I. Gentles, *The English Revolution and the Wars in the Three Kingdoms, 1638–1652* (Harlow: Pearson Longman, 2007), p. 437.

7 http://practitioners.exeter.ac.uk (accessed 1 May 2017).

8 M. Nevitt, 'Women in the business of revolutionary news: Elizabeth Alkin, "Parliament Joan", and the Commonwealth newsbook', *Prose Studies*, 21:2 (1998), 84–108; A. A. Hanham, 'Sir Thomas Clarges (1617–1695), politician', *ODNB*; P. Elmer, 'John Troutbeck (*bap.* 1612, *d.* 1684), physician and chemist', *ODNB*.

Select bibliography of secondary works

Alker, S., 'The soldierly imagination: narrating fear in Defoe's *Memoires of a Cavalier*, *Eighteenth-Century Fiction*, 19:1&2 (2006), 43–68

Appleby, D. J., 'Veteran politics in Restoration England, 1660–1670', *The Seventeenth Century*, 28:3 (2013), 323–42

Appleby, D. J., 'Unnecessary persons? Maimed soldiers and war widows in Essex, 1642– 62', *Essex Archaeology and History*, 32 (2001), 209–21

Atherton, I., 'Remembering (and forgetting) Fairfax's battlefields', in A. Hopper and P. Major (eds), *England's Fortress: New Perspectives on Thomas, 3rd Lord Fairfax* (Farnham: Ashgate, 2014), pp. 95–119

Bähr, A., 'Remembering fear: the fear of violence and the violence of fear in seventeenth-century war memories', in E. Kuijpers, J. Pollmann, J. Müller and J. van der Steen (eds), *Memory Before Modernity: Practices of Memory in Early Modern Europe* (Leiden: Brill, 2013), pp. 269–82

Beale, S., 'War widows and revenge in Restoration England', *The Seventeenth Century*, published online 14 August 2017, www.tandfonline.com/eprint/3MYx4WRejrXqhbNEFXhj/full (accessed 19 January 2018).

Beale, S., 'War widows and maimed soldiers in Northamptonshire after the English Civil Wars', *East Midlands History and Heritage*, 1 (2015), 18–20

Button, A., 'Royalist women petitioners in south-west England, 1655–62', *The Seventeenth Century*, 15:1 (2000), 53–66

Carlton, C., *Going to the Wars: The Experience of the British Civil Wars, 1638–1651* (London: Routledge, 1992)

Crumplin, M., *Men of Steel: Surgery in the Napoleonic Wars* (Shrewsbury: Quiller Press, 2007)

Daybell, J., *The Material Letter in Early Modern England Manuscript Letters and the Culture and Practices of Letter-Writing, 1512–1635* (Basingstoke: Palgrave Macmillan, 2012)

Dils, J. A., 'Epidemics, mortality and the Civil War in Berkshire, 1642–46', *Southern History*, 11 (1989), 40–52 and in R. C. Richardson (ed.), *The English Civil War: Local Aspects* (Stroud: Sutton, 1997), pp. 145–55

Donagan, B., *War in England, 1642–1649* (Oxford: Oxford University Press, 2008)

Donagan, B., 'The casualties of war: treatment of the dead and wounded in the English Civil War', in I. Gentles, J. Morrill and B. Worden (eds), *Soldiers, Writers and Statesmen of the English Revolution* (Cambridge: Cambridge University Press, 1998), pp. 114–32

Donagan, B., 'Prisoners in the English Civil War', *History Today*, 41:3 (1991), 28–35

Eales, J., *Community and Disunity: Kent and the English Civil Wars, 1640–1649* (Faversham: Keith Dickson Books, 2001)

Eddershaw D. and E. Roberts, *The Civil War in Oxfordshire* (Stroud: Sutton, 1995)

Edwards, D., P. Lenihan and C. Tait (eds), *Age of Atrocity: Violence and Political Conflict in Early Modern Ireland* (Dublin: Four Courts Press, 2007, reprinted 2010)

Elmer, P., 'Medicine, religion and the puritan revolution', in R. French and A. Wear (eds), *The Medical Revolution of the Seventeenth Century* (Cambridge: Cambridge University Press, 1989), pp. 10–45

Everitt, A., *The Community of Kent and the Great Rebellion, 1640–60* (Leicester: Leicester University Press, 1966)

Firth, C. H., 'The sick and wounded of the Great Civil War', *Cornhill Magazine*, 3rd series, 10 (1901), 289–99

Fissel, M. (ed.), *War and Government in Britain 1598–1650* (Manchester: Manchester University Press, 1991)

Fletcher, A., *A County Community in Peace and War: Sussex, 1600–1660* (London: Longman, 1975)

Foard, G., *Naseby: The Decisive Campaign* (Barnsley: Pen & Sword, 2004)

Furgol, E. M., *A Regimental History of the Covenanting Armies 1639–1651* (Edinburgh: John Donald, 1990)

Gabriel, R. A., *Between Flesh and Steel: A History of Military Medicine from the Middle Ages to the War in Afghanistan* (Washington DC: Potomac Books, 2013)

Gentles, I., *The English Revolution and the Wars in the Three Kingdoms 1638–1652* (Harlow: Pearson Longman, 2007)

Gentles, I., 'Political funerals in the English Revolution', in S. Porter (ed.), *London and the Civil War* (Basingstoke: Macmillan, 1996), pp. 205–24

Gentles, I., *The New Model Army in England, Ireland and Scotland, 1645–1653* (Oxford: Blackwell, 1991)

Gittings, C., *Death, Burial and the Individual in Early Modern England* (London: Routledge, 1988)

Gruber von Arni, E., *Justice to the Maimed Soldier: Soldier: Nursing, Medical Care and Welfare for Sick and Wounded Soldiers and their Families during the English Civil Wars and Interregnum, 1642–1660* (2nd edn, Nottingham: Partizan Press, 2015)

Gruber von Arni, E., '"Tempora mutantur et nos mutamur in illis": the experience of sick and wounded soldiers during the English Civil Wars and Interregnum, 1642–60', in J. Henderson, P. Horden and A. Pastore (eds), *The Impact of Hospitals, 300–2000* (Oxford: Peter Lang, 2007), pp. 317–40

Gruber von Arni, E., *Hospital Care and the British Standing Army, 1660–1714* (Aldershot: Ashgate, 2006)

Gruber von Arni, E., *Justice to the Maimed Soldier: Nursing, Medical Care and Welfare for Sick and Wounded Soldiers and their Families during the English Civil Wars and Interregnum, 1642–1660* (Aldershot: Ashgate, 2001)

Gruber von Arni, E. and A. Hopper, *'Battle-Scarred': Surgery, Medicine and Military Welfare during the British Civil Wars* (Leicester: University of Leicester, 2016)

Gruber von Arni, E. and A. Hopper, 'Welfare for the wounded', *History Today*, 66:7 (2016), 17–23

Hindle, S., *On the Parish? The Micro-Politics of Poor Relief in Rural England, c. 1550–1750* (Oxford: Oxford University Press, 2004)

Holmes, C., *The Eastern Association in the English Civil War* (Cambridge: Cambridge University Press, 1974)

Hopper, A., 'The armies', in M. Braddick (ed.), *The Oxford Handbook of the English Revolution* (Oxford: Oxford University Press, 2015), pp. 260–75

Hopper, A., *Turncoats and Renegadoes: Changing Sides during the English Civil Wars* (Oxford: Oxford University Press, 2012)

Hopper, A., *'Black Tom': Sir Thomas Fairfax and the English Revolution* (Manchester: Manchester University Press, 2007)

Hopper, A. and P. Major (eds), *England's Fortress: New Perspectives on Thomas, 3rd Lord Fairfax* (Farnham: Ashgate, 2014)

Hudson, G. L., 'The relief of English disabled ex-sailors, c. 1590–1680', in C. A. Fury (ed.), *The Social History of English Seamen, 1485–1680* (Woodbridge: Boydell, 2012), pp. 229–52

Hudson, G. L., 'Arguing disability: ex-servicemen's own stories in early modern England, 1590–1790', in R. Bivins and J. V. Pickstone (eds), *Medicine, Madness and Social History: Essays in Honour of Roy Porter* (Basingstoke: Palgrave Macmillan, 2007), pp. 105–17

Hudson, G. L. (ed.), *British Military and Naval Medicine 1600–1830* (Leiden: Brill, 2007)

Hudson, G. L., 'Disabled veterans and the state in early modern England', in D. A. Gerber (ed.), *Disabled Veterans in History* (Ann Arbor, MI: University of Michigan Press, 2000), pp. 117–44

Hudson, G. L., 'Negotiating for blood money: war widows and the courts in seventeenth-century England', in J. Kermode and G. Walker (eds), *Women, Crime and the Courts in Early Modern England* (London, University College, 1994), pp. 146–69

Hughes, A., *Politics, Society and Civil War in Warwickshire, 1620–1660* (Cambridge: Cambridge University Press, 1987)

Jennings, S. B., 'The anatomy of a civil war plague in a rural parish: East Stoke, Nottinghamshire, 1646', *Midland History*, 40:2 (2015), 201–19

Jennings, S. B., *'These Uncertaine Tymes': Newark and the Civilian Experience of the Civil Wars, 1640–1660* (Nottingham: Nottinghamshire County Council, 2009)

Jennings, S. B., '"A miserable, stinking infected town": pestilence, plague and death in a civil war garrison, Newark, 1640–1649', *Midland History*, 28 (2003), 51–70

Jones, W. R. D., *Thomas Rainborowe (c. 1610–1648), Civil War Seaman, Siegemaster and Radical* (Woodbridge: Boydell, 2005)

Kenyon, J. and J. Ohlmeyer (eds), *The Civil Wars: A Military History of England, Scotland and Ireland, 1638–1660* (Oxford: Oxford University Press, 1998), pp. 272–305.

Langley, C. R., 'Caring for soldiers, veterans and families in Scotland, 1638–1651', *History*, 102: 349 (2017), 5–23

Langley, C. R., *Worship, Civil War and Community, 1638–1660* (London: Routledge, 2016)

Laroche, R., *Medical Authority and Englishwomen's Herbal Texts, 1550–1650* (Farnham: Ashgate, 2009)

Mac Cuarta, B., 'Religious violence against settlers in south Ulster, 1641–2', in D. Edwards, P. Lenihan and C. Tait (eds), *Age of Atrocity: Violence and Political Conflict in Early Modern Ireland* (Dublin: Four Courts Press, 2007), pp. 154–75

McCallum, J., 'Charity and conflict: poor relief in mid-seventeenth-century Dundee', *Scottish Historical Review*, 95:1 (2016), 30–56

McCallum, J. E., *Military Medicine: From Ancient Times to the 21st Century* (Santa Barbara: ABC-CLIO, 2008)

McVaugh, M., 'Richard Wiseman and the medical practitioners of Restoration London', *Journal of the History of Medicine and Allied Sciences*, 62:2 (2007), 125–40

Morrill, J. S. (ed.), *The Impact of the English Civil War* (London: Collins & Brown, 1991)

Morrill, J. S., 'The ecology of allegiance in the English revolution', *Journal of British Studies*, 26:4 (1987), 451–79

Mortimer, I., *The Dying and the Doctors: The Medical Revolution in Seventeenth-Century England* (Woodbridge: Boydell, 2009)

Murphy, E., 'Atrocities at sea and the treatment of prisoners of war by the Parliamentary navy in Ireland, 1641–1649', *Historical Journal*, 53:1 (2010), 21–37

Newman, P. R., *Royalist Officers in England and Wales, 1642–1660* (New York: Garland Publishing, 1981)

Newman, P. R. and P. Roberts, *Marston Moor: The Battle of the Five Armies* (Pickering: Blackthorn Press, 2013)

Norri, J., *Dictionary of Medical Vocabulary in English, 1375–1550: Body Parts, Sicknesses, Instruments and Medicinal Preparations* (London: Routledge, 2016)

Peck, I., 'The great unknown: the negotiation and narration of death by English war widows, 1647–60', *Northern History*, 53:2 (2016), 220–35

Pelling, M., *The Common Lot: Sickness, Medical Occupations and the Urban Poor in Early Modern England* (Harlow: Longman, 1998)

Peters, E., 'Trauma narratives of the English Civil War', *Journal for Early Modern Cultural Studies*, 16:1 (2016), 78–94

Porter, R., *Disease, Medicine and Society in England 1500–1860* (Basingstoke: Macmillan, 1987)

Roy, I., 'The city of Oxford, 1640–1660', in R. C. Richardson (ed.), *Town and Countryside in the English Revolution* (Manchester: Manchester University Press, 1992), pp. 130–68

Scott, J., *England's Troubles: Seventeenth-Century English Political Instability in European Context* (Cambridge: Cambridge University Press, 2000)

Smyth, A., *Autobiography in Early Modern England* (Cambridge: Cambridge University Press, 2010)

Spurlock, R. S., *Cromwell and Scotland: Conquest and Religion 1650–1660* (Edinburgh: John Donald, 2007)

Stewart, L. A. M., *Rethinking the Scottish Revolution: Covenanted Scotland, 1637–1651* (Oxford: Oxford University Press, 2016)

Stoyle, M., 'The road to Farndon Field: explaining the massacre of the royalist women at Naseby', *English Historical Review*, 123:503 (2008), 895–923

Stoyle, M., 'Remembering the English Civil War', in P. Gray and O. Kendrick (eds), *The Memory of Catastrophe* (Manchester: Manchester University Press, 2004), pp. 19–30

Stoyle, M., '"Memories of the maimed": the testimony of Charles I's former soldiers, 1660–1730', *History*, 88:290 (2003), 204–26

Tarlow, S., *Ritual, Belief and the Dead in Early Modern Britain and Ireland* (Cambridge: Cambridge University Press, 2013)

Underdown, D., *Revel, Riot and Rebellion: Popular Politics and Culture in England 1603–1660* (Oxford: Clarendon Press, 1985)

Wallis P. and T. Pirohakul, 'Medical revolutions? The growth of medicine in England, 1660–1800', *Journal of Social History*, 49:3 (2016), 510–31

Walsham, A., *Providence in Early Modern England* (Oxford: Oxford University Press, 1999)

Walter, J., *Understanding Popular Violence in the English Revolution: The Colchester Plunderers* (Cambridge: Colchester University Press, 1999)

Wanklyn, M., *The Warrior Generals: Winning the British Civil Wars 1642–1652* (New Haven, CT: Yale University Press, 2010)

Wear, A. (ed.), *Medicine in Society: Historical Essays* (Cambridge: Cambridge University Press, 1992)

Webster, C., *The Great Instauration: Science, Medicine and Reform 1626–1660* (London: Duckworth, 1975)

Wood, A. C., *Nottinghamshire in the Civil War* (Oxford: Clarendon Press, 1937)

Worthen, H., 'Supplicants and guardians: the petitions of royalist war widows during the Civil Wars and Interregnum, 1642–1660', *Women's History Review*, 26:4 (2016), 528–40

Young, J. R., '"Escaping massacre": refugees in Scotland in the aftermath of the 1641 Ulster Rebellion', in D. Edwards, P. Lenihan and C. Tait (eds), *Age of Atrocity: Violence and Political Conflict in Early Modern Ireland* (Dublin: Four Courts Press, 2007), pp. 219–41

Zell, M. (ed.), *Early Modern Kent: 1540–1640* (Woodbridge: Boydell, 2000)

Zemon Davis, N., *Fiction in the Archives: Pardon Tales and their Tellers in Sixteenth-Century France* (Stanford, CA: Stanford University Press, 1987)

Index

Abbot, George, archbishop of
    Canterbury (1562–1633) 23
Aberystwyth Castle 29, 37
Abingdon 83, 97–9, 104, 105–7, 139, 145
Adolphus, Gustavus (1594–1632) 15
almshouses 96–7, 107
Alton, battle of (1643) 25, 105
American Civil War 4, 5, 12, 62
amputations 58, 70–1
antiseptics 61, 82
Antrim, marquis of *see* MacDonnell,
    Randal
apothecaries 12, 58, 85, 99, 105, 108, 113,
    121, 231
Aristotle 60
armour 11, 24, 63, 69, 78, 80
arrears of pay 144, 192, 199–202, 204
Ashburnham, John (1602/3–71) 105
Astley, Jacob, first baron Astley of
    Reading (1579–1652) 79
Atkinson, Thomas (*d.* 1661) 45

Bagot, Hervey (1618–74) 118
Bale, Benjamin 204
Ballingall, Sir George (1780–1855) 60
Banbury 26, 51–2, 125
Bannatyne, Robert 222–4
Barber-Surgeons' Company 12, 81–2
Basing House 12, 113, 146
Bedford, earl of *see* Russell, Francis,
    fourth earl; Russell, William,
    fifth earl

Beeston Castle 29, 32, 37
Bellasis, John, first baron Bellasis of
    Worlaby (1615–89) 43, 52
bereavement 13, 188
Berkhead, Thomas 180
Bertie, Peregrine, thirteenth baron
    Willoughby of Willoughby, Beck
    and Eresby (1555–1601) 82
Berwick 211, 213
Bethlem Hospital 81
billeting 40, 44–5, 48–9, 52, 97–8, 106,
    125, 141
Birmingham 28
Bishop, George 80, 87
Bishops' Wars (1638–40) 32, 81
Bissell, John 104, 106
blood-letting 58
bloody flux 122–4
Bolles, Richard (1590–1643) 25
Bolsover, Derbyshire 126
Bowman, Leonard 98, 103, 106
Boyle, Roger, first earl of Orrery
    (1621–79) 23
Breda, siege of 87
Brentford, storming of 96
Brereton, Sir William (1604–61) 25,
    197
Bridgewater, earl of *see* Egerton, John,
    first earl
Bristol 8, 48, 52, 104–5, 108–9, 125–6,
    165, 231
Brixworth, Northamptonshire 80–1, 85